Cardiovascular Diseases: From Basic Research to Clinical Application

Cardiovascular Diseases: From Basic Research to Clinical Application

Editors

Cristiana Bustea
Delia Mirela Tit

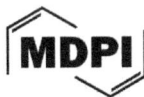

Basel • Beijing • Wuhan • Barcelona • Belgrade • Novi Sad • Cluj • Manchester

Editors
Cristiana Bustea
Department of Preclinical
Sciences
University of Oradea, Faculty
of Medicine and Pharmacy
Oradea
Romania

Delia Mirela Tit
Department of Pharmacy
University of Oradea, Faculty
of Medicine and Pharmacy
Oradea
Romania

Editorial Office
MDPI
St. Alban-Anlage 66
4052 Basel, Switzerland

This is a reprint of articles from the Special Issue published online in the open access journal *Life* (ISSN 2075-1729) (available at: www.mdpi.com/journal/life/special_issues/0UO87783VR).

For citation purposes, cite each article independently as indicated on the article page online and as indicated below:

Lastname, A.A.; Lastname, B.B. Article Title. *Journal Name* **Year**, *Volume Number*, Page Range.

ISBN 978-3-7258-0612-6 (Hbk)
ISBN 978-3-7258-0611-9 (PDF)
doi.org/10.3390/books978-3-7258-0611-9

© 2024 by the authors. Articles in this book are Open Access and distributed under the Creative Commons Attribution (CC BY) license. The book as a whole is distributed by MDPI under the terms and conditions of the Creative Commons Attribution-NonCommercial-NoDerivs (CC BY-NC-ND) license.

Contents

About the Editors vii

Preface ix

Andreea Catană, Cătălina Liliana Andrei, Suzana Guberna, Octavian Ceban and Crina Julieta Sinescu
Possible Correlations between Mean Platelet Volume and Biological, Electrocardiographic, and Echocardiographic Parameters in Patients with Heart Failure
Reprinted from: *Life* **2024**, *14*, 260, doi:10.3390/life14020260 1

Fabrizio Guarracini, Alberto Preda, Eleonora Bonvicini, Alessio Coser, Marta Martin, Silvia Quintarelli, et al.
Subcutaneous Implantable Cardioverter Defibrillator: A Contemporary Overview
Reprinted from: *Life* **2023**, *13*, 1652, doi:10.3390/life13081652 25

Marcello Baroni, Silvia Beltrami, Giovanna Schiuma, Paolo Ferraresi, Sabrina Rizzo, Angelina Passaro, et al.
In Situ Endothelial SARS-CoV-2 Presence and PROS1 Plasma Levels Alteration in SARS-CoV-2-Associated Coagulopathies
Reprinted from: *Life* **2024**, *14*, 237, doi:10.3390/life14020237 42

Rajni Singh, Prerna Gautam, Chhavi Sharma and Alexander Osmolovskiy
Fibrin and Fibrinolytic Enzyme Cascade in Thrombosis: Unravelling the Role
Reprinted from: *Life* **2023**, *13*, 2196, doi:10.3390/life13112196 54

Jin Jung, Su-Nam Lee, Sung-Ho Her, Ki-Dong Yoo, Keon-Woong Moon, Donggyu Moon and Won-Young Jang
Long-Term Clinical Impact of Patients with Multi-Vessel Non-Obstructive Coronary Artery Disease
Reprinted from: *Life* **2023**, *13*, 2119, doi:10.3390/life13112119 81

Cristiana Bustea, Delia Mirela Tit, Alexa Florina Bungau, Simona Gabriela Bungau, Vlad Alin Pantea, Elena Emilia Babes and Larisa Renata Pantea-Roşan
Predictors of Readmission after the First Acute Coronary Syndrome and the Risk of Recurrent Cardiovascular Events—Seven Years of Patient Follow-Up
Reprinted from: *Life* **2023**, *13*, 950, doi:10.3390/life13040950 93

Flavius-Alexandru Gherasie and Alexandru Achim
TAVR Interventions and Coronary Access: How to Prevent Coronary Occlusion
Reprinted from: *Life* **2023**, *13*, 1605, doi:10.3390/life13071605 110

Alberto Preda, Claudio Montalto, Michele Galasso, Andrea Munafò, Ilaria Garofani, Matteo Baroni, et al.
Fighting Cardiac Thromboembolism during Transcatheter Procedures: An Update on the Use of Cerebral Protection Devices in Cath Labs and EP Labs
Reprinted from: *Life* **2023**, *13*, 1819, doi:10.3390/life13091819 123

Christos S. Katsouras, Alexandros Tousis, Georgios Vasilagkos, Arsen Semertzioglou, Athanassios Vratimos, Ioanna Samara, et al.
Safety and Efficacy of an Innovative Everolimus-Coated Balloon in a Swine Coronary Artery Model
Reprinted from: *Life* **2023**, *13*, 2053, doi:10.3390/life13102053 142

Attila Nemes, Gergely Rácz, Árpád Kormányos, Zoltán Ruzsa, Alexandru Achim and Csaba Lengyel
The Relationship between Tricuspid Annular Longitudinal and Sphincter-Like Features of Its Function in Healthy Adults: Insights from the MAGYAR-Healthy Study
Reprinted from: *Life* **2023**, *13*, 2079, doi:10.3390/life13102079 . . . . **155**

Cristiana Bustea, Alexa Florina Bungau, Delia Mirela Tit, Diana Carina Iovanovici, Mirela Marioara Toma, Simona Gabriela Bungau, et al.
The Rare Condition of Left Ventricular Non-Compaction and Reverse Remodeling
Reprinted from: *Life* **2023**, *13*, 1318, doi:10.3390/life13061318 . . . . **165**

About the Editors

Cristiana Bustea

Dr. Cristiana Bustea is currently an Associate Professor at the Department of Preclinical Sciences, Faculty of Medicine and Pharmacy, University of Oradea, Romania. Additionally, she works as a senior cardiologist at the Intensive Coronary Unit at the Emergency Clinical Hospital of Bihor County. Her primary research interests focus on the pathophysiology of cardiovascular diseases, particularly acute coronary syndrome, oxidative stress and translational research.

Delia Mirela Tit

Delia Mirela Tit is a former student of the University of Oradea. She became a full professor in 2020, and was awarded the diploma of Doctor of Medicine in 2014, presenting her Habilitation Thesis in 2019. Her career has mostly taken place at the University of Oradea. She is supervisor of PhD degrees in the field of pharmacy, having over 100 works indexed in the Web of Science and 4 books published in Romania. Her primary area of interest is focused on pharmaceutical topics, including those relating to public health and sustainability.

Preface

Cardiovascular disease is currently the most prominent menace to human health. As it continues to be the leading cause of death, research in the field of cardiovascular diseases is critical. Although recent decades have seen tremendous progress regarding the identification of cardiovascular disease risk factors, the molecular basis of atherosclerosis, coronary revascularization and treatment of heart failure (among many other research areas), much remains to be done and the prospects are promising. In order to improve the quality and length of life for those at risk of cardiovascular disease, research for better predictors of cardiovascular disease and better means for prevention and treatment must be the target.

The purpose of this Special Issue was to identify several important advances in clinical and basic research relating to cardiovascular disease, providing tools for further progress in disease prevention and treatment. We hope that you will enjoy reading the included articles which cover only a fraction of the vast field of cardiovascular disease.

Finally, we would like to express our gratitude to MDPI and Ms. Nancy Ni for granting us the opportunity to produce this Special Issue and their support throughout the entire process.

Cristiana Bustea and Delia Mirela Tit
Editors

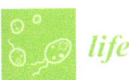

Article

Possible Correlations between Mean Platelet Volume and Biological, Electrocardiographic, and Echocardiographic Parameters in Patients with Heart Failure

Andreea Catană [1,*], Cătălina Liliana Andrei [1,*], Suzana Guberna [1], Octavian Ceban [2] and Crina Julieta Sinescu [1]

1. Department of Cardiology, University of Medicine and Pharmacy "Carol Davila", Emergency Hospital "Bagdasar-Arseni", 020021 Bucharest, Romania; sguberna@yahoo.com (S.G.); crina.sinescu@umfcd.ro (C.J.S.)
2. Economic Cybernetics and Informatics Department, The Bucharest University of Economic Studies, 010552 Bucharest, Romania; octavianceban1995@gmail.com
* Correspondence: catanaandreea91@yahoo.com (A.C.); ccatalina97@yahoo.com (C.L.A.); Tel.: +40-0745469489 (A.C.)

Citation: Catană, A.; Andrei, C.L.; Guberna, S.; Ceban, O.; Sinescu, C.J. Possible Correlations between Mean Platelet Volume and Biological, Electrocardiographic, and Echocardiographic Parameters in Patients with Heart Failure. *Life* **2024**, *14*, 260. https://doi.org/10.3390/life14020260

Academic Editor: João Morais

Received: 19 January 2024
Revised: 7 February 2024
Accepted: 14 February 2024
Published: 16 February 2024

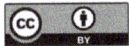

Copyright: © 2024 by the authors. Licensee MDPI, Basel, Switzerland. This article is an open access article distributed under the terms and conditions of the Creative Commons Attribution (CC BY) license (https://creativecommons.org/licenses/by/4.0/).

Abstract: (1) Background: Despite advancements in medical research and discoveries, heart failure (HF) still represents a significant and prevalent public health challenge. It is characterized by persistently high mortality and morbidity rates, along with increased rates of readmissions, particularly among the elderly population. (2) Methods: This study was conducted retrospectively on 260 patients with stable or decompensated chronic HF. The parameter of interest in the study population was the mean platelet volume (MPV), and the main objective of the research was to identify a possible relationship between MPV and several variables—biological (NT-proBNP, presepsin, red cell distribution width (RDW)), electrocardiographic (atrial fibrillation (AFib) rhythm, sinus rhythm (SR)), and echocardiographic (left ventricle ejection fraction (LVEF), left atrial (LA) diameter, left ventricle (LV) diameter, pulmonary hypertension (PH)). (3) Results: By applying logistic and linear regression models, we assessed whether there is a correlation between MPV and biological, electrocardiographic, and echocardiographic variables in patients with HF. The results revealed linear relationships between MPV and NT pro-BNP values and between MPV and RDW values, and an increased probability for the patients to have an AFib rhythm, reduced LVEF, dilated LA, dilated LV, and PH as their MPV value increases. The results were deemed statistically relevant based on a p-value below 0.05. (4) Conclusions: Through regression model analyses, our research revealed that certain negative variables in HF patients such as increased levels of NT-proBNP, increased levels of RDW, AFib rhythm, reduced LVEF, dilated LA, dilated LV, and PH, could be predicted based on MPV values.

Keywords: mean platelet volume; heart failure; NT-proBNP; atrial fibrillation; left ventricular ejection fraction

1. Introduction

Cardiovascular diseases still represent a leading cause of mortality globally. The incidence of diagnosed cases is on the rise across all countries, irrespective of their socioeconomic status. Furthermore, the global prevalence of cardiovascular diseases doubled in 2019 in comparison with 1990 [1,2].

Despite the increasingly efficient methods of investigations and the most complex treatment schemes worldwide through treatment guidelines, the number of deaths from cardiovascular causes has increased by approximately 66% [3].

The increase in life expectancy worldwide is one of the causes of the situations presented above. This has caused the burden of cardiovascular disease for each individual to increase [3].

Within the large spectrum of cardiovascular diseases, heart failure (HF) stands out as a significant and prevalent public health concern, with high rates of mortality, morbidity, and hospitalization. It maintains a leading position among cardiovascular conditions with a substantial negative impact on quality of life. This is evident through diminished exercise capacity and constraints on individual physical exertion, marking it as one of the cardiovascular diseases associated with the greatest degree of disability [4].

The role of platelets in hemostasis is very well known, but they also have an important role in the pathogenesis of atheroma plaque and atherothrombosis, and among platelet indices, mean platelet volume (MPV) is a biomarker through which platelet reactivity can be quantified [5–7].

The size of a platelet is directly correlated with its level of activity, hence larger platelets are inherently more metabolically active and contain a greater quantity of prothrombotic material [5–7]. Research studies have demonstrated a noteworthy relationship between MPV and cardiovascular risk factors, as well as an association with the risk of cardiovascular disease and cardiovascular-related mortality [5–7].

Platelet irregularities and dysfunction observed in individuals with heart failure are a consequence of elevated P-selectin expression, platelet aggregation, the presence of platelet-derived adhesion molecules, and increased mean platelet volume [8,9].

An elevated mean platelet volume in individuals with heart failure could be explained by an increase in platelet activity because of the activation of compensatory mechanisms launched in heart failure, which are represented by increased catecholaminergic secretion, increased activity of the renin–angiotensin system, and increased activity of the inflammatory system [10,11]. The link between MPV elevation and the activation of compensatory mechanisms in heart failure is outlined in a study conducted by Karabacak et al., who investigated the effects of beta-blockers on MPV and on the prognosis of heart failure. The results of the aforementioned study revealed that patients with heart failure who received beta-blockers experienced a decrease in their MPV levels and a better outcome, the possible explanation for this phenomenon being that beta-blockers decrease catecholaminergic activity and thus decrease the levels of MPV [12].

And since these compensatory mechanisms are launched in heart failure patients at risk of decompensation, this explains why the mean platelet volume (MPV) appears increased in those individuals. This hypothesis was tested in a study conducted by Hakki Kaya on patients with heart failure, which revealed that MPV was increased in the group of patients who were rehospitalized for decompensation [3].

Another possible hypothesis for why mean platelet volume increases in heart failure could be explained by the fact that heart failure patients are frequently predisposed to paroxysmal episodes of atrial fibrillation, an arrhythmia that is correlated with increased levels of MPV according to the study conducted by Turgut O et al. [13].

Studies on the relationship between the MPV value and certain biological (presepsin, NT-proBNP, red cell distribution width (RDW)), echocardiographic (left ventricle ejection fraction (LVEF), left atrium (LA) dimensions, left ventricle (LV) dimensions, presence of pulmonary hypertension (PH)), and electrocardiographic (sinus rhythm (SR), atrial fibrillation (AFib) rhythm) parameters in groups of subjects with HF are limited.

Using the MPV value as a predictor for certain negative variables in patients with HF such as reduced LVEF, increased NT-proBNP value, dilated LA, dilated LV, the presence of PH, and the presence of AFib rhythms is an element of novelty that could assist practitioners in identifying HF patients predisposed to a negative prognosis. Consequently, it may enable the implementation of more effective and potentially aggressive therapeutical plans for these individuals.

Based on the limited available medical literature concerning this issue, through our research, we aim to identify possible correlations between MPV and certain biological, electrocardiographic, and echocardiographic variables in patients with HF. Based on the above correlations that we aim to find, MPV could be used as a prognostic parameter in populations of patients with HF, and through this, we could gain the possibility to identify patients with HF at risk of having a negative prognosis. This finding could represent a new element of interest brought to the medical literature regarding new prognostic parameters that could be used in HF patients.

2. Methods

2.1. Design of the Study and Patient Selection

Our study was conducted retrospectively on patients with stable or decompensated chronic heart failure (HF) who were admitted to the Cardiology Department of the "Bagdasar-Arseni" Emergency Clinical Hospital. The main variable of interest in this study population was the mean platelet volume (MPV), and the main objective of our research was to identify a possible relationship between MPV and certain variables of interest that will be described in the paragraphs below.

According to the 2021 ESC Guidelines for HF [14], decompensated chronic HF is defined as the worsening of patients' clinical status, being included in NYHA functional classes III/IV, which are defined by a sum of symptoms and signs represented by symptoms at rest and signs of congestion, whereas patients with stable chronic HF are defined as individuals with a personal history of heart failure, who are asymptomatic or who have slight limitations of physical activity (NYHA functional classes I/II).

Regarding the sample size estimation, we included in our database all patients with heart failure admitted to the Cardiology Department of the Emergency Clinical Hospital Bagdasar-Arseni between January 2017 and January 2019, of which we selected 260 patients who met the inclusion criteria, which were as follows: patients with chronic HF (stable or decompensated), patients whose MPV value was available, and patients for which data on biological (RDW, NT-proBNP, presepsin), electrocardiographic (AFib, SR), and echocardiographic parameters (LA diameter, LV diameter, LVEF, PH) were available.

The patients with heart failure admitted in that period who were not included in the study met the exclusion criteria, which were as follows: patients without heart failure, subjects on which biological, electrocardiographic, and echocardiographic data for the variables of interest were not available, and patients who had diseases with a low survival time, active cancer, acute or chronic kidney disease, acute coronary syndrome, stroke, acute pulmonary embolism, or abnormal platelets levels/hematological diseases.

2.2. Data Collection

Our prime objective was to explore whether MPV could serve as a potential predictor factor in a study population consisting of patients with HF. Using logistic and linear regression models, our statistical analyses aimed to determine if there is a relevant relationship between the MPV value and specific categories of variables including biological factors (NT-proBNP, presepsin, RDW), electrocardiographic measures (AFib rhythm, SR), and echocardiographic measures (LVEF, LA diameter, LV diameter, PH).

Clinical and paraclinical data of patients with HF were obtained through medical records and by using the System Database of the "Bagdasar-Arseni" Emergency Clinical Hospital when the needed data were not available in the medical records.

Data regarding biological (NT-proBNP, presepsin, RDW), electrocardiographic (heart rhythm), and echocardiographic markers (left and right cavities' dimensions, left ventricular ejection fraction (LVEF), presence or absence of pulmonary hypertension) were obtained from the hospital's medical records.

The values of NT-proBNP considered significant for cardiac decompensation according to the ESC 2021 Guideline of HF [14] are as follows: over 450 pg/mL in patients under the age of 55, over 900 pg/mL in patients over the age of 55 but under 75 years, and over 1800 pg/mL in patients over 75 years old. A presepsin value that is considered significant for a possible infection is any value above 300 mg/dl. The RDW value is considered high over a value of 14%.

Regarding the cavity dimensions, according to the EACVI (European Association of Cardiovascular Imaging) guidelines [15], a left ventricle (LV) in men is considered dilated at an LV end-diastolic diameter (LVTDD) of more than 50 mm, and in women, at an LVTDD of more than 40 mm; the left atrium (LA) is considered dilated if the indexed LA volume is over 34 mL/sc, regardless of the patient's sex. According to EACVI guidelines [16], the LVEF is considered preserved at over 51%, slightly reduced at 41–50%, moderately reduced at 30–40%, and severely reduced when below 30%. Regarding pulmonary hypertension (PH), according to the ESC 2022 Guidelines on PH [17], a patient is considered to have an intermediate probability of PH in the presence of a peak tricuspid velocity (PTV) of 2.9–3.4 m/s or a PTV under 2.9 m/s plus other echo PH signs, and a patient is considered to have a high probability of PH in the presence of a PTV of 2.9–3.4 m/s plus other PH echo signs, or in the presence of a PTV over 3.4 m/s.

The basal values of some of these variables are presented in Table 1.

Table 1. Normal values of biological and echocardiographic variables.

Variable	Normal Value
NT-proBNP	<125 pg/mL
Presepsin	<300 mg/dL
RDW	<14%
MPV	7–8 fl
Reduced LVEF	<50%
Preserved LVEF	>50%
LA diameter	22–41 mm
LV diameter	37–50 mm

2.3. Statistical Analyses

The database was conceived using the Excel program, and the statistical analyses were performed based on logistic and linear regression models, which were processed in Python 3.10.

We used linear regression for cases where the dependent variable was continuous: NT-proBNP, presepsin, RDW, LVEF, LA diameter, LV diameter; and logistic regression where it was a classification problem (binary outcome): AFib, SR, reduced LVEF, LVEF preserved, dilated LA, dilated LV, PH.

In the case of the linear regression, we estimate a model in the form of $y = \beta_0 + \beta_1 * x_1 + \varepsilon$, where y is the dependent continuous variable and x_1 is the MPV (independent variable). β_0 and β_1 are the parameters that are going to be estimated on the sample data. By fitting a model like this, we can come up with interpretations about the relationship between x and y: for example, by testing the significance of β_1, which tells us whether we have reason to believe that there is a true relationship in the population level between x and y.

For the logistic regression, the obtained model is similar, and is defined as $score = \beta_0 + \beta_1 * x_1 + \varepsilon$, where $score$ is the probability that the event will happen (y = dependent binary variable), x_1 is the MPV value (independent variable), and β_0 and β_1 are the parameters that are going to be estimated on the sample data (β_0 = the coefficient for the dependent variable, β_1 = the coefficient for the MPV).

The logistic interpretations are very similar to those for the linear regression, except for the fact that, since we are predicting the outcome of an event, it is very useful to compute the estimated probability of that event to happen. Therefore, the probability of an event happening y is estimated based on the following equation: $probability = \frac{1}{1+e^{-score}}$.

The model was deemed statistically relevant at a p-value less than 0.05.

We have attached an Appendix A below that reveals all of the variables used in our research.

3. Results

Among the patients with heart failure admitted between 2017 and 2019, we included 260 patients who met the inclusion criteria mentioned above.

Regarding the patients' characteristics, of the 260 patients with heart failure, 71% had NYHA class IV heart failure, 15% had NYHA class III, and 14% had NYHA class I/II; 58% were female patients and 42% were male patients; 3% were aged between >40 and <50 years, 12% were aged between $\geq$50 and <60 years, 24% were aged between $\geq$60 and <70 years, and 61% were aged $\geq$70 years.

Concerning the correlation between the MPV value and biological (NT-proBNP, presepsin, RDW), electrocardiographic (AFib rhythm, SR), and echocardiographic parameters (LVEF, LA diameter, LV diameter, PH), detailed statistical data are presented in the subsequent paragraphs.

3.1. Biological Variables (NT-proBNP, Presepsin, RDW)

3.1.1. MPV–NT-proBNP Relationship

Concerning the relationship between MPV and the NT-proBNP value in our study population, our findings indicated that an elevated MPV is associated with a higher NT-proBNP value. This association was established using the linear regression model and the data regarding the MPV coefficients are revealed in Table 2.

Table 2. The relation between the MPV value and NT-proBNP value in the studied population.

Biomarker:	NT-proBNP	R-Squared:	0.091			
	Coefficient	Standard Error	t	p Value > |t|	[0.025	0.975]
Intercept	−17,610	4730.928	−3.721	0	[−26,900	−8288.88]
MPV	**2677.3154**	527.613	5.074	0	[1638.339	3716.291]

The data presented in Table 2 reveal the following key insights:

(1) The value of 0.091 associated with the R-square signifies that the changes in the value of NT-proBNP by 9.1% are explained by the changes in the value of MPV.
(2) The value of 2677.3154 associated with the MPV coefficient indicates that when the MPV increases by one unit, the NT-proBNP value increases by 2677 pg/mL.
(3) The p-value = 0.000, thus the model is statistically relevant, signifying that a higher MPV value is indeed linked to a higher NT-proBNP value.

This hypothesis, according to which there is a linear relationship between MPV and NT-proBNP, is depicted in Figure 1. The graph shows a tendency for the NT-proBNP value to rise as the MPV value increases. As an example, in a patient with an MPV value of 10.5 fl, an associated NT-proBNP value over 10.000 pg/mL can be anticipated.

3.1.2. MPV–Presepsin Relationship

Concerning the relationship between MPV and the presepsin value in patients with HF, by using the linear regression model, whose estimated coefficients are revealed in Table 3, our results show that there was not a relevant correlation between MPV and presepsin values. In this case, the p-value is at the limit of the threshold value of a statistically significant p-value (0.05), therefore we cannot assert with sufficient certainty that a higher MPV value is associated with an elevated presepsin value. These results can also be explained by the fact that the presepsin blood sample was not available for all of our patients, with the number of patients for whom presepsin data were available being 39.

Due to the fact that in our sample of patients with HF there was not a very large number of patients with available presepsin data, it was not possible to identify the existence of a relevant linear relationship between the MPV value and presepsin value. The depicted figure (Figure 2) illustrates somewhat contradictory findings. Contrary to our expectations, patients with higher MPV values exhibited a tendency towards lower presepsin values, rather than the anticipated trend of higher presepsin values. This observation contradicts the statistical results commonly reported in the medical literature regarding the correlation between MPV and sepsis.

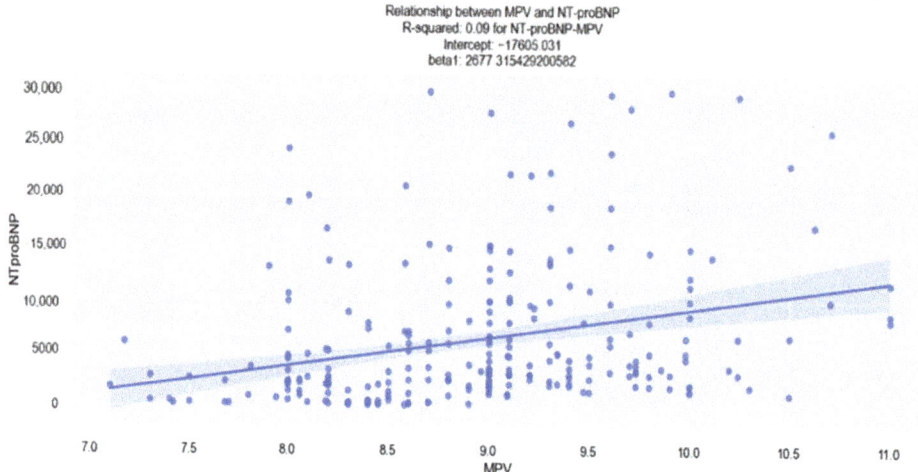

Figure 1. Linear relationship between MPV and NT-proBNP value in HF patients.

Table 3. The relation between MPV and presepsin values in the studied population.

Biomarker: No. of Observations:	Presepsin 39					
	Coefficient	Standard Error	t	p-Value > |t|	[0.025	0.975]
Intercept	2272.6483	835.742	2.719	0.01	[579.275	3966.022]
MPV	−182.7411	90.047	−2.029	**0.05**	[−365.195	−0.288]

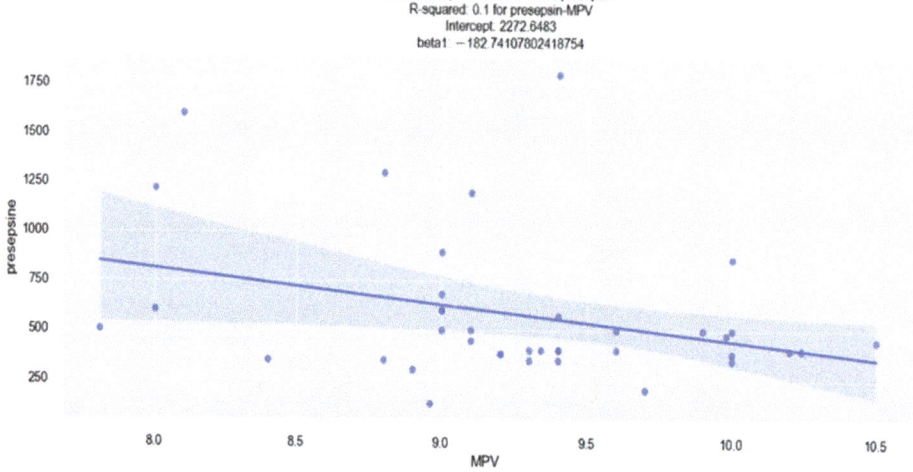

Figure 2. Linear relationship between MPV and presepsin value in HF patients.

3.1.3. RDW–MPV Relationship

Concerning the relationship between the MPV and red cell distribution width (RDW) values in our study, our findings indicate that an elevated MPV is associated with a higher RDW value. This association was established through the application of the linear regression method, and the data regarding the MPV coefficients are revealed in Table 4.

Table 4. MPV–RDW value relationship, determined with the linear regression model, in HF patients.

Biomarker:	RDW	R-Squared:	0.037			
	Coefficient	Standard Error	t	p-Value > |t|	[0.025	0.975]
Intercept	9.5573	1.244	7.685	0	[7.108	12.006]
MPV	0.4377	0.139	3.156	0.002	[0.165	0.711]

The data presented in Table 4 reveal the following key insights:

(1) The value of 0.037 associated with the R-square signifies that the change in the value of RDW by 3.7% are explained by the change in the value of MPV.
(2) The value of 0.43 associated with the MPV coefficient indicates the following: an increase of one unit in the MPV value is associated with an average increase of 0.4377% in the RDW value.
(3) The p-value associated with the MPV coefficient (0.43) is 0.002, which equals a high level of confidence in stating that patients with a higher MPV value upon admission had a higher RDW value.

The linear relationship between the MPV value and the RDW value is visually depicted in Figure 3. The graph illustrates a slight tendency for the RDW to increase as the MPV value rises. For instance, in a patient with an MPV value of 10 fl, an associated RDW value of 14% can be expected.

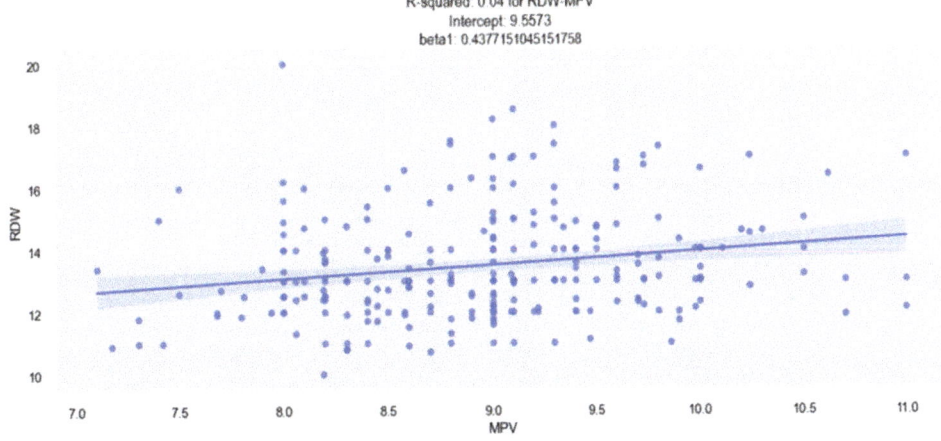

Figure 3. Linear relationship between MPV and RDW value in HF patients.

3.2. Electrocardiographic Parameters—Atrial Fibrillation and Sinus Rhythm

3.2.1. MPV–Atrial Fibrillation Relationship

Concerning the relationship between MPV and atrial fibrillation (AFib), statistical results showed that patients discovered at admission to have an AFib rhythm had a higher MPV value compared to those without AFib. These data are graphically represented in Figure 4. In the first graph of Figure 4, it can be seen that patients with an AFib rhythm

(AFib 1) had a higher MVP value (9 fl) compared to those without AFib (AFib 0), who had MPV values below 9 fl. Similar results are represented in the following two graphs, where it is observed that there is a tendency for patients with AFib (AFib 1) to be distributed more to the right, thus more towards higher values of MPV.

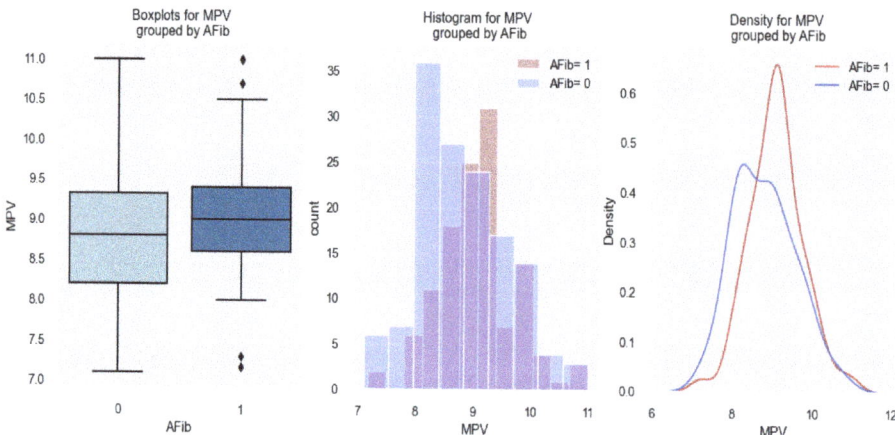

Figure 4. Differences in MPV values between subjects with AFib (1) and without AFib (0).

The findings from the above results are effectively explained through the application of the logistic regression model. The estimated coefficients of this model are presented in Table 5. This model allowed us to estimate the probability of a patient with HF having an AFib rhythm based on their MPV value.

Table 5. The relation between MPV value and the probability of AFib, determined with the logistic regression model, in HF patients.

Variable:	AFib	No. of Observations:	260			
	Coefficient	Standard Error	Z	p-Value > $|z|$	[0.025	0.975]
Intercept	−4.8282	1.573	−3.069	0.002	[−7.912	−1.745]
MPV	**0.5261**	0.175	3.002	**0.003**	[0.183	0.87]

The applied model, in this case, is represented as follows: score (event occurrence = AFib) = −4.8282 + 0.5261*MPV. Using this formula, if we consider having a patient with an MPV of 7 fl, we obtain a score of −1.14, and if we consider having a patient with an MPV of 10 fl, we obtain a score of 0.43. By applying the following equation: $probability = \frac{1}{1+e^{-score}}$, we can convert these results into probabilities. Therefore, in a patient with an MPV of 7 fl, the chances of having AFib are low (0.24 or 24%), and in a patient with an MPV of 10 fl, the chances of having AFib are high (0.60 or 60%). The p-value associated with this model is 0.003; thus, the mathematical model described above is considered relevant.

Therefore, based on the arguments presented, we may assert that the MPV value allows us to estimate the likelihood of a patient with HF having an AFib rhythm and that the higher their MPV value, the higher the likelihood of patients with HF having AFib rhythms. While the pseudo-R-squared is 2.6%, indicating that a relatively small proportion of AFib events can be explained by the MPV value, there is still a statistically significant correlation between MPV values and AFib rhythms.

The conclusions derived from the results above are also depicted in Figure 5, illustrating an increasing probability trend of AFib presence as the MPV value rises.

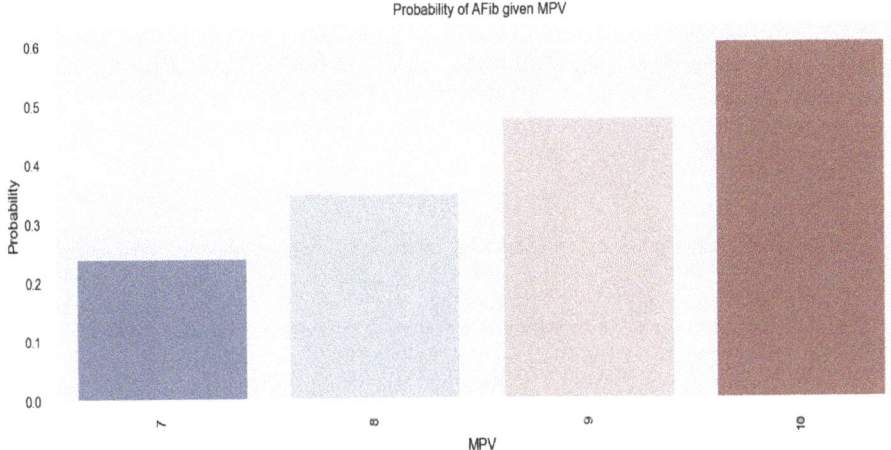

Figure 5. Estimated probability of having AFib depending on MPV value in the studied population.

3.2.2. MPV–Sinus Rhythm Relationship

In our investigation of the relationship between MPV and sinus rhythm (SR) in the studied population, our study results exhibited an opposite trend in comparison to patients with AFib rhythms. The data from our research revealed that patients with SR on admission exhibited lower MPV values in comparison to those without SR: these results are practically "mirror-like" compared to the patients with AFib on admission. The data obtained regarding this phenomenon are represented graphically in Figure 6. From the first graph of Figure 6, it is observed that patients with SR (SR 1) have a lower value of MPV compared to those without SR (SR 0)—8.8 versus 9 fl—and in the following two graphs, patients with SR (SR 1) are distributed more to the left, i.e., towards lower values of MPV (below 9 fl).

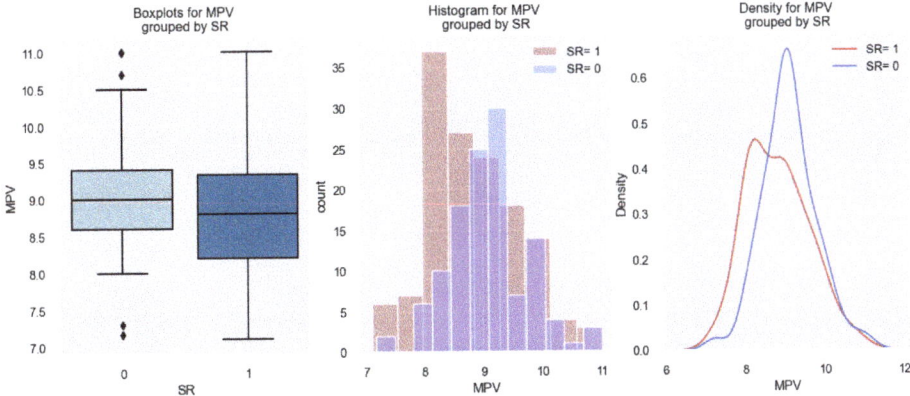

Figure 6. Differences in MPV values between subjects with SR (1) and without SR (0).

The above results are outlined through the application of the logistic regression model, and Table 6 shows the data regarding the model coefficients. This model allowed us to determine the likelihood of a patient in the studied population having SR depending on their value of MPV.

Table 6. The relation between MPV value and the likelihood of SR, determined with the logistic regression model, in HF patients.

Variable:	SR	No. of Observations:	260			
	Coefficient	Standard Error	Z	p-Value > |z|	[0.025	0.975]
Intercept	4.9591	1.578	3.143	0.002	[1.866	8.052]
MPV	−0.5372	0.176	−3.057	**0.002**	[−0.882	−0.193]

The model in this case is represented as follows: (event occurrence = SR) = 4.9591 − 0.5372*MPV. Using this formula, if we consider having an MPV of 7 fl, we obtain a score of −0.40. By applying the following equation: $probability = \frac{1}{1+e^{-score}}$, we can convert these results into probabilities. Therefore, for a patient with an MPV of 7 fl, the chances of them having SR are high (0.78 or 78%). The *p*-value associated with this model is 0.002; therefore, the mathematical model described above is considered relevant. The data derived from this model are also illustrated in Figure 7, which reveals that a decreased MPV in the study population is associated with a high chance of having SR. In summary, based on the results above, we deduced that MPV allows us to estimate the likelihood of having SR in our studied population and that the lower the MPV value, the greater the likelihood of HF patients having SR.

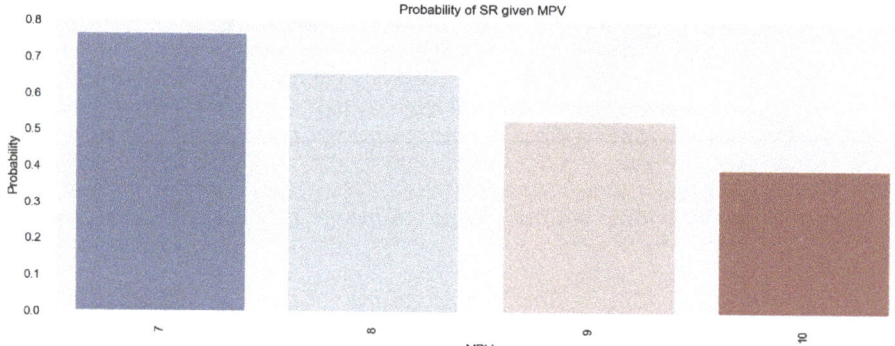

Figure 7. Estimated probability of having SR depending on MPV value in the studied population.

3.3. Echocardiographic Parameters (Left Ventricular Ejection Fraction, Left Atrium, Left Ventricle, Pulmonary Hypertension)

3.3.1. MPV–Left Ventricular Ejection Fraction Relationship

Regarding the relationship between the MPV value and the left ventricular ejection fraction (LVEF), the statistical data revealed promising results. The linear relationship between MPV and the LVEF value in patients with HF in our study was identified by applying the linear regression model (Table 7), through which we found that as the MPV value increases, the LVEF value decreases. This finding was derived from an analysis of the data presented in the table below (Table 7), revealing the following:

(1) The value of 0.053 associated with the R-square signifies that the changes in the value of LVEF by 5.3% are explained by the changes in the value of MPV.
(2) The value of −3.9016 associated with the MPV coefficient indicates that when the MPV increases by one unit, the LVEF value decreases by 3.9016%.
(3) The *p*-value = 0.000, thus the model is statistically relevant.

Table 7. The relation between MPV and LVEF, determined with the linear regression model, in HF patients.

Variable:	LVEF	R-Squared:	0.053			
	Coefficient	Standard Error	T	p-Value > |t|	[0.025	0.975]
Intercept	80.9093	9.228	8.768	0	[62.738	99.08]
MPV	−3.9016	1.029	−3.791	0	[−5.928	−1.875]

Therefore, based on the linear regression model, it can be concluded that there is a relevant relationship between the MPV value and LVEF value in patients with HF.

The conclusion obtained from the analysis of the above data is depicted in Figure 8, which is a graphical representation of the linear relationship between the MPV and LVEF values, and from which we can observe the tendency of the LVEF value to decrease as the MPV value increases (for example, an MPV value of 11 fl corresponds to an LVEF value, on average, below 40%).

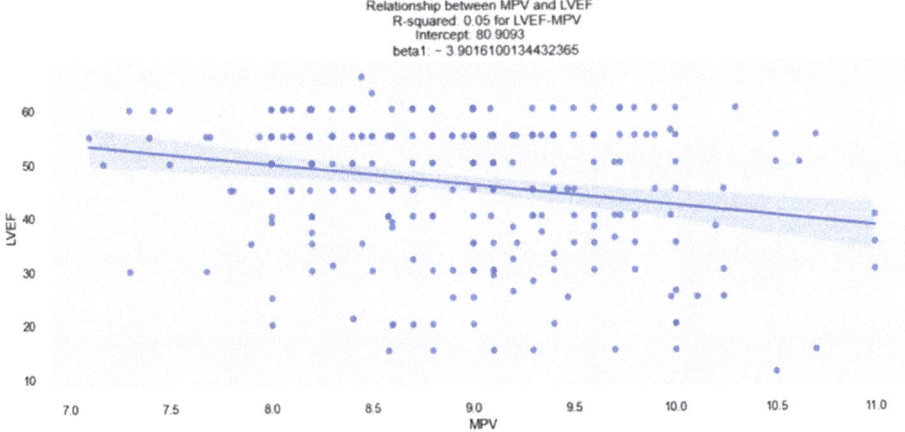

Figure 8. Linear relationship between MPV and LVEF in patients with HF.

MPV–Reduced LVEF Relationship

According to the ESC 2021 HF Guidelines [14], HF cases are classified according to the LVEF value as HF with a preserved LVEF (LVEF > 50%), HF with a medium-reduced LVEF (LVEF > 40–<50%), or HF with a severely reduced LVEF (LVEF < 40%).

In addition to the statistically significant relationship between the MPV and LVEF values, the statistical data of our study revealed varied and significant results regarding the type of LVEF (reduced versus preserved) and MPV value, the results being presented in the paragraphs below.

Regarding the relationship between MPV and the presence of a reduced LVEF (r LVEF) in patients with HF, it was found that patients with r LVEF had a higher value of MPV compared to those without r LVEF; these data are represented graphically in Figure 9.

In the first graph of Figure 9, it can be seen that patients with r LVEF (1) had a higher MPV value (approximately 9.2 fl) in comparison to those without r LVEF (0), who had MPV values below 9 fl. From the following two graphs, a tendency can be observed for the patients with r LVEF (1) to be distributed more to the right, thus towards higher values of MPV.

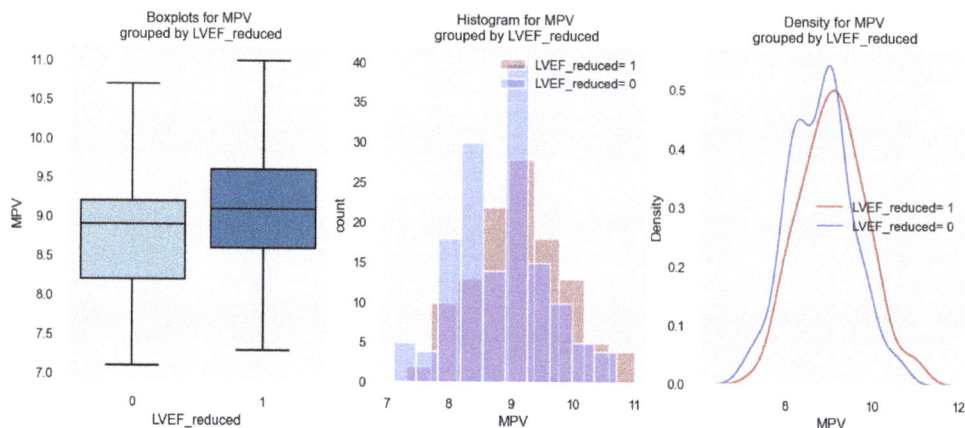

Figure 9. Reported MPV values in HF patients with a reduced LVEF (LVEF reduced = 1) versus HF patients without a reduced LVEF (LVEF reduced = 0).

The above results are outlined through the application of the logistic regression model, and Table 8 shows the data regarding the model coefficients. This model allowed us to determine the possibility of a patient having a reduced LVEF in our studied population depending on their value of MPV.

Table 8. The relation between MPV value and reduced LVEF, determined with the logistic regression model, in HF patients.

Variable:	Reduced LVEF	No. of Observations:	260			
	Coefficient	Standard Error	z	p-Value > |z|	[0.025	0.975]
Intercept	−5.1414	1.587	−3.24	0.001	[−8.251	−2.032]
MPV	**0.5485**	0.176	3.109	**0.002**	[0.203	0.894]

The model, in this case, is represented as follows: (event occurrence = reduced LVEF) = −5.1414 + 0.5485*MPV. Using this formula, if we consider having an MPV of 10 fl, we obtain a score of 0.34. By applying the following equation: $probability = \frac{1}{1+e^{-score}}$, we can convert these results into probabilities. Hence, for a patient with an MPV of 10 fl, the chances of them having a reduced LVEF are high (0.59 or 59%).

The above mathematical model is statistically relevant (p-value = 0.002). The data derived from this model are also illustrated in Figure 10, where it is observed that an increased MPV in this study population is associated with a high chance of having a reduced LVEF. In summary, based on the results above, we deduced that the MPV allows us to estimate the probability of having a reduced LVEF in our studied population and that the higher the MPV value, the greater the likelihood of an HF patient having a reduced LVEF.

MPV–Preserved LVEF Relationship

Regarding the statistical data related to the relationship between MPV and preserved LVEF (p LVEF), the results are opposite to those obtained in the case of patients with a reduced LVEF. The results of our study showed that patients with p LVEF had a lower value of MPV compared to those without p LVEF, as can be seen in the graphs represented in Figure 11. From the first graph of Figure 11, it can be seen that patients with p LVEF (1) had a lower MPV value (8.8 fl) compared to those without p LVEF (0), who had MPV values above 9 fl, and on the following two graphs, the distribution tendency of the patients with p LVEF (1) can be observed as veering towards the left, so towards lower MPV values.

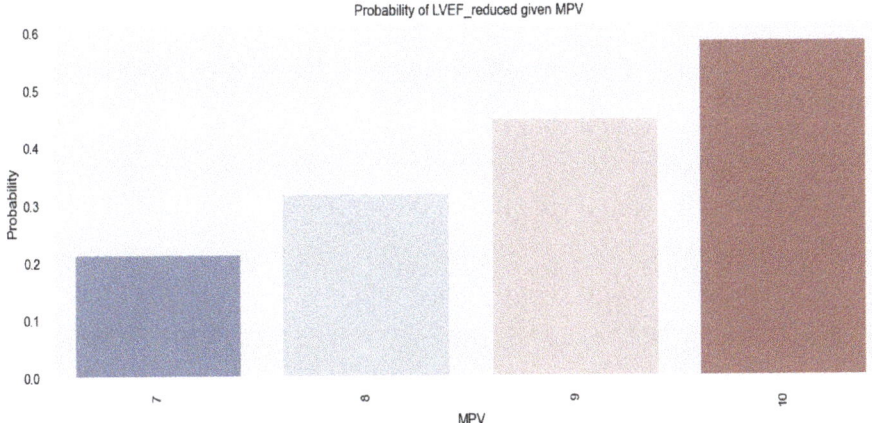

Figure 10. Estimated probability of having reduced LVEF depending on MPV value in the studied population.

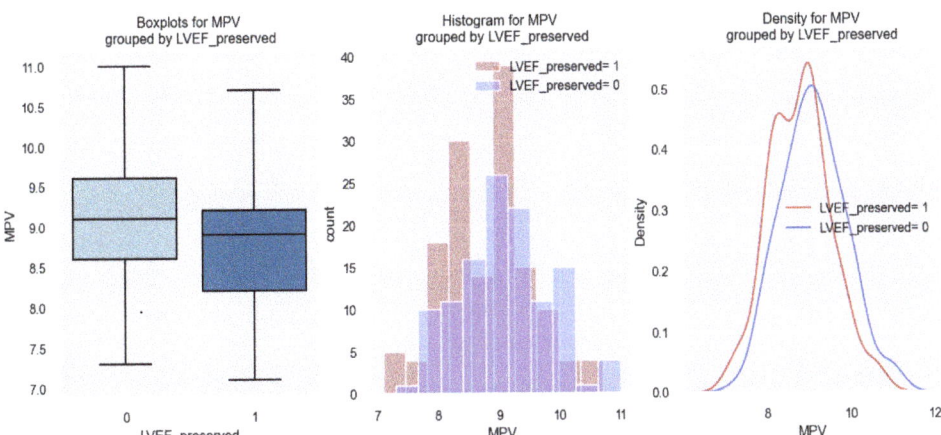

Figure 11. Reported MPV values in patients with HF with a preserved LVEF (LVEF preserved = 1) versus patients with HF without a preserved LVEF (LVEF preserved = 0).

The graphical representation of the above findings was delineated through the application of the logistic regression model. The estimated coefficients for this model are presented in Table 9. This model allows us to assess the chance of an HF patient having a preserved LVEF, depending on their MPV.

Table 9. The relation between MPV value and preserved LVEF, determined with the logistic regression model, in HF patients.

Variable:	Preserved LVEF	No. of Observations:	260			
	Coefficient	Standard Error	Z	p-Value > $|z|$	[0.025	0.975]
Intercept	5.4001	1.595	3.386	0.001	[2.275	8.526]
MPV	−0.581	0.177	−3.275	**0.001**	[−0.929	−0.233]

The applied model in this instance is expressed as follows: score (event occurrence = preserved LVEF) = 5.4001 − 0.581*MPV. Given this model, we can consider that, for example, a patient with an MPV of 8 fl has a score of 0.7521. In order to convert these scores into probabilities, we use the following equation: $probability = \frac{1}{1+e^{-score}}$. Consequently, the probability of a patient with an MPV of 8 fl having p LVEF is calculated to be 0.69, or 69%. The mathematical model applied to HF patients is relevant in this case (p-value = 0.001).

Figure 12 illustrates the previously derived results, indicating a trend wherein HF patients exhibit an increased probability of having a preserved LVEF as their MPV value decreases.

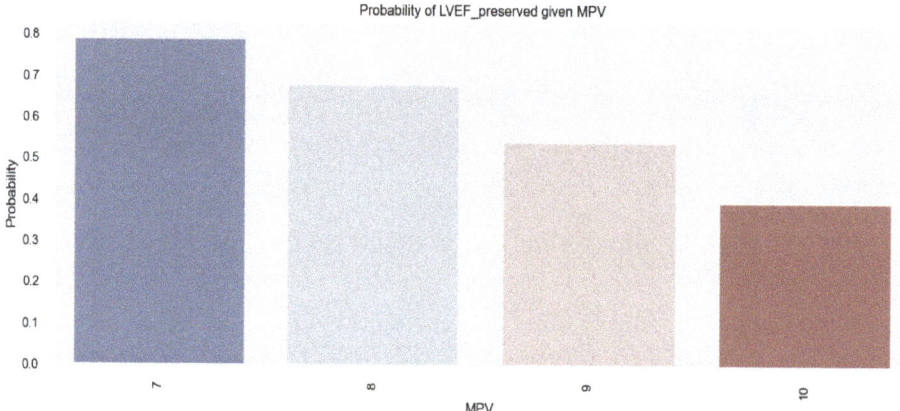

Figure 12. Estimated probability of having a preserved LVEF depending on MPV value in the studied population.

Corroborating the previously mentioned statistical data, we may assert that based on the value of a patient's MPV, we can predict the possibility of them having a preserved LVEF: the lower the value of MPV, the higher the probability of a patient with HF having a preserved LVEF.

3.3.2. MPV–Left Atrium Size Relationship

The linear relationship between the MPV value and the dimensions of the left atrium (LA), expressed in mm, in patients with HF in our study was identified by applying the linear regression method (Table 10), which showed that as the MPV value increases, the dimensions of the LA also increase. This finding was obtained from our analysis of the data presented in Table 10, which shows the following:

(1) The coefficient for MPV is 2.3035, indicating that, on average, when the MPV increases by one unit, the LA diameter increases, on average, by 2.3 mm.
(2) The associated *p-value* for the MPV coefficient is 0.000, signifying a statistically relevant result. Therefore, it can be affirmed that there exists a noteworthy relationship between the MPV value and the LA diameter in HF patients.

Table 10. The relation between MPV value and LA diameter, determined with the linear regression model, in HF patients.

Variable: No. of Observations:	LA Diameter (mm) 260	R-Squared: AIC:	0.069 1700			
	Coefficient	Standard Error	T	*p*-Value > |t|	[0.025	0.975]
Intercept	27.5822	4.727	5.835	0	[18.273	36.891]
MPV	**2.3035**	0.527	4.369	0	[1.265	3.342]

The conclusion obtained from the analysis of the above data is outlined in Figure 13, which depicts a graphical representation of the linear relationship between the MPV value and the LA diameter, and which shows that there is a tendency of the LA diameter to increase as the MPV value increases.

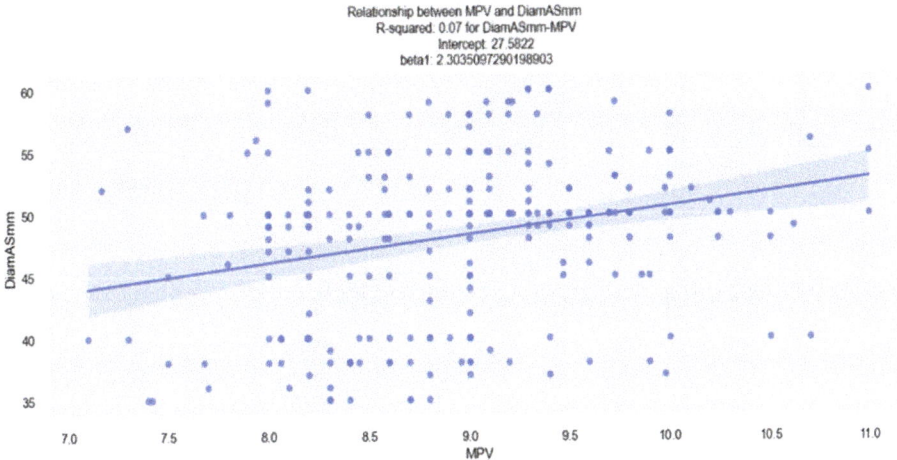

Figure 13. Linear relationship between MPV and LA diameter in patients with HF.

At the same time, the relationship between a higher MPV value and a dilated LA is exemplified clearly in the figures below (Figures 14 and 15).

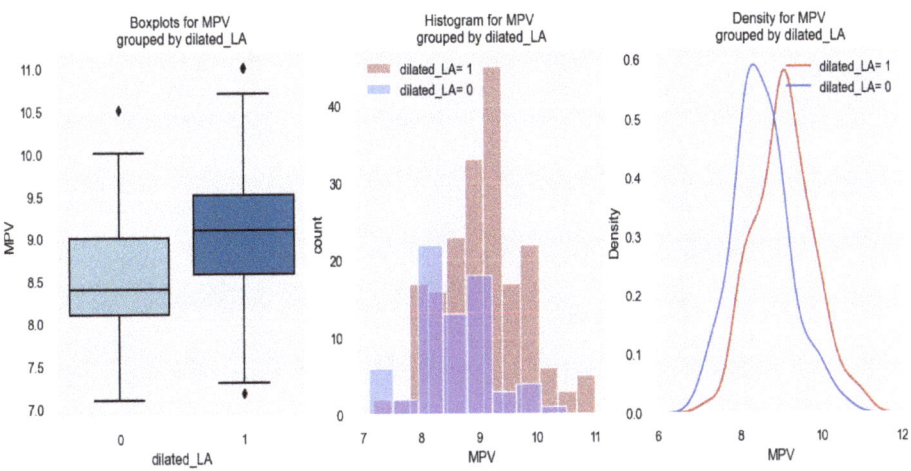

Figure 14. MPV values reported in HF patients with a dilated LA (dilated LA = 1) versus HF patients without a dilated LA (dilated LA = 0).

In the first graph of Figure 14, it can be seen that patients with a dilated LA (1) had a higher MPV value (about 9.1 fl) in comparison to those with a non-dilated LA (0), who had MPV values below 9 fl (8.4 fl), and in the following two graphs, a tendency was observed for patients with a dilated LA (1) to be distributed more to the right, thus towards higher values of MPV.

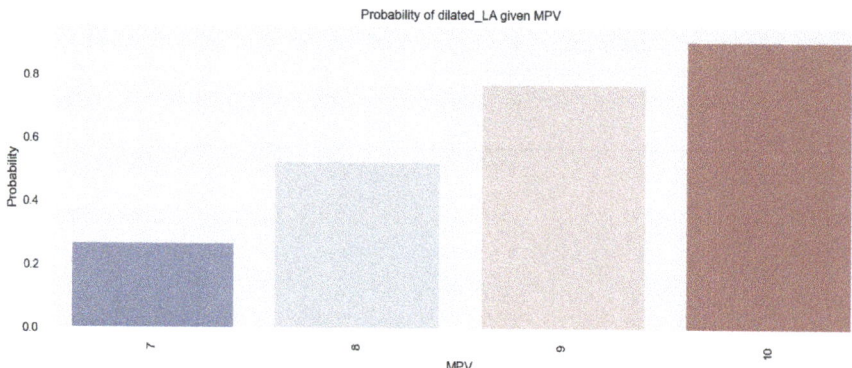

Figure 15. Estimated probability of HF patients having a dilated LA based on their MPV value, using the logistic regression method.

The aforementioned results are more effectively illustrated through the application of the logistic regression model. The graphical representation of this model is depicted in Figure 15, which reveals that for HF patients with an increased MPV, there is a tendency of an increased probability of them having a dilated LA (for example, there is an over 80% chance for a patient with an MPV of 10 fl to have a dilated LA, versus a patient with an MPV of 8 fl, for whom this chance is under 60%).

In summary, considering the arguments presented, it can be affirmed that the MPV value serves as a predictor for the probability of an HF patient to have a dilated LA. Moreover, our results reveal that the higher the value of their MPV, the greater the probability that a patient with HF will have a dilated LA.

3.3.3. MPV–LV Dimension Relationship

The linear relationship between the MPV and the dimensions of the left ventricle (LV), expressed in mm, in patients with HF in our study was identified by applying the linear regression method (Table 11), which showed that as the MPV value increases, the LV dimensions also increase. This finding was obtained from an analysis of the data in the table below (Table 11), which shows the following:

(1) The coefficient for the MPV is 1.6395, meaning that when the MPV increases by one unit, the LV diameter increases, on average, by 1.63 mm.
(2) The associated *p-value* for the MPV coefficient is 0.000, signifying a statistically relevant result. Thus, it can be affirmed that there exists a significant relationship between the MPV value and the LV diameter in HF patients from our study.

Table 11. The relation between MPV value and LV diameter, determined with the linear regression model, in HF patients.

Variable: No. of Observations:	LV Diameter (mm) 260	R-Squared: AIC:	0.048 1622			
	Coefficient	Standard Error	T	*p*-Value > |t|	[0.025	0.975]
Intercept	36.1691	4.067	8.893	0	[28.16	44.178]
MPV	**1.6395**	0.454	3.614	0	[0.746	2.533]

The conclusions obtained from the analysis of the data above are depicted in Figure 16, which is a graphical representation of the linear relationship between the MPV value and the LV diameter, and from which we can observe a tendency of the LV diameter to increase as the MPV value increases.

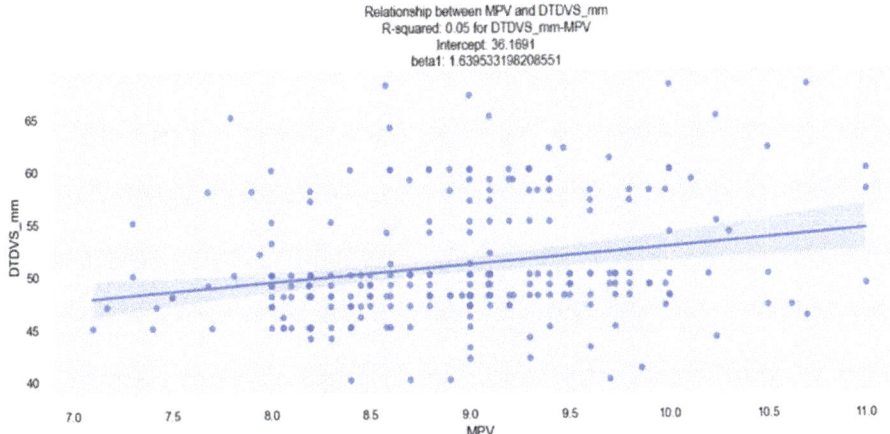

Figure 16. Linear relationship between MPV and LV diameter in patients with HF.

At the same time, the identification of a relationship between a higher MPV value and a dilated LV is exemplified clearly in the figures below (Figures 17 and 18). From the graphic representations in Figure 17, we can observe that patients with a dilated LV had higher MPV values (over 9 fl) in comparison to those without a dilated LV.

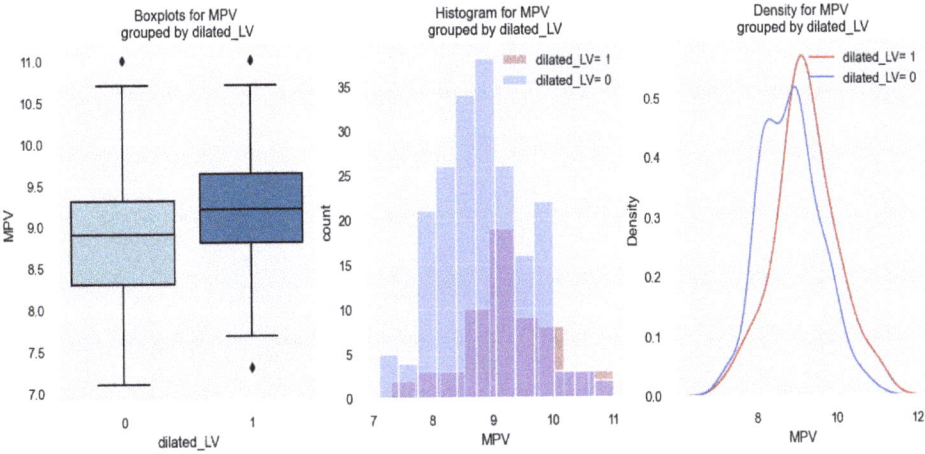

Figure 17. MPV values reported in patients with a dilated LV (dilated LV = 1) versus HF patients with a non-dilated LV (dilated LV = 0).

These results are better delineated through the application of the logistic regression model, whose data are graphically represented in Figure 18. Through this model, we can estimate the possibility of an HF patient having a dilated LV based on their MPV value. So, the figure below (Figure 18) reveals that there is an increased tendency for a patient with HF to have a dilated LV as their MPV value increases (for example, in patients with an MPV of 10 fl, there is a 35% chance of them having a dilated LV, in comparison to patients with an MPV value of 7 fl, for whom this chance is below 10%).

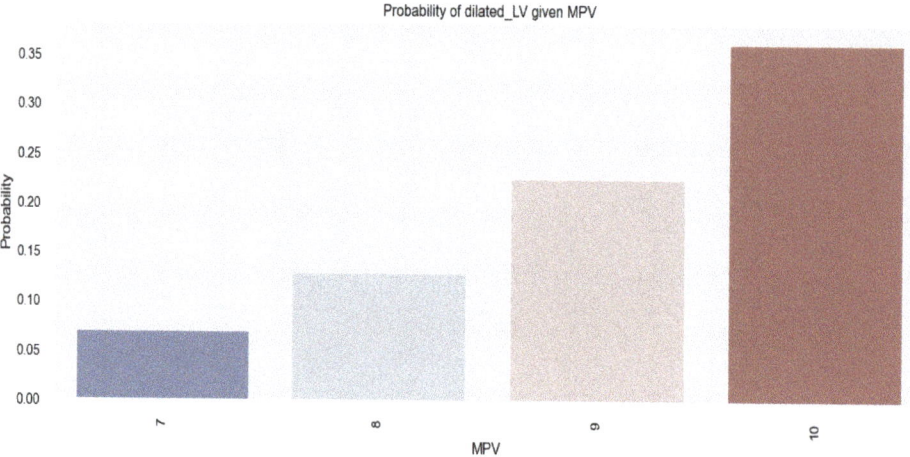

Figure 18. Estimated probability of HF patients having a dilated LV based on their MPV value, using the logistic regression method.

In summary, considering the arguments presented above, it can be affirmed that the MPV value serves as a predictor for the probability of an HF patient having a dilated LV. Furthermore, our study reveals that the higher the MPV value, the greater the probability of a patient with HF having a dilated LV.

3.3.4. Relationship between MPV and PH

Our study revealed that patients with pulmonary hypertension (PH) had a higher value of MPV compared to those without PH. This phenomenon is exemplified in the figures below (Figures 19 and 20).

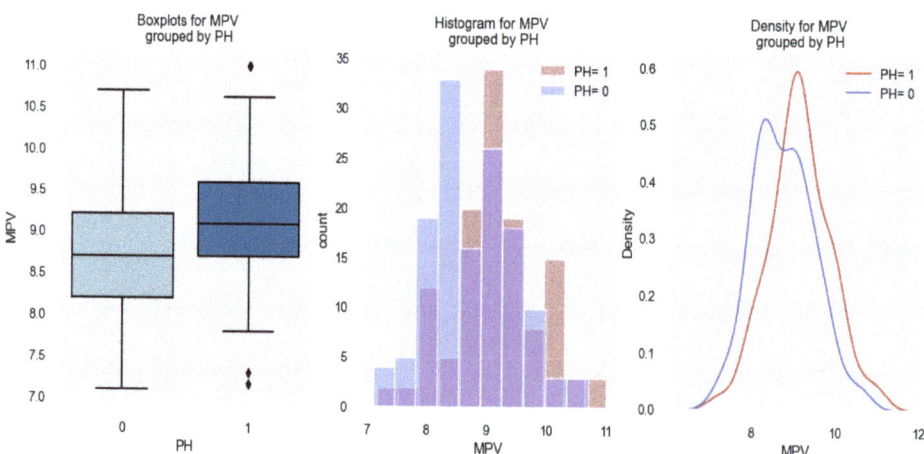

Figure 19. MPV values in HF patients with PH (PH = 1) versus HF patients without PH (PH = 0).

In the first graph of Figure 19, it can be observed that the presence of PH (PH = 1) is associated with an increased MPV value in comparison to the absence of PH (PH = 0) in our studied population, and from the following two graphs, it can be seen that patients with PH are distributed more towards the right, so towards higher MPV values, hence there is a slight tendency for MPV values to be higher for patients with PH.

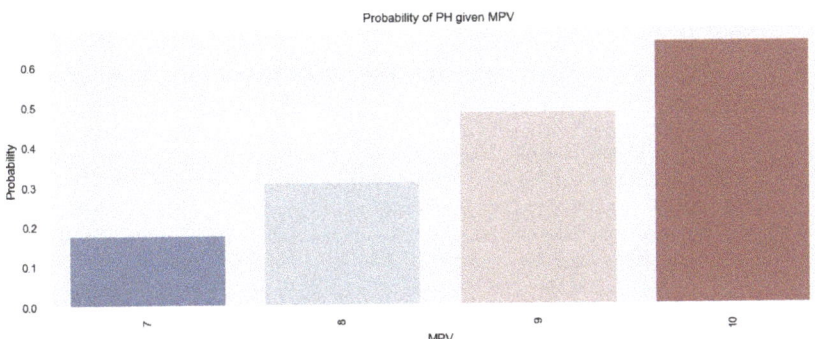

Figure 20. Estimated probability of having PH depending on MPV value in the studied population.

The insights derived from the above results are better described through the logistic regression model, whose data are represented in Figure 20. This model provides an estimation of the probability of an HF patient having PH based on their MPV value. Figure 20 highlights an increased tendency for PH to be present in HF patients with high MPV values. For instance, there is an over 60% chance that PH will be present in patients with an MPV of 10 fl in comparison to patients with an MPV of 8 fl (where there is a 31% chance of PH presence). In conclusion, based on the results presented above, it can be asserted that the MPV value can be used to predict the probability of an HF patient having PH. Moreover, in Figure 20, it can be observed that the higher the MVP value, the greater the probability of an HF patient having PH.

4. Discussion

Through our research, we aimed to add novelty to the current medical research regarding MPV as a prognostic parameter in HF patients by identifying correlations between MPV values and certain parameters, such as increased NT-proBNP, increased RDW, and the presence of an AFib rhythm, reduced LVEF, dilated LA and LV, and PH, which are considered negative prognostic variables in HF patients.

Based on the above correlations, MPV could be used as a prognostic parameter in populations of patients with HF, and through it, we could gain the ability to identify patients with HF at risk of having a negative prognosis.

Regarding the identification of a statistical link between the value of NT-proBNP and the value of MPV, our study confirms the results of the research conducted by Budak and his collaborators [17], which focused on patients with HF, and which revealed that BNP values were positively correlated with MPV values. The results of our research showed that HF patients with higher NT-proBNP values had higher MPV values, with the differences between our research and the study conducted by Budak being as follows: (1) our study focused on the relationship between NT-proBNP and MPV values; (2) the relationship between MPV and NT-proBNP values was demonstrated by applying the linear regression model, which revealed that by increasing the MPV value by one unit, NT-proBNP is increased by 2677 pg/mL.

A possible explanation for the correlation between increased levels of MPV and increased levels of NT-proBNP is that since NT-proBNP is a biomarker released as a consequence of the activation of compensatory neurohormonal mechanisms in decompensated heart failure, and thus is a biomarker linked to the aggravation of the clinical status in HF patients, this is the reason why HF patients with increased levels of NT-proBNP may also have increased levels of MPV.

Regarding the MPV–presepsin relationship in patients with HF, the studies are lacking, and the only ones available in the current medical literature are those that refer to the correlation between patients with sepsis and increased values of MPV, as shown by the study conducted by J. Van Der Lelie [18], who, however, did not target a population of patients with HF and did not follow the interrelation between presepsin and MPV. The explanation according to which patients with sepsis would have an increased MPV value is that the infection is predisposed to induce the appearance of immune complexes and the release of cytokines, which determines, through a compensatory mechanism, the occurrence of thrombocytopenia, expressed biologically by increased levels of MPV [9]. However, regarding our statistical results regarding the relationship between presepsin and MPV values, our study did not find a statistically significant relationship between these variables, the most plausible cause of this phenomenon being the reduced number of patients for which presepsin data were available.

Regarding the relationship between MPV and LVEF, two studies are cited in the literature: the one conducted by Nassiba M. et al. [19] and the one conducted by Schu-ichi Fujita et al. [20]. The study conducted by Nassiba M. [19] revealed that patients with a preserved LVEF had a higher MPV and that a larger MPV is considered a negative prognostic marker in HF patients with a preserved LVEF. The novelties brought by our research in contrast to the study conducted by Nassiba M. are as follows: (1) our research was focused on a population of HF patients regardless of their LVEF value; (2) our statistical results outlined that HF patients with a reduced LVEF had increased MPV values in comparison to those with a preserved LVEF, who had low values of MPV. The study conducted by Schu-ichi Fujita et al. [20] concentrated on a population of patients with both systolic and diastolic LV dysfunction, revealing that MPV is an independent factor associated with both systolic and diastolic LV dysfunction. The differences brought by our study are that patients with LV diastolic dysfunction (preserved LVEF) had a lower MPV value compared to patients with LV systolic dysfunction (reduced LVEF), who had higher MPV values, and that our results were obtained based on the application of logistic regression models, through which it was demonstrated that as their MPV value increases, an HF patient will be more likely to have a reduced LVEF. The possible reason for which MPV levels may be higher in patients with a reduced LVEF is that a lower LVEF is correlated to increased filling pressures in the left ventricle; this activates the neurohormonal compensatory mechanism, which is linked to a greater status of decompensation in heart failure, and as a consequence, the levels of MPV increase.

Regarding the relationship between MPV and AFib rhythms, the results of our research confirm other data from the medical literature according to the studies conducted by Yucel Colkesen [21] and by Okan Turgut et al. [13], according to which patients with a higher MPV value are at higher risk of paroxysmal AFib, and patients with an AFib rhythm had a higher MPV compared to patients with SR, respectively. The novelty of our study is the study population (patients with HF), as well as the statistical methodology applied (logistic regression models), through which we demonstrated that the higher the MPV value, the higher the probability of a patient with HF having AFib. The possible mechanism behind this link between the presence of AFib and increased levels of MPV in heart failure patients is because the AFib rhythm is one of the atrial arrhythmias associated with increased filling pressures in the left atrium and left ventricle, which in turn increase the pressure in pulmonary veins and capillaries, which consequently will be responsible for pulmonary congestions. The above chain of reactions will be responsible for a greater risk of decompensation in heart failure and for the activation of the neurohormonal and inflammatory compensatory systems, which in turn will produce platelet dysfunction, expressed by increased levels of MPV.

Extrapolating our statistical results according to which patients with a dilated LA had a higher value of MPV compared to patients with a non-dilated LA, we can link them to the statistical results obtained in the case of the relationship between the presence of an AFib rhythm and the value of MPV, taking into account that it is well known in the medical literature that patients with an AFib rhythm have a dilated LA due to the remodeling process through which their LA undergoes.

At the same time, by extrapolating the statistical results according to which patients with a dilated LV had a higher value of MPV compared to patients with a non-dilated LV, these interesting data can be linked to the statistical results obtained in the case of the relationship between LVEF and the value of MPV, taking into account that it is known in the medical literature that the majority of patients with a dilated LV have a reduced LVEF.

Regarding the results from our study according to which patients with HF with increased MPV values had a higher probability of having higher RDW values, this represents a novelty in the medical literature since the available studies related to this aspect are limited, and the existing studies on HF and MPV or HF and RDW did not study the possible statistical correlation between MPV and RDW values in patients with HF.

The current available medical research regarding the impact of RDW on HF patients is cited in two studies: one of them is a review-type study conducted by Andrew Xanthopoulos et al. [22], who revealed that patients with a higher RDW were more likely to have decompensated HF, and the second one is a type of a meta-analysis study conducted by Yuan-Lan Huang et al. [23], which revealed that HF patients with high RDW values had a more reserved prognosis, represented by frequent hospitalizations or increased mortality. The novelty that our study adds to the medical field in this context is that our research focused on MPV value–RDW value correlation in the HF population, revealing that patients with increased MPV values had increased RDW values. Therefore, the results from our study regarding the identification of a linear relationship between MPV and RDW values are promising. The reason why our findings revealed a link between elevated RDW values and elevated MPV values is probably because, like MPV, RDW also increases as a result of activation of the neurohormonal and inflammatory compensatory systems in heart failure patients, which in turn is responsible for anisocytosis, the latter one being responsible for increased levels of RDW [22,23].

The main strengths of our research are provided by the statistical analysis used, which was represented by regression model analyses. Through the above statistical analyses, we could determine significant correlations between MPV values and certain biological, electrocardiographic, and echocardiographic variables that are considered negative prognostic parameters in HF patients. Based on these promising results, we could consider that the MPV value may be a negative prognostic parameter in HF patients, and based on its value, we could target HF patients at risk of a poor outcome.

Since increased NT-proBNP, reduced LVEF, increased RDW, AFib, PH, and dilated LV and LA are variables associated with a worse clinical status and outcome in heart failure patients according to the available medical literature, and since our results revealed correlations between increased MPV values and these variables, we could expect that an increased MPV may predict negative changes in these biological, electrocardiographic, and echocardiographic parameters, and thus predict a negative prognosis in heart failure patients.

MPV is a parameter that is easy to obtain and because it is incorporated in any hemogram, it is available for any practitioner. The fact that a single parameter such as MPV could predict changes in the variables mentioned above and hence enable estimations of the probability of poor prognoses in heart failure patients represents an element of novelty for clinical practices, because through it we can label a patient at risk of a poor outcome and start a premature aggressive treatment to prevent future decompensations.

There are several limitations associated with our study:

(1) Retrospective design: this study was conducted retrospectively, involving data collection from the system database of the hospital; this approach introduces the potential of biased patient selection, as retrospective studies rely on pre-existing data, and the selection of patients may not be randomized.

(2) Influence of blood sample collection: NT-proBNP, RDW, and mean platelet volume values may be impacted by the retrospective method of blood sample collection; human error during these procedures may introduce variations in the recorded values, potentially affecting the accuracy and reliability of the results.

5. Conclusions

Based on the results from our study, we can conclude that there is a statistically significant relationship between increased values of MPV (over 9 fl) and biological (increased NT-proBNP, increased RDW), electrocardiographic (presence of AFib rhythm), and echocardiographic variables (reduced LVEF, dilated LV, dilated LA, presence of PH) in the studied population of patients with HF. Therefore, we could consider that MPV may be used as a negative prognostic parameter in HF patients, and based on its value, we may be able to identify heart failure patients susceptible to a negative prognosis.

Author Contributions: Conceptualization, A.C.; methodology, A.C.; software, O.C.; validation, A.C. and C.L.A.; formal analysis, A.C. and C.L.A.; investigation, A.C.; resources, C.L.A. and C.J.S.; data curation, A.C.; writing—original draft preparation, A.C.; writing—review and editing, A.C., C.L.A. and O.C.; visualization, C.J.S., C.L.A. and S.G.; supervision, C.J.S., C.L.A. and S.G. All authors have read and agreed to the published version of the manuscript.

Funding: This research received no external funding.

Institutional Review Board Statement: No emotional or physical harm was inflicted upon the patients throughout the research process. Our investigation solely involved the collection and analysis of data from medical records and the hospital's medical database system. It is noteworthy that our study operated within the specific guidelines established by the Ethical Committee of the University of Medicine and Pharmacy "Carol Davila", Bucharest. According to these guidelines, ethical approval was not deemed necessary for our non-interventional study, which solely entailed data collection and analysis. The Ethical Committee waived the need for ethical review and approval since our study utilized existing patient data.

Informed Consent Statement: Given the retrospective nature of this study and the assurance that the waiver of informed consent would not compromise the rights and welfare of the subjects, the requirement for written informed consent from the patients was waived. This decision was based on the fact that all data used in the study were fully anonymized and aggregated. This approach aligns with ethical considerations, ensuring the privacy and confidentiality of patient information while permitting the study to proceed without the need for individual informed consent.

Data Availability Statement: The data presented in this study are available on request from the corresponding author. The data are not publicly available due to ethical restrictions.

Conflicts of Interest: The authors declare no conflicts of interest.

Appendix A. Types of Variables Used

Independent Variable	Dependent Variable	Type of Variable	Regression Type
MPV	NT-proBNP	Continuous	Linear
MPV	Presepsin	Continuous	Linear
MPV	RDW	Continuous	Linear
MPV	AFib	Binary	Logistic
MPV	SR	Binary	Logistic
MPV	LVEF	Continuous	Linear
MPV	Reduced LVEF	Binary	Logistic
MPV	Preserved LVEF	Binary	Logistic
MPV	LA diameter_(mm)	Continuous	Linear
MPV	LV diameter (mm)	Continuous	Linear
MPV	Dilated LV	Binary	Logistic
MPV	Dilated LA	Binary	Logistic
MPV	PH	Binary	Logistic

References

1. Chu, S.G.; Becker, R.C.; Berger, P.B.; Bhatt, D.L.; Eikelboom, J.W.; Konkle, B.; Mohler, E.R.; Reilly, M.P.; Berger, J.S. Mean platelet volume as a predictor of cardiovascular risk: A systematic review and meta-analysis. *J. Thromb. Haemost.* **2010**, *8*, 148–156. [CrossRef]
2. Greisenegger, S.; Endler, G.; Hsieh, K.; Tentschert, S.; Mannhalter, C.; Lalouschek, W. Is Elevated Mean Platelet Volume Associated with a Worse Outcome in Patients with Acute Ischemic Cerebrovascular Events? *Stroke* **2004**, *35*, 1688–1691. [CrossRef]
3. Hakki, K.; Mustafa, K.Y.; Recep, K.; Osman, B.; Mehmet, B.Y. Mean Platelet Volume as a Predictor of Heart Failure-Related Hospitalizations in Stable Heart Failure Outpatients with Sinus Rhythm. *Acta Cardiol. Sin.* **2017**, *33*, 292–300.
4. Slavka, G.; Perkmann, T.; Haslacher, H.; Greisenegger, S.; Marsik, C.; Wagner, O.F.; Endler, G. Mean Platelet Volume May Represent a Predictive Parameter for Overall Vascular Mortality and Ischemic Heart Disease. *Arterioscler. Thromb. Vasc. Biol.* **2011**, *31*, 1215–1218. [CrossRef]
5. Martin, J.F.; Trowbridge, E.A.; Salmon, G.; Plumb, J. The biological significance of platelet volume: Its relationship to bleeding time, platelet thromboxane B2 production and megakaryocyte nuclear DNA concentration. *Thromb. Res.* **1983**, *32*, 443–460. [CrossRef]
6. Noris, P.; Melazzini, F.; Balduini, C.L. New roles for mean platelet volume measurement in the clinical practice? *Platelets* **2016**, *27*, 607–612. [CrossRef]
7. Serebruany, V.L.; Murugesan, S.R.; Pothula, A.; Atar, D.; Lowry, D.R.; O'Connor, C.M.; Gurbel, P.A. Increased soluble platelet/endothelial cellular adhesion molecule-1 and osteonectin levels in patients with severe congestive heart failure. Independence of disease etiology, and antecedent aspirin therapy. *Eur. J. Heart Fail.* **1999**, *1*, 243–249. [CrossRef] [PubMed]
8. Serebruany, V.L.; McKenzie, M.E.; Meister, A.F.; Fuzaylov, S.Y.; Gurbel, P.A.; Atar, D.; Gattis, W.A.; O'Connor, C.M. Whole blood impedence aggregometry for the assessment of platelet function in patients with congestive heart failure (EPCOT Trial). *Eur. J. Heart Fail.* **2002**, *4*, 461–467. [CrossRef] [PubMed]
9. Chung, I.; Choudhury, A.; Lip, G.Y.H. Platelet activation in acute, decompensated congestive heart failure. *Thromb. Res.* **2007**, *120*, 709–713. [CrossRef] [PubMed]
10. Jafri, S.M.; Ozawa, T.; Mammen, E.; Levine, T.B.; Johnson, C.; Goldstein, S. Platelet function, thrombin, and fibrinolytic activity in patients with heart failure. *Eur. Heart J.* **1993**, *14*, 205–212. [CrossRef] [PubMed]
11. Aukrust, P.; Ueland, T.; Müller, F.; Andreassen, A.K.; Nordøy, I.; Aas, H.; Kjekshus, J.; Simonsen, S.; Frøland, S.S.; Gullestad, L. Elevated Circulating Levels of C-C Chemokines in Patients with Congestive Heart Failure. *Circulation* **1998**, *97*, 1136–1143. [CrossRef] [PubMed]
12. Karabacak, M.; Dogan, A.; Aksoy, F.; Ozaydin, M.; Erdogan, D.; Karabacak, P. Both Carvedilol and Nebivolol May Improve Platelet Function and Prothrombotic State in Patients with Nonischemic Heart Failure. *Angiology* **2014**, *65*, 533–537. [CrossRef] [PubMed]
13. Turgut, O.; Zorlu, A.; Kilicli, F.; Cinar, Z.; Yucel, H.; Tandogan, I.; Dokmetas, H.S. Atrial fibrillation is associated with increased mean platelet volume in patients with type 2 diabetes mellitus. *Platelets* **2013**, *24*, 493–497. [CrossRef] [PubMed]
14. McDonagh, T.A.; Metra, M.; Adamo, M.; Gardner, R.S.; Baumbach, A.; Böhm, M.; Burri, H.; Butler, J.; Čelutkienė, J.; Chioncel, O.; et al. 2021 ESC Guidelines for the diagnosis and treatment of acute and chronic heart failure: Developed by the Task Force for the diagnosis and treatment of acute and chronic heart failure of the European Society of Cardiology (ESC) with the special contribution of the Heart Failure Association (HFA) of the ESC. *Eur. Heart J.* **2021**, *42*, 3599–3726. [PubMed]
15. Lancellotti, P.; Zamorano, J.L.; Habib, G.; Badano, L. (Eds.) *The EACVI Textbook of Echocardiography*; Editura Oxford: Oxford, UK, 2016.
16. Budak, Y.U.; Huysal, K.; Demirci, H. Correlation between mean platelet volume and B-type natriuretic peptide concentration in emergency patients with heart failure. *Biochem. Med.* **2015**, *25*, 97–102. [CrossRef] [PubMed]
17. Humbert, M.; Kovacs, G.; Hoeper, M.M.; Badagliacca, R.; Berger, R.M.; Brida, M.; Carlsen, J.; Coats, A.J.; Escribano-Subias, P.; Ferrari, P.; et al. 2022 ESC/ERS Guidelines for the diagnosis and treatment of pulmonary hypertension: Developed by the task force for the diagnosis and treatment of pulmonary hypertension of the European Society of Cardiology (ESC) and the European Respiratory Society (ERS). Endorsed by the International Society for Heart and Lung Transplantation (ISHLT) and the European Reference Network on rare respiratory diseases (ERN-LUNG). *Eur. Heart J.* **2022**, *43*, 3618–3731. [PubMed]
18. Van der Lelie, J.; Von dem Borne, A.K. Increased mean platelet volume in septicaemia. *J. Clin. Pathol.* **1983**, *36*, 693–696. [CrossRef] [PubMed]
19. Menghoum, N.; Beauloye, C.; Lejeune, S.; Badii, M.C.; Gruson, D.; van Dievoet, M.A.; Pasquet, A.; Vancraeynest, D.; Gerber, B.; Bertrand, L.; et al. Mean platelet volume: A prognostic marker in heart failure with preserved ejection fraction. *Platelets* **2023**, *34*, 2188965. [CrossRef]
20. Fujita, S.I.; Takeda, Y.; Kizawa, S.; Ito, T.; Sakane, K.; Ikemoto, Y.; Okada, Y.; Sohmiya, K.; Hoshiga, M.; Ishizaka, N. Platelet volume indices are associated with systolic and diastolic cardiac dysfunction and left ventricular hypertrophy. *BMC Cardiovasc. Disord.* **2015**, *15*, 52. [CrossRef]
21. Colkesen, Y.; Acil, T.; Abayli, B.; Yigit, F.; Katircibasi, T.; Kocum, T.; Demircan, S.; Sezgin, A.; Ozin, B.; Muderrisoglu, H. Mean platelet volume is elevated during paroxysmal atrial fibrillation: A marker of increased platelet activation? *Blood Coagul. Fibrinolysis* **2008**, *19*, 411–414. [CrossRef]

22. Xanthopoulos, A.; Giamouzis, G.; Dimos, A.; Skoularigki, E.; Starling, R.C.; Skoularigis, J.; Triposkiadis, F. Red Blood Cell Distribution Width in Heart Failure: Pathophysiology, Prognostic Role, Controversies and Dilemmas. *J. Clin. Med.* **2022**, *11*, 1951. [CrossRef] [PubMed]
23. Huang, Y.L.; Hu, Z.D.; Liu, S.J.; Sun, Y.; Qin, Q.; Qin, B.D.; Zhang, W.W.; Zhang, J.R.; Zhong, R.Q.; Deng, A.M. Prognostic Value of Red Blood Cell Distribution Width for Patients with Heart Failure: A Systematic Review and Meta-Analysis of Cohort Studies. *PLoS ONE* **2014**, *9*, e104861. [CrossRef] [PubMed]

Disclaimer/Publisher's Note: The statements, opinions and data contained in all publications are solely those of the individual author(s) and contributor(s) and not of MDPI and/or the editor(s). MDPI and/or the editor(s) disclaim responsibility for any injury to people or property resulting from any ideas, methods, instructions or products referred to in the content.

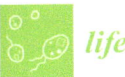

life

Review

Subcutaneous Implantable Cardioverter Defibrillator: A Contemporary Overview

Fabrizio Guarracini [1,*], Alberto Preda [2], Eleonora Bonvicini [1], Alessio Coser [1], Marta Martin [1], Silvia Quintarelli [1], Lorenzo Gigli [2], Matteo Baroni [2], Sara Vargiu [2], Marisa Varrenti [2], Giovanni Battista Forleo [3], Patrizio Mazzone [2], Roberto Bonmassari [1], Massimiliano Marini [1] and Andrea Droghetti [4]

1. Department of Cardiology, S. Chiara Hospital, 38122 Trento, Italy; eleonorabonvicini@yahoo.it (E.B.); alessio.coser@apss.tn.it (A.C.); marta.martin@apss.tn.it (M.M.); silvia.quintarelli@apss.tn.it (S.Q.); roberto.bonmassari@apss.tn.it (R.B.); massimiliano.marini@apss.tn.it (M.M.)
2. Electrophysiology Unit, Cardio-Thoraco-Vascular Department, ASST Grande Ospedale Metropolitano Niguarda, 20162 Milan, Italy; preda.alberto@hsr.it (A.P.); lorenzo.gigli@ospedaleniguarda.it (L.G.); matteo.baroni@ospedaleniguarda.it (M.B.); sara.vargiu@ospedaleniguarda.it (S.V.); marisa.varrenti@ospedaleniguarda.it (M.V.); patrizio.mazzone@ospedaleniguarda.it (P.M.)
3. Department of Thoracic Surgery, Candiolo Cancer Institute, FPO-IRCCS, Candiolo, 10060 Turin, Italy; forleo@me.com
4. Cardiology Unit, Luigi Sacco University Hospital, 20157 Milan, Italy; adroghetti@libero.it
* Correspondence: fabrizio.guarracini@apss.tn.it; Tel.: +39-(0)461-903121; Fax: +39-(0)461-903122

Abstract: The difference between subcutaneous implantable cardioverter defibrillators (S-ICDs) and transvenous ICDs (TV-ICDs) concerns a whole extra thoracic implantation, including a defibrillator coil and pulse generator, without endovascular components. The improved safety profile has allowed the S-ICD to be rapidly taken up, especially among younger patients. Reports of its role in different cardiac diseases at high risk of SCD such as hypertrophic and arrhythmic cardiomyopathies, as well as channelopathies, is increasing. S-ICDs show comparable efficacy, reliability, and safety outcomes compared to TV-ICD. However, some technical issues (i.e., the inability to perform anti-bradycardia pacing) strongly limit the employment of S-ICDs. Therefore, it still remains only an alternative to the traditional ICD thus far. This review aims to provide a contemporary overview of the role of S-ICDs compared to TV-ICDs in clinical practice, including technical aspects regarding device manufacture and implantation techniques. Newer outlooks and future perspectives of S-ICDs are also brought up to date.

Keywords: subcutaneous implantable cardioverter defibrillator; ventricular tachycardia; sudden death; cardiomyopathy

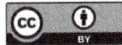

1. Introduction

The development of S-ICDs from concept to their initial commercialization was a journey lasting 19 years. Only in 2009 and 2012 did the first generation of S-ICDs receive the CE mark and US FDA approval, respectively. The S-ICD was developed as a possible alternative to transvenous ICDs (TV-ICDs), trying to achieve the same effectiveness as TV-ICDs in terms of detecting and treating both ventricular fibrillation (VF) and ventricular tachycardia (VT) [1,2]. Several studies were performed in order to evaluate the efficacy and safety of these devices and rapid advances were made in the following years, leading to the development of a second generation of S-ICDs in 2015 and a third generation in 2016.

S-ICDs are structurally similar to TV-ICDs, being made of a pulse generator and a defibrillator coil. The advantage of S-ICDs concerns the components, which are completely outside of the chest. This substantial difference minimizes the risk of lead fractures or systemic infections, some of the most feared complications of TV-ICDs [3], as well as making any extraction procedure much simpler and less dangerous [4]. Consequently, the outlook for S-ICDs is stronger in two scenarios: when used in younger patients, who are usually affected by genetic heart diseases and are at high risk of sudden cardiac death (SCD) such as hypertrophic cardiomyopathy (HCM), dilated cardiomyopathy (DCM), and genetic arrhythmia syndromes [5–7]; and in instances in which the transvenous route is inaccessible. Nevertheless, S-ICDs present several limitations compared to TV-ICDs: due to the lack of an endocardial electrode, S-ICDs are only able to deliver post-shock ventricular pacing for 30 s. For this reason, for patients who need anti-bradycardia pacing or resynchronization therapy, S-ICD implants are contraindicated [8]. Another issue concerns the alloy of which the coil is composed, which contains a small amount of nickel (around 16%). However, the device is registered as nickel free and no cases of allergic reactions have been reported in allergic patients so far.

In recent years, larger studies confirmed the role of S-ICDs as a valuable alternative to TV-ICDs (Table 1). In both prospective trials [9–12] and registries [13,14], S-ICDs showed remarkable safety in the short and medium term, which was associated with a relatively low inappropriate shock rate in populations with different clinical characteristics and cardiovascular diseases, as well as indications of primary or secondary prevention of SCD. In this review, we provide an overview of the current role of S-ICDs in clinical practice compared to TV-ICDs, as well as updates to surgical techniques, medical management, and future perspectives of this increasingly used technology.

Table 1. Major studies on S-ICD.

Study	Year	Type	Aim of Study	Primary Endpoints	Secondary Endpoints	Results
IDE (Investigational Device Exemption) Trial [15]	2013	Prospective, non-randomized, multicenter clinical study	Safety and effectiveness of S-ICD	-Shock effectiveness in converting induced VF in conversion test -Complication-free Rate at 180 days	//	-100% VF conversion rate at 180 days -92–99% complications-free rate at 180 days
EFFORTLESS (Evaluation of factors impacting clinical outcome and cost effectiveness of the S-ICD) Registry [13]	2017	Prospective, non-randomized, multicenter observational registry	Early, mid- and long-term clinical effectiveness	-Complication-free rate at 30 days -Complication-free rate at 360 days -Inappropriate shocks-free rate for AF/SVT	//	-97% complication-free rate at 30 days -94% complication-free rate at 360 days -7% inappropriate shock rate (94% oversensed episodes)
S-ICD post approval Study [14]	2017	Prospective, non-randomized, multicenter registry	Safety and effectiveness of S-ICD	-Complication-free rate at 60 months -Shock effectiveness in converting spontaneous VT/VF at 60 months	-Electrode-related complications-free rate at 60 months -First shock effectiveness i converting induced and spontaneous VT/VF at 60 months	-96.2% complication-free rate at 30 days -98.7% successful conversion rate of induced VT/VF at 60 months
PRAETORIAN (Prospective randomized comparison of subcutaneous and transvenous implantable cardioverter defibrillator therapy) Study [11]	2020	Prospective, randomized, international, controlled trial	Comparison of safety and effectiveness in TV-ICD and S-ICD (non-inferiority)	-Adverse event rate at 48 months	-MACE, appropriate and inappropriate shocks, time to successful therapy, first shock conversion efficacy, implant procedure time, hospitalization rate, fluoroscopy time, cardiac (pre)-syncope events, cross over to the other arm, cardiac decompensation at 48 months -Quality of life at 30 months	-No difference in overall and arrhythmic mortality -Four times lead-related complications rate in TV-ICD -Two times infection rate in TV-ICD -No difference in complications rate in 4 years -No difference in inappropriate shock rate

Table 1. *Cont.*

Study	Year	Type	Aim of Study	Primary Endpoints	Secondary Endpoints	Results
UNTOUCHED (Understanding outcomes with the S-ICD in primary prevention patients with low ejection fraction) Study [10]	2021	Prospective, non-randomized, multinational trial	Safety and effectiveness of S-ICD	-Inappropriate shocks free rate at 18 months	-Freedom from system and procedure related complication at 30 days -All cause shock free rate at 18 months	-95.9% inappropriate shock-free rate at 18 months -90.6% all-cause shock-free rate at 18 months -92.7% complications-free rate at 18 months
ATLAS (Avoid transvenous leads in appropriate subjects) Trial [12]	2022	Prospective, randomized, multicenter controlled study	Comparison of safety and effectiveness in TV-ICD and S-ICD (superiority)	-Lead-related complications at 6 months -Other complications at 6 months	-Late device-related complications after 6 months -Arrhythmic deaths, visits, inappropriate shocks, all-cause mortality, economic analysis, patients acceptance after 6 months	-12 times lead-related complications in TV-ICD

2. Subcutaneous ICD: What We Know So Far

2.1. Pre-Implant Screening

S-ICDs consists of a completely extra-thoracic device without the registration of intracardiac electrograms. For this reason, when a S-ICD implant is planned, it is necessary to ensure optimal sensing through a pre-implant screening [16]. The pre-implant screening aims to evaluate the amplitude of the sensed R wave and if the available three sensing vectors (primary from the proximal electrode ring to can, secondary from the distal electrode ring to can, and the third from the distal to the proximal electrode) are able to differentiate the R wave from the T wave in order to ensure appropriate sensing of VT and avoid inappropriate ICD shocks (IAS) [17]. The electrogram analyzed by the S-ICD is more similar to a standard 12-lead electrocardiogram (ECG) than to an intracavitary electrogram, with a distinct P-wave, T-wave and QRS-complex. A dedicated tool is used to measure the amplitude of the three sensing vectors from the standard 12-lead ECG in both a supine and a sitting/standing position. The screening is passed if at least one of the vectors works in both positions. Different studies demonstrated that 8% to 15% of the individuals are excluded from the implant of S-ICD after the screening [18–20]. Because many IAS are observed during exercise, some studies have suggested the possibility of conducting the screening during exercise to evaluate the three vectors in a dynamic way [21,22]. The most frequent cause of IAS in implanted S-ICD is T waves oversensing; therefore, in such cases, prolonged screening periods and a more detailed study of the T variation in different contexts are needed to improve the screening phase [23,24]. Exercise screening should be recommended in specific diseases with higher incidence of screening failure, such as HCM [25].

2.2. Implant Technique

The implant of S-ICD differs from a TV-ICD. S-ICD is made of a case pulse generator that is placed in a subcutaneous pocket between the anterior and the mid-axillary lines at the level of the V-VI intercostal space. Currently, a third-generation S-ICD device provided by Boston Scientific (EMBLEM; Boston Scientific, Marlborough, MA, USA) is used. It weighs 130 g and it measures $83.1 \times 69.1 \times 12.7$ mm. It is magnetic resonance (MRI) compatible.

There is a single 45 cm lead with sensing ring electrodes at its extremities. One extremity is tunneled in the subcutaneous plane from the case to the sternum, where it is fixed 1 cm cranial to the xiphoid process while the other extremity is rounded and tunneled vertically parallel to the left side of the sternum.

To optimize the implant, different techniques have been tested. The first cases used a three-incision technique with two incisions at the extremities, one for the lead and one for the case. After that, a two-incision technique was developed using just the inferior incision for the placement of the lead and eliminating the superior one. Several studies demonstrated that the two-incision technique is as safe and efficacious as the three-incision one, providing a faster and less complicated procedure [26,27]. A high probability of effective defibrillation with a two-incision procedure was also reported [28].

Regarding the placement of the pulse generator, different sites of implant were evaluated. An intermuscular implant in the virtual space between the anterior surface of the serratus anterior muscle and the posterior surface of the latissimus dorsi muscle was demonstrated to reduce the risk of infections [29]. This technique could be also useful when insufficient subcutaneous tissue is available, such as in thin patients with a low body mass index or for cosmetic reasons [30]. In one study, the intermuscular implant reduced the shock impedance in obese patients [31]. Finally, a sub-serratus implant, by reducing the distance between the generator and the heart, may improve device efficacy and provide a better cosmetic effect, but only a few studies of this nature have been conducted [32].

Fluoroscopy is not necessary during an S-ICD implant, except in the pre-procedural step when finding the landmarks used for implantation. The procedure is mainly performed under deep sedation or general anesthesia [13] and the total duration of the procedure is demonstrated to be just a little longer than that of the transvenous one [27].

The S-ICD implant has a lower rate of severe complications compared to TV-ICD. Despite a slightly higher frequency of pocket hematoma, it strongly reduces the risk of pneumothorax, traumatic pericardial effusion, and lead dislodgment, with lower rates of re-intervention [27]. In the IDE study, no cases of cardiac perforation, tamponade, pneumothorax, or subclavian vein stenosis were registered [9].

The implant technique has been improved over the last 10 years of experience. In particular, it has been demonstrated that there is a steep learning curve for physicians who perform S-ICD implants, with only around 13 implants needed to acquire good autonomy. Increased experience with implantation techniques also led to a significant reduction in complication rates [33].

2.3. Inappropriate Shocks

ICD shocks are potentially associated with myocardial injury, altered hemodynamic, apoptosis, and inflammatory signaling [34]. Several studies demonstrated a positive relation between the burden of ICD shocks and development or worsening of heart failure, as well as increased risk of heart failure hospitalizations and mortality [35–37]. Moreover, shocks have non-negligible psychological and physical impact on patients, with the risk of seriously affecting their quality of life for decades [38]. Older studies reported that up to 17% of people with TV-ICD could receive an IAS, usually due to misinterpretation of supraventricular tachycardias (SVT), including sinus tachycardia, atrial fibrillation (AF), and atrial flutter or device malfunction [39,40]. This issue has been appreciated a lot in recent years and led to the development of newer optimized and focused diagnostic strategies, which progressively lessened the rate of IAS over time up to 1.9%, according to recent studies [41]. Regarding S-ICD, inappropriate T oversensing and myopotentials are the main cause of IAS [42,43]. On the contrary, S-ICD's performance in discriminating AF seems higher than TV-ICD, according to a recent metanalysis [44]. In the IDE study, IAS was performed in 13.1% [15], while in the EFFORTLESS registry it was performed in 11.7% of cases, in addition to 2.3% of cases involving non-recognized SVT [13]. A more recent post approval study stated that 6.5% of cases involved IAS [14].

In the START study, the S-ICD algorithm was found to be effective for SVT discrimination, even better than TV-ICD [16]. Initial devices used single zone programming that was only capable of monitoring the cardiac rate. Improvements were made with the development of a second zone capable of conditional discrimination for rates between 170–240 beats/min. This zone is programmed to recognize rate and differentiate between SVT and VT with the possibility of achieving early diagnosis of AF. Dual zone programming strongly demonstrated a reduction in IAS incidence (11.7% vs. 20.5%) compared to single-zone programming [13,14].

The UNTOUCHED study reported the lowest rate of IAS for SVT among S-ICD controlled trials, with an IAS-free rate of 95.9% ($p < 0.001$) at 18 months (against a standard performance goal of 91.6% of TV-ICDs) [10]. Data from the UNTOUCHED study greatly differed from the data of the PRAETORIAN TRIAL [11], which reported higher rate of IAS in the S-ICD group, despite the absence of statistical significance. The reason for this discrepancy may be due to the higher prevalence of the third-generation S-ICD in the UNTOUCHED group compared to the PRAETORIAN one. Indeed, among the most important innovations of third-generation S-ICDs was the introduction of the SMART PASS filter (since 2018), which was designed to reduce the amplitude of lower-frequency signals (such as T-waves), maintaining unchanged signals from R-waves, VT or VF [45]. The introduction of SMART PASS effectively reduced the rate of IAS in another study [46]. This highlights the importance of morphology discrimination algorithms applied in the conditional shock zone in reducing IAS in S-ICDs as opposed to the initial use of interval criteria before applying morphology criteria in TV-ICDs [47].

2.4. Infections

The S-ICD Post Approval Study examined by Gold and colleagues [48] in order to evaluate the incidence and predictors of infections in a 3-year follow-up period observed an infection prevalence of 3.3% (69% within 90 days, 92.7% within 1 year, and none after 2 years). No lead extraction was needed. The mortality rate was 0.6%/year with no systemic infections. The results were similar to those of other previous studies.

Several meta-analyses reported no significant differences in the occurrence of device-related infections (OR = 1.57; 95% CI: 0.67–3.68) compared to TV-ICDs [49,50]. According to these data, the rates of all types of infection are the same between S-ICDs and TV-ICDs. However, a more accurate analysis identified a greater rate of high-risk infections (i.e., systemic infections) in the TV-ICD group. On the contrary, the S-ICD group was more prone to pocket infections, which are associated with a significantly lower risk of death [51].

In both cases, device removal is needed, although extractions of TV-ICD are significantly harder and have a higher risk of severe complications compared to S-ICDs extractions [52,53]. Patients at high risk of infection, such as dialyzed or immunocompromised patients, could benefit from S-ICD.

2.5. Lead Complications

Transvenous leads are the weakest elements of the TV-ICD system, causing dislocation, fracture, or infections. Lead fracture accounted for the first case of abandoned lead in the population with cardiac implantable electronic devices (CIEDs) [54]. The term "lead fracture" refers to a fracture in the lead's conductor coil and typically accounts for less than 2% of IAS per year [55]. The risk increases in younger people and in females and becomes greater over time [56]. Lead fractures often occur in correspondence with stress points, such as near the pulse generator, at the venous access site, or at the lead tip, where repetitive motion places stress on the conductor coil. Lead fracture or displacement are often investigated when loss of sensing or pacing are detected during routine checks of the device. In ICDs, lead fractures are among the most frequent causes of IAS due to artifacts oversensing [57]. Moreover, a fracture of the high-voltage conductor coil may compromise the ability to deliver therapy when needed. In most cases of lead fracture, lead interrogation will show an increase in lead impedance, which may arise slowly or abruptly. Transvenous leads complications also include new or worsened tricuspid regurgitation, pericardial effusion or pericarditis, cardiac perforation with or without tamponade, hemothorax/pneumothorax, and upper-extremity vein thrombosis [58].

These conditions must be taken into account when a new device is implanted, especially in young individuals. New prospects have been offered by the S-ICD for this population, mainly due to the significant reduction in lead-related complications. In the PRAETORIAN trial, the primary endpoint consisted of a composite endpoint of device-related complications or inappropriate shocks at 4 years. The occurrence of lead-related complications was significantly higher in TV-ICD patients (6.6% in the TV-ICD arm versus 1.4% in the S-ICD arm; $p = 0.001$) [11]. The ATLAS trial reported 4.8% lead complications in the TV-ICD group compared to 0.6% in the S-ICD group at six months [12].

A recent meta-analysis conducted by Fong et al. substantially confirmed these data [44]. In particular, despite a similar rate of whole complications between the two groups (RR, 0.59 [95% CI, 0.33–1.04]; $p = 0.070$), a significant drop in the lead-related complications was found in the S-ICD group (RR, 0.14 [95% CI, 0.07–0.29]; $p < 0.0001$).

It is worth noticing that S-ICD lead-related complications are different from the ones of the TV-ICD groups because of the different conformation and position (Table 2). Indeed, the most frequent S-ICD lead-related complications happened in the early post-implant phase, consisting of lead movement and suboptimal lead position that usually only needed to be repositioned [49].

Table 2. Transvenous ICD vs. subcutaneous ICD.

	TV-ICD	S-ICD
Pre-implant Screening	Not needed	Needed
Implant Technique	Transvenous	Subcutaneous
Sedation	Local	Deep/general anesthesia
Fluoroscopy	Needed	Not needed
Electrocardiogram	Intracavitary ECG	12-lead ECG
Inappropriate shocks	SVT	T oversensing, myopotential, discrimination error
Anti-tachycardia pacing	Possible	Not possible
SHOCK threshold	5–30 J	80 J
Infections	Systemic infections	Pocket infections
Lead complications	Dislocations/fractures; tricuspid regurgitation, pericardial effusion or pericarditis, cardiac perforation	Lead movement/suboptimal lead position

Data on long-term complications are still needed to perform a comprehensive comparison between the two devices.

2.6. Appropriate Therapies

The S-ICD has a reproducible good capacity for detection of VAs. In the IDE study, all VAs were successfully converted, with the exception of a self-interrupted monomorphic VT [15]. Similar data have been registered in the post-approval study, where only 5.3% of patients showed a VA with a conversion rate of 100% [9].

The START trial systematically compared the discrimination capacities between S-ICD and TV-ICD. In particular, at the end of S-ICD or TV-ICD implant, a VT was simulated and an appropriate detection rate (>99%) was registered in both groups [16]. On the contrary, in the PRAETORIAN trial, Knops et al. reported a higher rate of appropriate shocks in the S-ICD group. This result can be easily explained by the lack of S-ICDs to provide an anti-tachycardia pacing (ATP) therapy [59]. It must be considered that in the 4-year follow up of the PRAETORIAN trial, a switch from S-ICD to a TV-ICD was reported in 0.9% of cases. The reason was the need for anti-bradycardia pacing (0.7%) and the need for ATP therapy (0.2%) [11].

In conclusion, the efficacy of shock therapy was evaluated, with similar results between the two groups. The first shock efficacy was 93.8% in the S-ICD group and 91.6% in the TV-ICD group ($p = 0.40$) while efficacy of the last shock was 97.9% and 98.4%, respectively ($p = 0.70$) [59]. Accordingly, a 98% successful conversion rate was registered by Bardy and colleagues in one of the first observational studies [2].

S-ICD can deliver up to five consecutive biphasic shocks. The recharge lasts 14 s. The shock polarity can vary from coil to generator (standard) or generator to coil (reverse). The system is able to keep the last effective one in its memory. In cases of failure, the system automatically switches to an alternative mode. S-ICDs have a higher defibrillation threshold compared to TV-ICDs and deliver a biphasic shock of 80 J (versus 40 J of TV-ICDs). A study showed a lower increase in myocardial injury biomarkers in patients with S-ICD compared to TV-ICD after shock delivery [60].

3. Indications for S-ICD Implant

The current AHA/ACC/HRS guidelines (2017) indicate, in class I, the implant of S-ICD in patients who meet the criteria for an ICD when a high risk of infection or inadequate vascular access is present, but only if there is no expected need for anti-bradycardia pacing, cardiac resynchronization therapy, or VAs termination [61]. Instead, the latest ESC guidelines (2022) give the same indication with a IIa level of evidence.

According to current guidelines, the major reason to withhold an S-ICD implantation is the need for pacing. The need for anti-bradycardia pacing and cardiac resynchronization therapy (CRT) is the most frequent reason for excluding S-ICD. However, the inability of

S-ICD to deliver ATP therapy is another non-negligible concern. Indeed, the history of monomorphic VT or non-sustained ventricular tachycardia (NSVT) increases the chance of appropriate ATP therapy in 1 out of 10 patients and 1 out of 3 patients, respectively [62]. This condition may be considered among all discriminant factors in the choice between S-ICD and TV-ICD. Alternatively, in cases of monomorphic VT or NSVT and contraindications for TV-ICD, the coupling of the S-ICD implant and VT ablation was shown to reduce the need of ATP [63].

Along with anti-bradycardia pacing, the battery longevity is another matter of concern when a S-ICD is considered. The first generation of S-ICD had a median battery longevity of 5 years [64] and, despite recent advances, the longevity of the third-generation S-ICD remains shorter than TV-ICD, with a median of 6 years.

In addition, S-ICD is incapable of direct sensing of atrial arrythmia and, although it features the possibility of remote monitoring, the data broadcast is not automated, but patient induced. Another limitation of S-ICD regards the cost, which is significantly higher than TV-ICD.

Despite the above-mentioned limitations, the implant of S-ICD should be considered as the first choice for a specific group of patients. In children and young people, S-ICD is safe and effective [65] and could be useful due to these patients' long life expectancy and more active lifestyle. Indeed, transvenous lead-related complications are reported to be very high in this population and have been linked to a relevant risk of IASs [66]. In the ATLAS trial, which enrolled younger patients compared to other studies, a lower rate of major lead-related complication in S-ICD patients was noted [12]. Although there might be a mismatch between the size of the generator case compared to the available anatomical location in the lateral axilla in infants and small children, subcutaneous leads are better suited to body growth changes and therefore more adaptable for young people who are still growing.

Patients on dialysis may be also good candidates for S-ICD due to limited vascular access or partial obstruction of central veins, as well as the higher risk of systemic infections and complications related to the extraction [67,68]. Koman et al. reported similar procedural outcomes and inappropriate and appropriate shocks in hemodialysis patients with S-ICD compared to a control TV-ICD group [69].

In conclusion, patients at high risk of infections may benefit from a subcutaneous device: this group include patients with a previous device infection, patients with renal disease, and patients who are chronically immunosuppressed [63,68]. Figure 1 summarizes the advantages of S-ICD over TV-ICD.

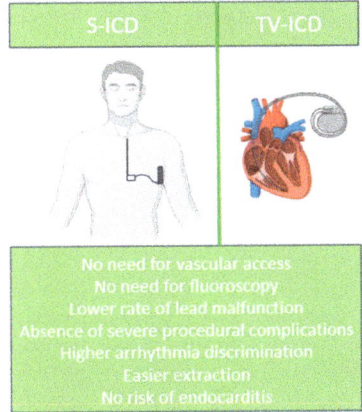

Figure 1. Advantages of S-ICD over TV-ICD.

4. Particular Set of Patients according to the Underlying Cardiomyopathy

4.1. Hypertrophic Cardiomyopathy

Patients with hypertrophic cardiomyopathy (HCM) may need ICD therapy from adolescence. As previously explained, since the risk of lead-related complications increases with age, S-ICD could be a good option in these patients [70]. The majority of HCM patients were found to be eligible for S-ICD implant after the screening step [71] and the safety and efficacy of S-ICD in HCM patients was similar to that of TV-ICD with a similar rate of post operative complications (92.7% vs. 89.5%), final shock conversion efficacy (100% vs. 98%), and IAS (12.5% vs. 10.3%, mainly due to T wave oversensing) [72]. Anti-bradycardia pacing is rarely needed in individuals affected by HCM. In cases of advanced disease or severe left ventricle outflow tract obstruction without other therapeutic opportunities, an intravenous device could be useful for resynchronization therapy or to reduce the outflow tract obstruction [7]. Notably, according to one study, patients with HCM and S-ICD had significantly fewer ICD interventions (due to an inability to deliver ATP) than patients with TV-ICD but without differences in shock delivery rate and mortality at follow-up [72,73]. These data suggest that among all ATP therapies delivered from the TV-ICD, a consistent number may be potentially unnecessary.

4.2. Brugada Syndrome, Long QT Syndrome and Arrhythmogenic Right Ventricular Cardiomyopathy

Young people with channelopathies such as Brugada syndrome (BrS) and long QT syndrome (LQTS) or those affected by genetic cardiomyopathies such as arrhythmogenic right ventricular cardiomyopathy (ARVC) may be good candidates for S-ICD due to its high safety profile [74,75]. However, while BrS and LQTS patients are not strictly dependent on ATP therapy due to more frequent incidence of polymorphic VTs [76,77], in arrhythmogenic cardiomyopathies the choice between a TV-ICD or S-ICD should be evaluated case by case through integration of clinical and genetic data [78]. Indeed, several arrhythmogenic cardiomyopathies including ARVC may have significantly higher incidence of sustained monomorphic TVs [79]. Consequently, this category of patients could have greater benefit from a device capable of delivering ATP therapies. Another non-negligible concern of ARVC is related to its evolutionary nature, leading to reduction in myocardial voltages over time and subsequent risk of IAS due to non-cardiac oversensing [80]. Therefore, a careful assessment of the risk–benefit ratio in this category of young individuals with higher risk of SCD should be performed, considering the higher risk of lead-related complications as well as the risk of an increase in the sensing and pacing threshold [81]. In BrS, the typical morphology of the ST tract could lead to oversensing on the T wave, interfering with the functioning of the device [82]. In these cases, careful screening is needed.

4.3. Congenital Heart Disease

Several studies have documented the safety and feasibility of S-ICD implantation in patients with congenital heart disease (CHD) or with vascular abnormalities [83,84]. An analysis of IDE study and EFFORTLESS registry showed similar rates of complications in the CHD versus the non-CHD group (10.5% vs. 9.6% [$p = 0.89$]) as well as IAS (10.5% vs. 10.9% [$p = 0.96$]) [83]. However, in this category of patients with higher rates of both SVT and VT, as well as macroscopic anatomical alterations, more studies are needed.

5. Future Perspectives

The use of S-ICD is rapidly spreading, particularly due to the absence of transvenous leads in this procedure and its significantly lower risk of long-term complications such as lead fracture and infections. However, several pitfalls must be considered and are summarized in Table 3. Of these, the most important limitation of the device is its inability to provide anti-bradycardia pacing or ATP. To overcome these limitations, the association of S-ICD with leadless pacemakers (with or without ATP capabilities) was proposed as an alternative to TV-ICDs. Only one case report of a combined implantation of S-

ICD and a leadless pacemaker (without ATP capabilities) has been reported in human models [85]. According to the study, the two implants were safe even if not used at the same time. The authors declared no risk of oversensing detected by the S-ICD even with the maximum pacing output. Moreover, no concern about the potential for leadless pacemaker dysfunction after delivery of an S-ICD shock was reported and no device interactions were noted.

Table 3. Indications and pitfalls of S-ICD.

Indications	Pitfalls
Indication for ICD when pacing for bradycardia, cardiac resynchronization or ATP is not needed	Disease progression with need for anti-bradycardia pacing, cardiac resynchronization or enhancement of antiarrhythmic medical therapy
Congenital heart disease	Frequent development of conduction system disfunction overtime
Anatomical barriers to IV-ICD implantation (i.e., venous occlusion)	Aesthetic defect in thin women
History of IV lead infection	Only defibrillation therapy provided
Immunocompromised individuals	Large surgical wound, need for large disinfection area
Hemodialysis	\\
Young patients	Aesthetic defect, contact sports forbidden
Ion channelopathies	Polymorphic or monomorphic VTs not treatable
Hypertrophic cardiomyopathy	Increased risk of T oversensing
Dilated cardiomyopathy	Usually manifested with VTs of variable cardiac frequency (slower VTs not treated by the device)

A second generation of leadless pacemakers capable of delivering ATP has been designed to work in combination with S-ICD. This association between two devices (EMPOWER™ Modular Pacing System and EMBLEM™ S-ICD [Boston Scientific, St. Paul, MN, USA]), known as the Modular CRM (mCRM) therapy system, avoids transvenous leads while providing the option to pace or deliver ATP. Some preclinical studies have been already conducted to test the correct device–device communication, as well as the ability to perform correct sensing, right ventricular stimulation, and ATP, reporting encouraging results even in the long term [86–88]. To further explore the safety, performance, and effectiveness of mCRM, the MODULAR ATP study was designed and started (ClinicalTrials.gov Identifier: NCT04798768).

Another strategy designed to integrate ATP therapy in non-TV-ICDs consists of placing a substernal lead in contact with the pericardium on top of the right ventricle, allowing for registration of direct cardiac signal [89]. So far, the only device with this characteristic available in commerce is the Extravascular-ICD Aurora (Medtronic). After Tung et al. successfully implanted a substernal lead in three patients for the first time [89], additional cases were published [90]. In the ASD2 study, the pacing, sensing, and defibrillating capability of a substernal lead was studied in 79 patients; ventricular pacing was effective in 97.4% patients, with a defibrillation threshold of 30 J needed to terminate 104 out of 128 episodes (81.3%) of VF [91]. Although only a few complications have been reported, tunneling the lead under the sternum requires extensive practice. More studies are needed to evaluate the long-term implications.

Unlike that of TV-ICD, the test of the defibrillation threshold (DFT) is still indicated after every S-ICD implant [92]. However, DFT testing is not without risks, as DFT testing-related death, stroke and prolonged resuscitation have been reported in small series [93]. For this reason, the possibility of a DFT-free implant is being considered. In a study involving 1290 patients, DFT performance was not associated with significant differences in cardiovascular mortality and ineffective shocks, suggesting that its omission may be safe [94]. The PRAETORIAN score is an algorithm developed to identify patients with high defibrillation thresholds using a routine chest radiograph and provides feedback to implanters on S-ICD positioning. The score is calculated by integrating the distance between the device and the thoracic wall and the distance between the device and the midline [95]. A low PRAETORIAN score means a low risk of conversion failure. The ongoing randomized PRAETORIAN DFT trial (ClinicalTrials.gov Identifier: NCT03495297) will evaluate avoidance of the DFT testing in well-positioned S-ICD [96].

The automatization of the remote monitoring transmission of CIEDs is of paramount importance and must be considered in future perspectives due to its crucial role in early interventions [97]. At present, remote transmission happens only by pressing a button on the receiver and not when an alert is registered. A reduction in patients' compliance during follow up is reported [98].

Finally, results are expected from the 8-year follow up of the PRAETORIAN trial (PRATERORIAN XL). The primary objective is to establish the superiority of S-ICDs to TV-ICDs regarding acute and chronic complications.

6. Conclusions

S-ICD has proven to be safe and effective compared to TV-ICD. Innovations in pre-implant screening, implant technique, programming algorithm, and monitoring have already been developed, but further improvements are needed. New alternatives to overcome the limitations of S-ICD are in development. So far, S-ICD seems to be a valuable alternative to TV-ICD in some specific cases, such as those of young people or those with difficult vascular access, a high risk of infection, and no need for anti-bradycardia pacing or ATP.

Author Contributions: Conceptualization, F.G., E.B. and A.P.; writing—original draft preparation, F.G., A.C., M.M. (Marta Martin) and S.Q.; writing—review and editing, L.G., M.B., S.V., G.B.F. and M.V.; supervision, F.G., R.B., P.M., M.M. (Massimiliano Marini). and A.D.; All authors have read and agreed to the published version of the manuscript.

Funding: This research received no external funding.

Institutional Review Board Statement: Not applicable.

Informed Consent Statement: Not applicable.

Data Availability Statement: Not applicable.

Conflicts of Interest: The authors declare no conflict of interest.

References

1. Alter, P.; Waldhans, S.; Plachta, E.; Moosdorf, R.; Grimm, W. Complications of implantable cardioverter defibrillator therapy in 440 consecutive patients. *Pacing Clin. Electrophysiol.* **2005**, *28*, 926–932. [CrossRef] [PubMed]
2. Bardy, G.H.; Smith, W.M.; Hood, M.A.; Crozier, I.G.; Melton, I.C.; Jordaens, L.; Theuns, D.; Park, R.E.; Wright, D.J.; Connelly, D.T.; et al. An Entirely Subcutaneous Implantable Cardioverter–Defibrillator. *N. Engl. J. Med.* **2010**, *363*, 36–44. [CrossRef] [PubMed]
3. Dabiri Abkenari, L.; Theuns, D.A.; Valk, S.D.; Van Belle, Y.; de Groot, N.M.; Haitsma, D.; Muskens-Heemskerk, A.; Szili-Torok, T.; Jordaens, L. Clinical experience with a novel subcutaneous implantable defibrillator system in a single center. *Clin. Res. Cardiol.* **2011**, *100*, 737–744. [CrossRef] [PubMed]
4. De Filippo, P.; Migliore, F.; Palmisano, P.; Nigro, G.; Ziacchi, M.; Rordorf, R.; Pieragnoli, P.; Di Grazia, A.; Ottaviano, L.; Francia, P.; et al. Procedure, management, and outcome of subcutaneous implantable cardioverter–defibrillator extraction in clinical practice. *EP Eur.* **2023**, *25*, euad158. [CrossRef]
5. Kuschyk, J.; Müller-Leisse, J.; Duncker, D.; Tülümen, E.; Fastenrath, F.; Fastner, C.; Kruska, M.; Akin, I.; Liebe, V.; Borggrefe, M.; et al. Comparison of transvenous vs subcutaneous defibrillator therapy in patients with cardiac arrhythmia syndromes and genetic cardiomyopathies. *Int. J. Cardiol.* **2021**, *323*, 100–105. [CrossRef]
6. Migliore, F.; Pelliccia, F.; Autore, C.; Bertaglia, E.; Cecchi, F.; Curcio, A.; Bontempi, L.; Curnis, A.; De Filippo, P.; D'Onofrio, A.; et al. Subcutaneous implantable cardioverter defibrillator in cardiomyopathies and channelopathies. *J. Cardiovasc. Med.* **2018**, *19*, 633–642. [CrossRef]

7. Weinstock, J.; Bader, Y.H.; Maron, M.S.; Rowin, E.J.; Link, M.S. Subcutaneous Implantable Cardioverter Defibrillator in Patients With Hypertrophic Cardiomyopathy: An Initial Experience. *J. Am. Heart Assoc.* **2016**, *5*, e002488. [CrossRef]
8. Willy, K.; Doldi, F.; Reinke, F.; Rath, B.; Wolfes, J.; Wegner, F.K.; Leitz, P.; Ellermann, C.; Lange, P.S.; Köbe, J.; et al. Bradycardia in Patients with Subcutaneous Implantable Defibrillators—An Overestimated Problem? Experience from a Large Tertiary Centre and a Review of the Literature. *RCM* **2022**, *23*, 352. [CrossRef]
9. Burke, M.C.; Gold, M.R.; Knight, B.P.; Barr, C.S.; Theuns, D.; Boersma, L.V.A.; Knops, R.E.; Weiss, R.; Leon, A.R.; Herre, J.M.; et al. Safety and Efficacy of the Totally Subcutaneous Implantable Defibrillator: 2-Year Results From a Pooled Analysis of the IDE Study and EFFORTLESS Registry. *J. Am. Coll. Cardiol.* **2015**, *65*, 1605–1615. [CrossRef]
10. Gold, M.R.; Lambiase, P.D.; El-Chami, M.F.; Knops, R.E.; Aasbo, J.D.; Bongiorni, M.G.; Russo, A.M.; Deharo, J.-C.; Burke, M.C.; Dinerman, J.; et al. Primary Results From the Understanding Outcomes With the S-ICD in Primary Prevention Patients With Low Ejection Fraction (UNTOUCHED) Trial. *Circulation* **2021**, *143*, 7–17. [CrossRef]
11. Knops, R.E.; Olde Nordkamp, L.R.A.; Delnoy, P.-P.H.M.; Boersma, L.V.A.; Kuschyk, J.; El-Chami, M.F.; Bonnemeier, H.; Behr, E.R.; Brouwer, T.F.; Kääb, S.; et al. Subcutaneous or Transvenous Defibrillator Therapy. *N. Engl. J. Med.* **2020**, *383*, 526–536. [CrossRef]
12. Rordorf, R. The ATLAS Randomised Clinical Trial: What do the Superiority Results Mean for Subcutaneous ICD Therapy and Sudden Cardiac Death Prevention as a Whole? *Arrhythm Electrophysiol. Rev.* **2022**, *11*. [CrossRef]
13. Boersma, L.; Barr, C.; Knops, R.; Theuns, D.; Eckardt, L.; Neuzil, P.; Scholten, M.; Hood, M.; Kuschyk, J.; Jones, P.; et al. Implant and Midterm Outcomes of the Subcutaneous Implantable Cardioverter-Defibrillator Registry: The EFFORTLESS Study. *J. Am. Coll. Cardiol.* **2017**, *70*, 830–841. [CrossRef]
14. Burke, M.C.; Aasbo, J.D.; El-Chami, M.F.; Weiss, R.; Dinerman, J.; Hanon, S.; Kalahasty, G.; Bass, E.; Gold, M.R. 1-Year Prospective Evaluation of Clinical Outcomes and Shocks: The Subcutaneous ICD Post Approval Study. *JACC Clin. Electrophysiol.* **2020**, *6*, 1537–1550. [CrossRef]
15. Weiss, R.; Knight, B.P.; Gold, M.R.; Leon, A.R.; Herre, J.M.; Hood, M.; Rashtian, M.; Kremers, M.; Crozier, I.; Lee, K.L.; et al. Safety and efficacy of a totally subcutaneous implantable-cardioverter defibrillator. *Circulation* **2013**, *128*, 944–953. [CrossRef]
16. Gold, M.R.; Theuns, D.A.; Knight, B.P.; Sturdivant, J.L.; Sanghera, R.; Ellenbogen, K.A.; Wood, M.A.; Burke, M.C. Head-to-head comparison of arrhythmia discrimination performance of subcutaneous and transvenous ICD arrhythmia detection algorithms: The START study. *J. Cardiovasc. Electrophysiol.* **2012**, *23*, 359–366. [CrossRef]
17. Chang, S.C.; Patton, K.K.; Robinson, M.R.; Poole, J.E.; Prutkin, J.M. Subcutaneous ICD screening with the Boston Scientific ZOOM programmer versus a 12-lead ECG machine. *Pacing Clin. Electrophysiol.* **2018**, *41*, 511–516. [CrossRef]
18. Groh, C.A.; Sharma, S.; Pelchovitz, D.J.; Bhave, P.D.; Rhyner, J.; Verma, N.; Arora, R.; Chicos, A.B.; Kim, S.S.; Lin, A.C.; et al. Use of an electrocardiographic screening tool to determine candidacy for a subcutaneous implantable cardioverter-defibrillator. *Heart Rhythm* **2014**, *11*, 1361–1366. [CrossRef]
19. Olde Nordkamp, L.R.A.; Warnaars, J.L.F.; Kooiman, K.M.; de Groot, J.R.; Rosenmöller, B.; Wilde, A.A.M.; Knops, R.E. Which patients are not suitable for a subcutaneous ICD: Incidence and predictors of failed QRS-T-wave morphology screening. *J. Cardiovasc. Electrophysiol.* **2014**, *25*, 494–499. [CrossRef]
20. Randles, D.A.; Hawkins, N.M.; Shaw, M.; Patwala, A.Y.; Pettit, S.J.; Wright, D.J. How many patients fulfil the surface electrocardiogram criteria for subcutaneous implantable cardioverter-defibrillator implantation? *Europace* **2014**, *16*, 1015–1021. [CrossRef]
21. Ziacchi, M.; Corzani, A.; Diemberger, I.; Martignani, C.; Marziali, A.; Mazzotti, A.; Massaro, G.; Rapezzi, C.; Biffi, M.; Boriani, G. Electrocardiographic Eligibility for Subcutaneous Implantable Cardioverter Defibrillator: Evaluation during Bicycle Exercise. *Heart Lung. Circ.* **2016**, *25*, 476–483. [CrossRef] [PubMed]
22. Afzal, M.R.; Evenson, C.; Badin, A.; Patel, D.; Godara, H.; Essandoh, M.; Okabe, T.; Tyler, J.; Houmsse, M.; Augostini, R.; et al. Role of exercise electrocardiogram to screen for T-wave oversensing after implantation of subcutaneous implantable cardioverter-defibrillator. *Heart Rhythm* **2017**, *14*, 1436–1439. [CrossRef] [PubMed]
23. Dunn, A.J.; ElRefai, M.H.; Roberts, P.R.; Coniglio, S.; Wiles, B.M.; Zemkoho, A.B. Deep learning methods for screening patients' S-ICD implantation eligibility. *Artif. Intell. Med.* **2021**, *119*, 102139. [CrossRef] [PubMed]
24. Wiles, B.M.; Morgan, J.M.; Allavatam, V.; ElRefai, M.; Roberts, P.R. S-ICD screening revisited: Do passing vectors sometimes fail? *Pacing Clin. Electrophysiol.* **2022**, *45*, 182–187. [CrossRef] [PubMed]
25. Srinivasan, N.T.; Patel, K.H.; Qamar, K.; Taylor, A.; Bacà, M.; Providência, R.; Tome-Esteban, M.; Elliott, P.M.; Lambiase, P.D. Disease Severity and Exercise Testing Reduce Subcutaneous Implantable Cardioverter-Defibrillator Left Sternal ECG Screening Success in Hypertrophic Cardiomyopathy. *Circ. Arrhythmia Electrophysiol.* **2017**, *10*, e004801. [CrossRef]
26. El-Chami, M.; Weiss, R.; Burke, M.C.; Gold, M.R.; Prutkin, J.M.; Kalahasty, G.; Shen, S.; Mirro, M.J.; Carter, N.; Aasbo, J.D. Outcomes of two versus three incision techniques: Results from the subcutaneous ICD post-approval study. *J. Cardiovasc. Electrophysiol.* **2021**, *32*, 792–801. [CrossRef]
27. Knops, R.E.; Olde Nordkamp, L.R.; de Groot, J.R.; Wilde, A.A. Two-incision technique for implantation of the subcutaneous implantable cardioverter-defibrillator. *Heart Rhythm* **2013**, *10*, 1240–1243. [CrossRef]
28. Francia, P.; Biffi, M.; Adduci, C.; Ottaviano, L.; Migliore, F.; De Bonis, S.; Dello Russo, A.; De Filippo, P.; Viani, S.; Bongiorni, M.G.; et al. Implantation technique and optimal subcutaneous defibrillator chest position: A Praetorian score-based study. *Europace* **2020**, *22*, 1822–1829. [CrossRef]

29. Migliore, F.; Mattesi, G.; De Franceschi, P.; Allocca, G.; Crosato, M.; Calzolari, V.; Fantinel, M.; Ortis, B.; Facchin, D.; Daleffe, E.; et al. Multicentre experience with the second-generation subcutaneous implantable cardioverter defibrillator and the intermuscular two-incision implantation technique. *J. Cardiovasc. Electrophysiol.* **2019**, *30*, 854–864. [CrossRef]
30. Ferrari, P.; Giofrè, F.; De Filippo, P. Intermuscular pocket for subcutaneous implantable cardioverter defibrillator: Single-center experience. *J. Arrhythm* **2016**, *32*, 223–226. [CrossRef]
31. Smietana, J.; Frankel, D.S.; Serletti, J.M.; Arkles, J.; Pothineni, N.V.K.; Marchlinski, F.E.; Schaller, R.D. Subserratus implantation of the subcutaneous implantable cardioverter-defibrillator. *Heart Rhythm* **2021**, *18*, 1799–1804. [CrossRef]
32. Heist, E.K.; Belalcazar, A.; Stahl, W.; Brouwer, T.F.; Knops, R.E. Determinants of Subcutaneous Implantable Cardioverter-Defibrillator Efficacy: A Computer Modeling Study. *JACC Clin. Electrophysiol.* **2017**, *3*, 405–414. [CrossRef]
33. Knops, R.E.; Brouwer, T.F.; Barr, C.S.; Theuns, D.A.; Boersma, L.; Weiss, R.; Neuzil, P.; Scholten, M.; Lambiase, P.D.; Leon, A.R.; et al. The learning curve associated with the introduction of the subcutaneous implantable defibrillator. *Europace* **2016**, *18*, 1010–1015. [CrossRef]
34. Brewster, J.; Sexton, T.; Dhaliwal, G.; Charnigo, R.; Morales, G.; Parrott, K.; Darrat, Y.; Gurley, J.; Smyth, S.; Elayi, C.S. Acute Effects of Implantable Cardioverter-Defibrillator Shocks on Biomarkers of Myocardial Injury, Apoptosis, Heart Failure, and Systemic Inflammation. *Pacing Clin. Electrophysiol.* **2017**, *40*, 344–352. [CrossRef]
35. MacIntyre, C.J.; Sapp, J.L.; Abdelwahab, A.; Al-Harbi, M.; Doucette, S.; Gray, C.; Gardner, M.J.; Parkash, R. The Effect of Shock Burden on Heart Failure and Mortality. *CJC Open* **2019**, *1*, 161–167. [CrossRef]
36. Moss, A.J.; Hall, W.J.; Cannom, D.S.; Klein, H.; Brown, M.W.; Daubert, J.P.; Estes, N.A.M.; Foster, E.; Greenberg, H.; Higgins, S.L.; et al. Cardiac-Resynchronization Therapy for the Prevention of Heart-Failure Events. *N. Engl. J. Med.* **2009**, *361*, 1329–1338. [CrossRef]
37. Li, A.; Kaura, A.; Sunderland, N.; Dhillon, P.S.; Scott, P.A. The Significance of Shocks in Implantable Cardioverter Defibrillator Recipients. *Arrhythm Electrophysiol. Rev.* **2016**, *5*, 110–116. [CrossRef]
38. Sears, S.F.; Hauf, J.D.; Kirian, K.; Hazelton, G.; Conti, J.B. Posttraumatic Stress and the Implantable Cardioverter-Defibrillator Patient. *Circ. Arrhythmia Electrophysiol.* **2011**, *4*, 242–250. [CrossRef] [PubMed]
39. Fleeman, B.E.; Aleong, R.G. Optimal Strategies to Reduce Inappropriate Implantable Cardioverter-defibrillator Shocks. *J. Innov. Card Rhythm Manag.* **2019**, *10*, 3623–3632. [CrossRef]
40. Auricchio, A.; Hudnall, J.H.; Schloss, E.J.; Sterns, L.D.; Kurita, T.; Meijer, A.; Fagan, D.H.; Rogers, T. Inappropriate shocks in single-chamber and subcutaneous implantable cardioverter-defibrillators: A systematic review and meta-analysis. *Europace* **2017**, *19*, 1973–1980. [CrossRef]
41. Auricchio, A.; Schloss, E.J.; Kurita, T.; Meijer, A.; Gerritse, B.; Zweibel, S.; AlSmadi, F.M.; Leng, C.T.; Sterns, L.D. Low inappropriate shock rates in patients with single- and dual/triple-chamber implantable cardioverter-defibrillators using a novel suite of detection algorithms: PainFree SST trial primary results. *Heart Rhythm* **2015**, *12*, 926–936. [CrossRef] [PubMed]
42. Olde Nordkamp, L.R.; Brouwer, T.F.; Barr, C.; Theuns, D.A.; Boersma, L.V.; Johansen, J.B.; Neuzil, P.; Wilde, A.A.; Carter, N.; Husby, M.; et al. Inappropriate shocks in the subcutaneous ICD: Incidence, predictors and management. *Int. J. Cardiol.* **2015**, *195*, 126–133. [CrossRef] [PubMed]
43. Noel, A.; Ploux, S.; Bulliard, S.; Strik, M.; Haeberlin, A.; Welte, N.; Marchand, H.; Klotz, N.; Ritter, P.; Haïssaguerre, M.; et al. Oversensing issues leading to device extraction: When subcutaneous implantable cardioverter-defibrillator reached a dead-end. *Heart Rhythm* **2020**, *17*, 66–74. [CrossRef] [PubMed]
44. Fong, K.Y.; Ng, C.J.R.; Wang, Y.; Yeo, C.; Tan, V.H. Subcutaneous Versus Transvenous Implantable Defibrillator Therapy: A Systematic Review and Meta-Analysis of Randomized Trials and Propensity Score–Matched Studies. *J. Am. Heart Assoc.* **2022**, *11*, e024756. [CrossRef] [PubMed]
45. Conte, G.; Cattaneo, F.; de Asmundis, C.; Berne, P.; Vicentini, A.; Namdar, M.; Scalone, A.; Klersy, C.; Caputo, M.L.; Demarchi, A.; et al. Impact of SMART Pass filter in patients with ajmaline-induced Brugada syndrome and subcutaneous implantable cardioverter-defibrillator eligibility failure: Results from a prospective multicentre study. *Europace* **2022**, *24*, 845–854. [CrossRef]
46. Theuns, D.; Brouwer, T.F.; Jones, P.W.; Allavatam, V.; Donnelley, S.; Auricchio, A.; Knops, R.E.; Burke, M.C. Prospective blinded evaluation of a novel sensing methodology designed to reduce inappropriate shocks by the subcutaneous implantable cardioverter-defibrillator. *Heart Rhythm* **2018**, *15*, 1515–1522. [CrossRef]
47. Madhavan, M.; Friedman, P.A. Optimal Programming of Implantable Cardiac-Defibrillators. *Circulation* **2013**, *128*, 659–672. [CrossRef]
48. Gold, M.R.; Aasbo, J.D.; Weiss, R.; Burke, M.C.; Gleva, M.J.; Knight, B.P.; Miller, M.A.; Schuger, C.D.; Carter, N.; Leigh, J.; et al. Infection in patients with subcutaneous implantable cardioverter-defibrillator: Results of the S-ICD Post Approval Study. *Heart Rhythm* **2022**, *19*, 1993–2001. [CrossRef]
49. Rordorf, R.; Casula, M.; Pezza, L.; Fortuni, F.; Sanzo, A.; Savastano, S.; Vicentini, A. Subcutaneous versus transvenous implantable defibrillator: An updated meta-analysis. *Heart Rhythm* **2021**, *18*, 382–391. [CrossRef]
50. Su, L.; Guo, J.; Hao, Y.; Tan, H. Comparing the safety of subcutaneous versus transvenous ICDs: A meta-analysis. *J. Interv. Card Electrophysiol.* **2021**, *60*, 355–363. [CrossRef]
51. Knops, R.E.; Pepplinkhuizen, S.; Delnoy, P.; Boersma, L.V.A.; Kuschyk, J.; El-Chami, M.F.; Bonnemeier, H.; Behr, E.R.; Brouwer, T.F.; Kaab, S.; et al. Device-related complications in subcutaneous versus transvenous ICD: A secondary analysis of the PRAETORIAN trial. *Eur. Heart J.* **2022**, *43*, 4872–4883. [CrossRef]

52. Bongiorni, M.G.; Kennergren, C.; Butter, C.; Deharo, J.C.; Kutarski, A.; Rinaldi, C.A.; Romano, S.L.; Maggioni, A.P.; Andarala, M.; Auricchio, A.; et al. The European Lead Extraction ConTRolled (ELECTRa) study: A European Heart Rhythm Association (EHRA) Registry of Transvenous Lead Extraction Outcomes. *Eur. Heart J.* **2017**, *38*, 2995–3005. [CrossRef]
53. Behar, N.; Galand, V.; Martins, R.P.; Jacon, P.; Badenco, N.; Blangy, H.; Alonso, C.; Guy-Moyat, B.; El Bouazzaoui, R.; Lebon, A.; et al. Subcutaneous Implantable Cardioverter-Defibrillator Lead Extraction: First Multicenter French Experience. *JACC Clin. Electrophysiol.* **2020**, *6*, 863–870. [CrossRef]
54. Kusumoto, F.M.; Schoenfeld, M.H.; Wilkoff, B.L.; Berul, C.I.; Birgersdotter-Green, U.M.; Carrillo, R.; Cha, Y.M.; Clancy, J.; Deharo, J.C.; Ellenbogen, K.A.; et al. 2017 HRS expert consensus statement on cardiovascular implantable electronic device lead management and extraction. *Heart Rhythm* **2017**, *14*, e503–e551. [CrossRef]
55. Alt, E.; Völker, R.; Blömer, H. Lead fracture in pacemaker patients. *Thorac. Cardiovasc. Surg.* **1987**, *35*, 101–104. [CrossRef]
56. Kleemann, T.; Becker, T.; Doenges, K.; Vater, M.; Senges, J.; Schneider, S.; Saggau, W.; Weisse, U.; Seidl, K. Annual rate of transvenous defibrillation lead defects in implantable cardioverter-defibrillators over a period of >10 years. *Circulation* **2007**, *115*, 2474–2480. [CrossRef]
57. Occhetta, E.; Bortnik, M.; Magnani, A.; Francalacci, G.; Marino, P. Inappropriate implantable cardioverter-defibrillator discharges unrelated to supraventricular tachyarrhythmias. *EP Eur.* **2006**, *8*, 863–869. [CrossRef]
58. Pfeiffer, D.; Jung, W.; Fehske, W.; Korte, T.; Manz, M.; Moosdorf, R.; Lüderitz, B. Complications of pacemaker-defibrillator devices: Diagnosis and management. *Am. Heart J.* **1994**, *127*, 1073–1080. [CrossRef]
59. Knops, R.E.; Stuijt, W.v.d.; Delnoy, P.P.H.M.; Boersma, L.V.A.; Kuschyk, J.; El-Chami, M.F.; Bonnemeier, H.; Behr, E.R.; Brouwer, T.F.; Kääb, S.; et al. Efficacy and Safety of Appropriate Shocks and Antitachycardia Pacing in Transvenous and Subcutaneous Implantable Defibrillators: Analysis of All Appropriate Therapy in the PRAETORIAN Trial. *Circulation* **2022**, *145*, 321–329. [CrossRef]
60. Killingsworth, C.R.; Melnick, S.B.; Litovsky, S.H.; Ideker, R.E.; Walcott, G.P. Evaluation of acute cardiac and chest wall damage after shocks with a subcutaneous implantable cardioverter defibrillator in Swine. *Pacing Clin. Electrophysiol.* **2013**, *36*, 1265–1272. [CrossRef]
61. Al-Khatib, S.M.; Stevenson, W.G.; Ackerman, M.J.; Bryant, W.J.; Callans, D.J.; Curtis, A.B.; Deal, B.J.; Dickfeld, T.; Field, M.E.; Fonarow, G.C.; et al. 2017 AHA/ACC/HRS guideline for management of patients with ventricular arrhythmias and the prevention of sudden cardiac death: Executive summary: A Report of the American College of Cardiology/American Heart Association Task Force on Clinical Practice Guidelines and the Heart Rhythm Society. *Heart Rhythm* **2018**, *15*, e190–e252. [CrossRef] [PubMed]
62. Quast, A.B.E.; Brouwer, T.F.; Tjong, F.V.Y.; Wilde, A.A.M.; Knops, R.E. Clinical parameters to optimize patient selection for subcutaneous and transvenous implantable defibrillator therapy. *Pacing Clin. Electrophysiol.* **2018**, *41*, 990–995. [CrossRef] [PubMed]
63. Boersma, L.; Burke, M.C.; Neuzil, P.; Lambiase, P.; Friehling, T.; Theuns, D.A.; Garcia, F.; Carter, N.; Stivland, T.; Weiss, R. Infection and mortality after implantation of a subcutaneous ICD after transvenous ICD extraction. *Heart Rhythm* **2016**, *13*, 157–164. [CrossRef] [PubMed]
64. Lewis, G.F.; Gold, M.R. Safety and Efficacy of the Subcutaneous Implantable Defibrillator. *J. Am. Coll. Cardiol.* **2016**, *67*, 445–454. [CrossRef]
65. Sarubbi, B.; Colonna, D.; Correra, A.; Romeo, E.; D'Alto, M.; Palladino, M.T.; Virno, S.; D'Onofrio, A.; Russo, M.G. Subcutaneous implantable cardioverter defibrillator in children and adolescents: Results from the S-ICD "Monaldi care" registry. *J. Interv. Card Electrophysiol.* **2022**, *63*, 283–293. [CrossRef] [PubMed]
66. Olgun, H.; Karagoz, T.; Celiker, A.; Ceviz, N. Patient- and lead-related factors affecting lead fracture in children with transvenous permanent pacemaker. *Europace* **2008**, *10*, 844–847. [CrossRef]
67. Saad, T.F.; Hentschel, D.M.; Koplan, B.; Wasse, H.; Asif, A.; Patel, D.V.; Salman, L.; Carrillo, R.; Hoggard, J. Cardiovascular implantable electronic device leads in CKD and ESRD patients: Review and recommendations for practice. *Semin. Dial.* **2013**, *26*, 114–123. [CrossRef]
68. Brunner, M.P.; Cronin, E.M.; Duarte, V.E.; Yu, C.; Tarakji, K.G.; Martin, D.O.; Callahan, T.; Cantillon, D.J.; Niebauer, M.J.; Saliba, W.I.; et al. Clinical predictors of adverse patient outcomes in an experience of more than 5000 chronic endovascular pacemaker and defibrillator lead extractions. *Heart Rhythm* **2014**, *11*, 799–805. [CrossRef]
69. Koman, E.; Gupta, A.; Subzposh, F.; Saltzman, H.; Kutalek, S.P. Outcomes of subcutaneous implantable cardioverter-defibrillator implantation in patients on hemodialysis. *J. Interv. Card Electrophysiol.* **2016**, *45*, 219–223. [CrossRef]
70. Francia, P.; Olivotto, I.; Lambiase, P.D.; Autore, C. Implantable cardioverter-defibrillators for hypertrophic cardiomyopathy: The Times They Are a-Changin'. *Europace* **2022**, *24*, 1384–1394. [CrossRef]
71. Lambiase, P.D.; Gold, M.R.; Hood, M.; Boersma, L.; Theuns, D.; Burke, M.C.; Weiss, R.; Russo, A.M.; Kääb, S.; Knight, B.P. Evaluation of subcutaneous ICD early performance in hypertrophic cardiomyopathy from the pooled EFFORTLESS and IDE cohorts. *Heart Rhythm* **2016**, *13*, 1066–1074. [CrossRef]
72. Elliott, P.M.; Anastasakis, A.; Borger, M.A.; Borggrefe, M.; Cecchi, F.; Charron, P.; Hagege, A.A.; Lafont, A.; Limongelli, G.; Mahrholdt, H.; et al. 2014 ESC Guidelines on diagnosis and management of hypertrophic cardiomyopathy: The Task Force for the Diagnosis and Management of Hypertrophic Cardiomyopathy of the European Society of Cardiology (ESC). *Eur. Heart. J.* **2014**, *35*, 2733–2779. [CrossRef]

73. Jankelson, L.; Garber, L.; Sherrid, M.; Massera, D.; Jones, P.; Barbhaiya, C.; Holmes, D.; Knotts, R.; Bernstein, S.; Spinelli, M.; et al. Subcutaneous versus transvenous implantable defibrillator in patients with hypertrophic cardiomyopathy. *Heart Rhythm* **2022**, *19*, 759–767. [CrossRef]
74. Lambiase, P.D.; Eckardt, L.; Theuns, D.A.; Betts, T.R.; Kyriacou, A.L.; Duffy, E.; Knops, R. Evaluation of subcutaneous implantable cardioverter-defibrillator performance in patients with ion channelopathies from the EFFORTLESS cohort and comparison with a meta-analysis of transvenous ICD outcomes. *Heart Rhythm O2* **2020**, *1*, 326–335. [CrossRef]
75. Wang, W.; Gasperetti, A.; Sears, S.F.; Tichnell, C.; Murray, B.; Tandri, H.; James, C.A.; Calkins, H. Subcutaneous and Transvenous Defibrillators in Arrhythmogenic Right Ventricular Cardiomyopathy: A Comparison of Clinical and Quality-of-Life Outcomes. *JACC Clin. Electrophysiol.* **2022**, *9*, 394–402. [CrossRef]
76. Mizusawa, Y.; Wilde, A.A.M. Brugada Syndrome. *Circ. Arrhythmia Electrophysiol.* **2012**, *5*, 606–616. [CrossRef]
77. Passman, R.; Kadish, A. Polymorphic ventricular tachycardia, long Q-T syndrome, and torsades de pointes. *Med. Clin. North. Am.* **2001**, *85*, 321–341. [CrossRef]
78. Towbin, J.A.; McKenna, W.J.; Abrams, D.J.; Ackerman, M.J.; Calkins, H.; Darrieux, F.C.C.; Daubert, J.P.; de Chillou, C.; DePasquale, E.C.; Desai, M.Y.; et al. 2019 HRS expert consensus statement on evaluation, risk stratification, and management of arrhythmogenic cardiomyopathy. *Heart Rhythm* **2019**, *16*, e301–e372. [CrossRef]
79. Link, M.S.; Laidlaw, D.; Polonsky, B.; Zareba, W.; McNitt, S.; Gear, K.; Marcus, F.; Estes, N.A., 3rd. Ventricular arrhythmias in the North American multidisciplinary study of ARVC: Predictors, characteristics, and treatment. *J. Am. Coll. Cardiol.* **2014**, *64*, 119–125. [CrossRef]
80. Corrado, D.; van Tintelen, P.J.; McKenna, W.J.; Hauer, R.N.W.; Anastastakis, A.; Asimaki, A.; Basso, C.; Bauce, B.; Brunckhorst, C.; Bucciarelli-Ducci, C.; et al. Arrhythmogenic right ventricular cardiomyopathy: Evaluation of the current diagnostic criteria and differential diagnosis. *Eur. Heart J.* **2019**, *41*, 1414–1429. [CrossRef]
81. Watanabe, H.; Chinushi, M.; Izumi, D.; Sato, A.; Okada, S.; Okamura, K.; Komura, S.; Hosaka, Y.; Furushima, H.; Washizuka, T.; et al. Decrease in amplitude of intracardiac ventricular electrogram and inappropriate therapy in patients with an implantable cardioverter defibrillator. *Int. Heart. J.* **2006**, *47*, 363–370. [CrossRef]
82. Von Hafe, P.; Faria, B.; Dias, G.; Cardoso, F.; Alves, M.J.; Alves, A.; Rodrigues, B.; Ribeiro, S.; Sanfins, V.; Lourenço, A. Brugada syndrome: Eligibility for subcutaneous implantable cardioverter-defibrillator after exercise stress test. *Rev. Port. Cardiol.* **2021**, *40*, 33–38. [CrossRef] [PubMed]
83. D'Souza, B.A.; Epstein, A.E.; Garcia, F.C.; Kim, Y.Y.; Agarwal, S.C.; Belott, P.H.; Burke, M.C.; Leon, A.R.; Morgan, J.M.; Patton, K.K.; et al. Outcomes in Patients With Congenital Heart Disease Receiving the Subcutaneous Implantable-Cardioverter Defibrillator: Results From a Pooled Analysis From the IDE Study and the EFFORTLESS S-ICD Registry. *JACC Clin. Electrophysiol.* **2016**, *2*, 615–622. [CrossRef] [PubMed]
84. Bordachar, P.; Marquié, C.; Pospiech, T.; Pasquié, J.L.; Jalal, Z.; Haissaguerre, M.; Thambo, J.B. Subcutaneous implantable cardioverter defibrillators in children, young adults and patients with congenital heart disease. *Int. J. Cardiol.* **2016**, *203*, 251–258. [CrossRef] [PubMed]
85. Mondésert, B.; Dubuc, M.; Khairy, P.; Guerra, P.G.; Gosselin, G.; Thibault, B. Combination of a leadless pacemaker and subcutaneous defibrillator: First in-human report. *HearthRhytm Case Rep.* **2015**, *1*, 469–471. [CrossRef]
86. Tjong, F.V.Y.; Brouwer, T.F.; Koop, B.; Soltis, B.; Shuros, A.; Schmidt, B.; Swackhamer, B.; Quast, A.E.B.; Wilde, A.A.M.; Burke, M.C.; et al. Acute and 3-Month Performance of a Communicating Leadless Antitachycardia Pacemaker and Subcutaneous Implantable Defibrillator. *JACC Clin. Electrophysiol.* **2017**, *3*, 1487–1498. [CrossRef]
87. Tjong, F.V.Y.; Brouwer, T.F.; Kooiman, K.M.; Smeding, L.; Koop, B.; Soltis, B.; Shuros, A.; Wilde, A.A.M.; Burke, M.; Knops, R.E. Communicating Antitachycardia Pacing-Enabled Leadless Pacemaker and Subcutaneous Implantable Defibrillator. *J. Am. Coll. Cardiol.* **2016**, *67*, 1865–1866. [CrossRef]
88. Breeman, K.T.N.; Swackhamer, B.; Brisben, A.J.; Quast, A.B.E.; Carter, N.; Shuros, A.; Soltis, B.; Koop, B.E.; Burke, M.C.; Wilde, A.A.M.; et al. Long-term performance of a novel communicating antitachycardia pacing-enabled leadless pacemaker and subcutaneous implantable cardioverter-defibrillator system: A comprehensive preclinical study. *Heart Rhythm* **2022**, *19*, 837–846. [CrossRef]
89. Schneider, A.E.; Burkhart, H.M.; Ackerman, M.J.; Dearani, J.A.; Wackel, P.; Cannon, B.C. Minimally invasive epicardial implantable cardioverter-defibrillator placement for infants and children: An effective alternative to the transvenous approach. *Heart Rhythm* **2016**, *13*, 1905–1912. [CrossRef]
90. Hata, H.; Sumitomo, N.; Nakai, T.; Amano, A. Retrosternal Implantation of the Cardioverter-Defibrillator Lead in an Infant. *Ann. Thorac. Surg.* **2017**, *103*, e449–e451. [CrossRef]
91. Boersma, L.V.A.; Merkely, B.; Neuzil, P.; Crozier, I.G.; Akula, D.N.; Timmers, L.; Kalarus, Z.; Sherfesee, L.; DeGroot, P.J.; Thompson, A.E.; et al. Therapy From a Novel Substernal Lead: The ASD2 Study. *JACC Clin. Electrophysiol.* **2019**, *5*, 186–196. [CrossRef]
92. Stiles, M.K.; Fauchier, L.; Morillo, C.A.; Wilkoff, B.L. 2019 HRS/EHRA/APHRS/LAHRS focused update to 2015 expert consensus statement on optimal implantable cardioverter-defibrillator programming and testing. *Europace* **2019**, *21*, 1442–1443. [CrossRef]
93. Birnie, D.; Tung, S.; Simpson, C.; Crystal, E.; Exner, D.; Ayala Paredes, F.A.; Krahn, A.; Parkash, R.; Khaykin, Y.; Philippon, F.; et al. Complications associated with defibrillation threshold testing: The Canadian experience. *Heart Rhythm* **2008**, *5*, 387–390. [CrossRef]

94. Forleo, G.B.; Gasperetti, A.; Breitenstein, A.; Laredo, M.; Schiavone, M.; Ziacchi, M.; Vogler, J.; Ricciardi, D.; Palmisano, P.; Piro, A.; et al. Subcutaneous implantable cardioverter-defibrillator and defibrillation testing: A propensity-matched pilot study. *Heart Rhythm* **2021**, *18*, 2072–2079. [CrossRef]
95. Quast, A.B.E.; Baalman, S.W.E.; Brouwer, T.F.; Smeding, L.; Wilde, A.A.M.; Burke, M.C.; Knops, R.E. A novel tool to evaluate the implant position and predict defibrillation success of the subcutaneous implantable cardioverter-defibrillator: The PRAETORIAN score. *Heart Rhythm* **2019**, *16*, 403–410. [CrossRef]
96. Quast, A.B.E.; Baalman, S.W.E.; Betts, T.R.; Boersma, L.V.A.; Bonnemeier, H.; Boveda, S.; Brouwer, T.F.; Burke, M.C.; Delnoy, P.; El-Chami, M.; et al. Rationale and design of the PRAETORIAN-DFT trial: A prospective randomized CompArative trial of SubcutanEous ImplanTable CardiOverter-DefibrillatoR ImplANtation with and without DeFibrillation testing. *Am. Heart J.* **2019**, *214*, 167–174. [CrossRef]
97. Ganeshan, R.; Enriquez, A.D.; Freeman, J.V. Remote monitoring of implantable cardiac devices: Current state and future directions. *Curr. Opin. Cardiol.* **2018**, *33*, 20–30. [CrossRef]
98. De Filippo, P.; Luzi, M.; D'Onofrio, A.; Bongiorni, M.G.; Giammaria, M.; Bisignani, G.; Menardi, E.; Ferrari, P.; Bianchi, V.; Viani, S.; et al. Remote monitoring of subcutaneous implantable cardioverter defibrillators. *J. Interv. Card Electrophysiol.* **2018**, *53*, 373–381. [CrossRef]

Disclaimer/Publisher's Note: The statements, opinions and data contained in all publications are solely those of the individual author(s) and contributor(s) and not of MDPI and/or the editor(s). MDPI and/or the editor(s) disclaim responsibility for any injury to people or property resulting from any ideas, methods, instructions or products referred to in the content.

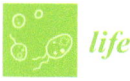 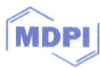

Article

In Situ Endothelial SARS-CoV-2 Presence and PROS1 Plasma Levels Alteration in SARS-CoV-2-Associated Coagulopathies

Marcello Baroni [1,†], Silvia Beltrami [2,†], Giovanna Schiuma [2], Paolo Ferraresi [1], Sabrina Rizzo [2], Angelina Passaro [3], Juana Maria Sanz Molina [2], Roberta Rizzo [2,*], Dario Di Luca [4] and Daria Bortolotti [2]

[1] Department of Life Sciences and Biotechnology (SVEB), University of Ferrara, 44121 Ferrara, Italy; marcello.baroni@unife.it (M.B.); paolo.ferraresi@unife.it (P.F.)
[2] Department of Chemical, Pharmaceutical and Agricultural Sciences, University of Ferrara, 44121 Ferrara, Italy; silvia.beltrami@unife.it (S.B.); giovanna.schiuma@unife.it (G.S.); sabrina.rizzo@unife.it (S.R.); juana.sanz@unife.it (J.M.S.M.); brtdra@unife.it (D.B.)
[3] Department of Translational Medicine, University of Ferrara, 44121 Ferrara, Italy; angelina.passaro@unife.it
[4] Department of Medical Sciences, University of Ferrara, 44121 Ferrara, Italy; ddl@unife.it
* Correspondence: rbr@unife.it
† These authors contributed equally to this work.

Abstract: Background: Coagulation decompensation is one of the complications most frequently encountered in COVID-19 patients with a poor prognosis or long-COVID syndrome, possibly due to the persistence of SARS-CoV-2 infection in the cardiovascular system. To date, the mechanism underlying the alteration of the coagulation cascade in COVID-19 patients remains misunderstood and the anticoagulant protein S (PROS1) has been described as a potential risk factor for complications related to COVID-19, due to PLpro SARS-CoV-2 enzyme proteolysis. Methods: Biopsies and blood samples were collected from SARS-CoV-2 positive and negative swab test subjects with coagulopathies (peripheral arterial thrombosis), and SARS-CoV-2 presence, ACE2 and CD147 expression, and plasmatic levels of PROS1 were evaluated. Results: We reported a significant decrease of plasmatic PROS1 in the coagulopathic SARS-CoV-2 swab positive cohort, in association with SARS-CoV-2 in situ infection and CD147 peculiar expression. These data suggested that SARS-CoV-2 associated thrombotic/ischemic events might involve PROS1 cleavage by viral PLpro directly in the site of infection, leading to the loss of its anticoagulant function. Conclusions: Based on this evidence, the identification of predisposing factors, such as CD147 increased expression, and the use of PLpro inhibitors to preserve PROS1 function, might be useful for COVID-19 coagulopathies management.

Keywords: coagulopathy; PROS1; PLpro; SARS-CoV-2; COVID-19

1. Introduction

The broad tropism of Severe Acute Respiratory Syndrome virus 2 (SARS-CoV-2) contributes to the manifestation of various diseases associated with this infection. This is attributed to the widespread presence of specific receptors for SARS-CoV-2 on human cells [1,2]. SARS-CoV-2 enters host cells by utilizing the angiotensin-converting enzyme 2 (ACE2), which is primarily expressed in lung cells, cardiac myocytes, vascular endothelium, kidney, heart, gastrointestinal tract, pancreas, and testicles [3]. Apart from ACE2, the CD147 receptor has also been identified as a potential receptor for the virus [4]. CD147, also known as extracellular matrix metalloproteinase inducer (EMMPRIN), is a member of the immunoglobulin superfamily and is expressed at varying levels in diverse cell types, including hematopoietic, epithelial, endothelial cells (ECs), and leukocytes [4].

Despite the widespread presence of SARS-CoV-2 receptors throughout the body, the virus primarily targets the upper and/or lower respiratory tract, resulting in fever, dry cough, fatigue, dyspnea, diarrhea, headache, and myalgia [5]. Some individuals recovering from COVID-19 may develop Long COVID-19 syndrome (LCS), leading to long-term complications [6,7] in various body systems beyond the respiratory tract [8,9]. LCS can impact respiratory, cardiovascular, renal, neurological, hematological, and digestive sites, but it remains poorly understood. Recent findings indicate the presence of SARS-CoV-2 in the gastrointestinal tract of individuals previously positive for the virus, particularly those hospitalized for abdominal thrombosis. This long-term manifestation of COVID-19 is associated with unique CD147 and VEGF expression, potentially contributing to hemostatic and vascular alterations [10,11]. Complications such as coagulopathies (thrombosis, disseminated intravascular coagulation), immune and inflammatory activation play a crucial role in the rapid deterioration of the patient's clinical condition [12], representing the second leading cause of death during SARS-CoV-2 infection [13,14].

At the basis of the manifestation of thrombotic events associated with COVID-19 disease there is an important imbalance of the hemostatic system, also due to the ability of SARS-CoV-2 to infect both vascular endothelial cells and platelets [15]. Although SARS-CoV-2 infection in endothelial cells is non-productive [16], it may induce cell modifications contributing to adverse cardiovascular events typical of COVID-19. In response to direct or indirect viral exposure, endothelial cells produce a pro-inflammatory response [17,18], that provokes an increased production of thrombin, blocking fibrinolysis thereby determining a hypercoagulability condition [18]. For this reason, COVID-19 hospitalized patients often showed alterations of several coagulation parameters, such as activated partial thromboplastin time (aPTT), prothrombin time (PT), fibrinogen, platelet count, fibrin degradation products (FDP), D-dimer, von Willebrand factor, factor VIII, factor V, factor II, tissue factor, antithrombin, thrombomodulin and protein S [19]. Moreover, COVID-19 patients present hyperactivated ACE2-positive [20] and CD147-positive [21] platelets, which supports the notion of SARS-CoV-2 directly participating in the observed thrombus formation and inflammation in COVID-19 subjects.

Recently, protein S1 (PROS1) has been described to be involved in the occurrence of coagulopathies associated with COVID-19 [22]. PROS1 is a vitamin K-dependent plasma glycoprotein that is primarily synthetized by the endothelium [23] and megakaryocytes [24] which plays a key role in natural anticoagulant processes. It functions as a cofactor for activated protein C (APC), enhancing APC's ability to inhibit blood clot formation by inactivating coagulation factors Va and VIIIa. PROS1 acts as a key regulator in maintaining a delicate balance between procoagulant and anticoagulant forces, preventing excessive blood clotting and thrombosis. Alterations in PROS1, whether due to genetic mutations or acquired deficiencies, can lead to an increased risk of venous thrombosis. When PROS1 is compromised, the anticoagulant activity of APC is impaired, allowing unchecked coagulation processes that may result in abnormal blood clot formation and a higher risk of thromboembolism development [25].

While the specific role of PROS1 in SARS-CoV-2 coagulopathies is an area of ongoing research, its potential involvement in the context of COVID-19-associated clotting disorders is noteworthy. SARS-CoV-2 infection has been linked to a heightened risk of coagulopathies, including thrombosis and disseminated intravascular coagulation (DIC). PROS1, as a key regulator of anticoagulant processes, may play a role in mitigating these coagulation abnormalities.

The impact of SARS-CoV-2 on PROS1 activity has been substantiated through the observation of reduced activity in 65% of COVID-19 patients [26]. This phenomenon is attributed to the papain-like protease (PLpro) of SARS-CoV-2, which has been identified as a potential contributor to thrombotic hypercoagulation and deregulation. PLpro modifies PROS1 antithrombotic and immunomodulatory properties by proteolytical cleavage [24,27]. The validity of this hypothesis was further confirmed through in vitro experiments, which demonstrated the cleavage of PROS1 occurring in proximity to viral replication complexes [26,28]. Therefore, the modification of PROS1 expression by PLpro within platelets could disturb thrombin formation and activate platelets, potentially contributing to the disruption of various platelet functions observed in COVID-19 patients, playing a role in the formation of thrombi [29].

As of now, there is no available information on the potential direct link between in situ vascular infection by SARS-CoV-2 and the impairment of PROS1 in COVID-19 patients with coagulopathies. Given the increasing focus on cardiovascular long-term effects of COVID-19, this study seeks to elucidate the potential connection between alterations in PROS1 plasma levels and the concomitant presence of the virus within cardiovascular tissues, following past or ongoing SARS-CoV-2 infection. The goal is to identify novel clinical biomarkers that can aid in the management of coagulopathies associated with COVID-19.

2. Materials and Methods

2.1. Patients and Samples Collection

The study was conducted on 18 patients affected by coagulopathies (peripheral arterial thrombosis) enrolled from May to December 2020 at the Internal Medicine Unit of the Sant'Anna University Hospital in Ferrara. All the patients showed arterial coagulation, 56% were subjected to thromboendarterectomy and 17% were subjected to amputation. All the subjects were free from any medication before the sample collection and patients with concomitant comorbidities, such as BCPO, diabetes or autoimmune diseases, were excluded. In particular, two cohorts were identified: 7 patients had at least one SARS-CoV-2 positive oropharyngeal swab within 6 months of the coagulopathy event, experiencing mild symptoms, and 11 patients had never reported a SARS-CoV-2 positive oropharyngeal swab. No subjects were vaccinated for SARS-CoV-2, or present previous comorbidities or treatments (e.g., anticoagulants, antiplatelet agents). The study was approved by our hospital's ethics committee (Number: 540/2020/Oss/AOUFe—20 May 2020). All the data were anonymized and no connection with the patient's identity was possible. For each patient we collected arterial (endothelial tissue) and thrombotic (endovascular thrombotic material) material. Tissue samples were used for total RNA extraction with TRIZOL or fixed in formalin and embedded in paraffin and processed to obtain 4 µm thick sections for histological evaluation and immunohistochemistry. Plasma samples were collected from all the patients and used for ELISA assay.

2.2. Histology and Immunohistochemistry

Immunohistochemical (IHC) analysis was performed on the collected samples for detection of SARS-CoV-2 NP (NB100-56576, Novus Biologicals, Centennial, CO, USA, Centennial, 1:250 dilution), CD147 (clone MEM-M6/1, dilution 1:100, Novus Biologicals) and ACE2 (clone EPR4435-2, 1:250 dilution, Abcam, Cambridge, UK), using the Ultratek kit (Histoline, Milan, Italy), as previously described [11]. After immunohistochemical staining, tissue images were analyzed by QuPath software v2.3 and scored based on the intensity and number of positively stained cells/mm^2 (H-score).

2.3. Real-Time PCR

The presence of SARS-CoV-2 genome, targeting the viral spike RBD (Receptor Binding Domain), ACE2 and CD147 in the histological tissues of thrombi and venous/arterial samples was detected by RT-qPCR. cDNA has been synthesized via reverse transcription using the High Capacity kit (ThermoFisher, Scientific, Waltham, MA, USA), from the extracted RNA and gene expression detected by amplification with QuantStudio3 (Thermo Fisher Scientific, Waltham, MA, USA), using PowerUp SYBR Green Master Mix. SARS-CoV-2 RBD domain were amplified using primer forward (5'-CAA TGG TTT AAC AGT CAC AGG-3') and reverse (5'-CTC AAG TGT CTG TGG ATC ACG-3'); ACE2, CD147 and GAPDH, as housekeeping gene, were detected using PrimeTime primer sets (ACE2: Hs.PT.58.27645939; CD147: Hs.PT.56a.39293590.g; GAPDH: Hs.PT.39.22214836), as previously described [11,30].

2.4. PROS1 ELISA Assay

Polyclonal sheep anti-human protein S (PS) antibody (4 mg/L, H.T.I., Huntington, VT, USA) was coated overnight at 4 °C to microtiter plate (Nunc, MaxiSorp®, ThermoFisher, Scientific, Waltham, MA, USA) in a 50 mM $Na_2CO_3/NaHCO_3$, 5 mM $CaCl_2$, pH 9.0 buffer, and incubated for 75′ at room temperature (r.t.) with increasing concentrations of PS (0–400 μg/L), from human pooled normal plasma. Bound PS, from 1/2000 diluted plasma samples, was detected with 60′ of incubation at r.t. with polyclonal rabbit anti-PS antibody (4 mg/L, Dako, Glostrup, Denmark) and with a polyclonal goat peroxidase-conjugated antibody (0.6 mg/L, Dako), both incubated at r.t for 60′. A 5 mg tablet OPD (Sigma-Merck, Darmstadt, Germany), dissolved in 12 mL of 50 mM citrate–phosphate buffer pH 5.0 and 7 μL of 30% H_2O_2, was added as substrate for peroxidase. After 5′, the reaction was quenched with the addition of 2.5 M H_2SO_4 and the color produced was quantified using a SpectraFluor Plus microplate reader (Tecan, Salzburg, Austria), measuring the absorbance at 492 nm. A mix of 50 mM Tris, 150 mM NaCl, 5 mM $CaCl_2$, pH 7.4 was used to prepare the blocking, or the sample diluent, or the washer buffers by the addition of 5% albumin from bovine serum (BSA, Sigma Merck, St. Louis, MO, USA), or 0.2% BSA, or 0.1% Tween 20 (Sigma-Merck), respectively. All buffers were 0.2 μm filtered. The assay showed very high sensitivity, it allows the recognition of PROS1 in plasma diluted up to 16,000 times (Supplementary Figure S1a) and the specificity is given to the assay by the double recognition based on two polyclonal antibodies (ELISA sandwich) [31]. No cross-reactivity was evident in thousands of samples (media and plasma) evaluated and no differences in PROS1 or PROS1-C4BP complex recognition (Supplementary Figure S1b). The inter-assay coefficient of variability (1.69%) was calculated by 3 independent assays performed with 3 samples, quantified in triplicate.

2.5. Statistical Analysis

Biological variables reported as frequency were analyzed by Fisher exact test or Chi square test. Biological variables reported as mean ± SD were compared between study groups by Student's t-test. The statistical analysis was performed by GraphPad Prism v.9 Software.

3. Results

3.1. Characterization of the Study Population

The patients were subdivided based on reported SARS-CoV-2 positive swabs (Table 1). The SARS-CoV-2 Alpha VOC (variant of concern) was detected in all the samples. As reported in Table 1, the patients with SARS-CoV-2 positive swab showed a higher mean age compared to patients with no SARS-CoV-2 positive swab ($p < 0.0001$; Student's t-test), while no significant differences in gender ratio was observed. Both cohorts underwent thromboendoarterectomy, with only two patients with previous SARS-CoV-2 positive swabs characterized by the need of amputation (Table 1, $p < 0.0001$; Fisher exact test).

Table 1. Demographical and clinical characterization of subjects enrolled in the study.

	SARS-CoV-2 Positive Swab ($N = 7$)	SARS-CoV-2 Negative Swab ($N = 11$)	p Values
Gender; N; %	M (5; 71%) F (2; 29%)	M (9; 82%) F (2; 18%)	0.51
Age; mean ± SD	85.0 ± 3.3	70.8 ± 6.7	<0.0001
Thromboendarterectomy	57% (4)	55% (6)	0.65
Amputation	29% (2)	0% (0)	<0.0001

3.2. SARS-CoV-2 In Situ Presence Correlates with Previous Infection in Coagulopathic COVID-19 Subjects

RNA samples were obtained from arterial biopsies, which were composed of the endothelial tissues and the thrombotic clots. The samples from subjects with previous SARS-CoV-2 positive swab tests were evaluated for the expression of viral RNA encoding spike protein RBD by RT-qPCR. We found the presence of SARS-CoV-2 RNA encoding spike protein RBD in the 50% of the endothelial tissue and in the totality of the thrombotic clots. (Figure 1a, $p < 0.0001$; Chi square test).

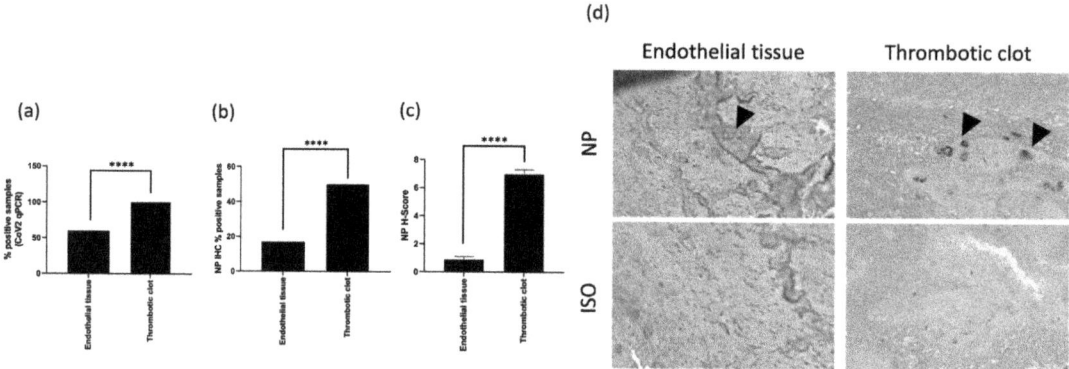

Figure 1. SARS-CoV-2 in situ infection evaluation: (**a**) percentage of positivity for SARS-CoV-2 RBD spike protein in tissues analyzed by Real-Time PCR; (**b**) percentage of positivity for SARS-CoV-2 NP in tissues analyzed by IHC staining and (**c**) corresponding H-Score; and (**d**) representative IHC images for SARS-CoV-2 NP (NP) and isotype control (ISO) in endothelial tissue and thrombotic clot. **** $p < 0.0001$, Chi square test.

We observed the expression of SARS-CoV-2 NP in the 15% of the endothelial tissues and in the 50% of the thrombotic clots (Figure 1b, 50%; $p < 0.0001$; Chi square test). The H score, accounting for the intensity and the proportion of NP expression, was higher in thrombotic clots than in endothelial tissues (Figure 1c; H-score 6.98 ± 0.34 vs. 0.88 ± 0.21, respectively; $p < 0.0001$ Student's t-test). The biopsies were analyzed for the expression of SARS-CoV-2 NP by IHC (Figure 1d).

The higher positivity rate found by RT-PCR analysis in all the specimens in comparison with IHC staining might be associated with both a higher sensibility of RT-PCR analysis, or with a lower SARS-CoV-2 protein translation.

3.3. CD147 Expression Correlates with SARS-CoV-2 In Situ Infection in Coagulopathic COVID-19 Subjects

The presence of both SARS-CoV-2 RNA and protein expression suggests the ability of the virus to infect the analyzed tissues. Since the viral infection of a host cell depends on the presence of specific receptors, we analyzed the expression of two of the main viral entry receptors, ACE2 and CD147 [4,32], at both the transcriptional and protein level (Figure 2).

The analysis of mRNA levels by "real time PCR revealed an increased expression of ACE2 mRNA in thrombotic clots of the subjects with previous SARS-CoV-2 positive swab tests in comparison with the subjects with negative SARS-CoV-2 swab tests (Figure 2a, $p < 0.0001$; Student's t-test). Interestingly, the analysis of ACE2 and CD147 protein expression by IHC showed the highest levels in subjects with previous SARS-CoV-2 positive swab tests, in the endothelial tissues for ACE2 and in thrombotic clots for CD147 (Figure 2c–e; $p < 0.01$; Student's t-test).

These data are in agreement with the in situ presence of SARS-CoV-2 RNA and NP protein (Figure 1), suggesting a possible in situ infection, as already described [15].

3.4. SARS-CoV-2 In Situ Infection Correlates with Lower Plasma Levels of PROS1

SARS-CoV-2 in situ endothelial infection is known to lead to an abortive infection [16], even affecting the proteome expression of the infected endothelial cells. The main effect seems to be on the inflammatory and angiogenetic processes, accounting for the presence of a basal viral protein expression that might alter cellular functions.

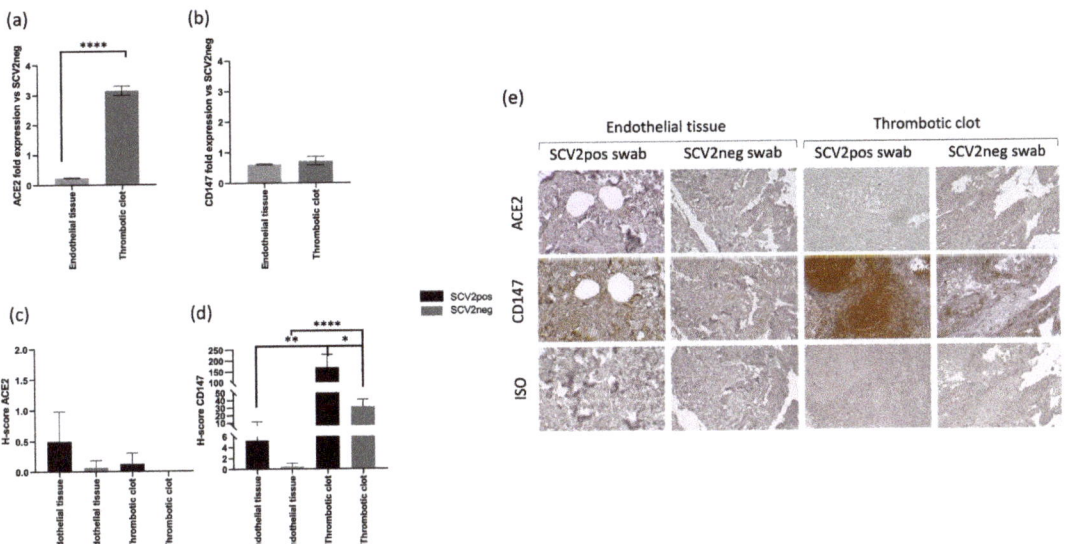

Figure 2. ACE2 (**a**) and CD147 (**b**) fold expression in endothelial tissues and thrombotic clots from SARS-CoV-2 swab positive coagulopathic subjects evaluated by Real Time PCR. The ACE2 and CD147 expression in endothelial tissues and thrombotic clots from SARS-CoV-2 swab negative patients (SCV2neg) were considered as reference levels; (**c**) ACE2 and (**d**) CD147 IHC staining intensity reported as H-Score in endothelial tissues and thrombotic clots from positive (SCV2pos) and negative (SCV2neg) SARS-CoV-2 swab coagulopathic subjects; (**e**) representative IHC staining for ACE2, CD147 and isotype control (ISO) in endothelial tissues and thrombotic clots from positive (SCV2pos) and negative (SCV2neg) SARS-CoV-2 swab coagulopathic subjects. * $p < 0.05$; ** $p < 0.01$; **** $p < 0.0001$, Student's *t*-test.

PROS1 has been demonstrated to affect hemostatic regulation, due to its interaction with protein C (APC) and tissue factor pathway inhibitor (TFPI), inducing an antithrombotic/anticoagulative pathway [24,27]. We evaluated the levels of PROS1 by ELISA in the plasma samples of SARS-CoV-2 positive and negative swab test patients.

PROS1 plasma levels were significantly lower in SARS-CoV-2 positive swab test patients in comparison with SARS-CoV-2 negative swab test patients (Figure 3a $p < 0.01$; Student's *t*-test). When the SARS-CoV-2 positive swab test patients were subdivided according with the in situ SARS-CoV-2 RBD spike protein RNA positivity or negativity, we observed significantly lower PROS1 plasma levels in patients with SARS-CoV-2 positivity (Figure 3b, $p < 0.05$; Student's *t*-test).

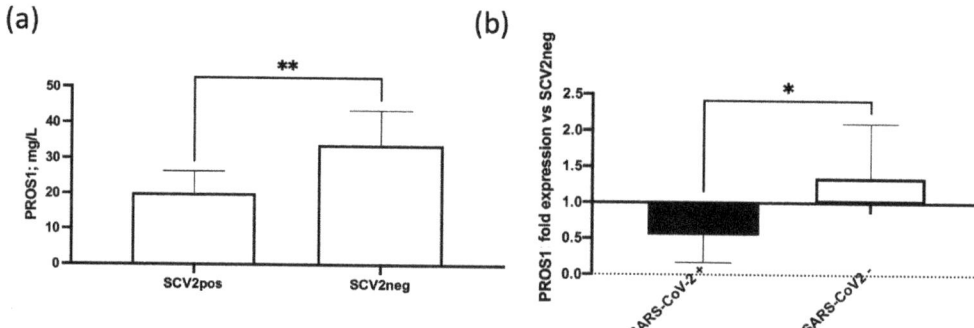

Figure 3. (**a**) Plasma concentration of PROS1 in SARS-CoV-2 positive (SCV2pos) and negative (SCV2neg) swab test patients; (**b**) PROS1 plasma levels in SARS-CoV-2 positive (SCV2pos) swab test patients, subdivided according to the positivity (SARS-CoV-2+) or negativity (SARS-CoV-2-) of the bioptic tissues for SARS-CoV-2 RBD spike RNA, in comparison with PROS1 plasma levels in SARS-CoV-2 positive (SCV2pos) swab test patients' fold difference considering the presence of SARS-CoV-2 (SARS-CoV-2+) or absence (SARS-CoV-2-) in the genome in the biopsies analyzed by Real Time PCR in comparison with the levels in plasma samples from SARS-CoV-2 negative (SCV2neg) swab test patients. * $p < 0.05$; ** $p < 0.01$, Student's t-test.

4. Discussion

Despite several evidence reporting SARS-CoV-2 tropism for the cardiovascular system [12,13], little is known about coagulopathies development. Recent findings reported that SARS-CoV-2 gastrointestinal in situ infection was related to abdominal bleeding and ischemia [33], suggesting that previous SARS-CoV-2 infection could develop a secondary effect at the vascular level, exploiting specific tissues as a reservoir of infection. Drawing from this understanding, it is conceivable to propose a chronological association between SARS-CoV-2 infection and the development of coagulopathies. This connection involves the individual susceptibility to viral infection, influenced by the expression of viral receptors and predisposition to coagulopathies, which may include potential mutations or functional alterations in PROS1. Additionally, the direct impact of viral infection on the coagulation cascade, including PLpro cleavage on PROS1, could collectively contribute to determining the risk of coagulopathies in COVID-19. These elements might underlie the cardiovascular events observed in LCS, where individuals, despite exhibiting mild symptoms during the acute infection, may experience the activation of prothrombotic pathways due to the persistent presence of the virus. In this study, we analyzed SARS-CoV-2 positive and negative swab patients, who experienced peripheral arterial thrombosis, to evaluate SARS-CoV-2 in situ presence and its possible role in vascular damage. Both groups of patients underwent thromboendoarterectomy, with SARS-CoV-2-positive swab patients characterized by a higher frequency of amputation. We enrolled patients with no previous comorbidities and treatments to avoid confounding variables. The development of coagulopathy is observed to occur subsequent to the confirmation of a positive swab result in individuals belonging to the group with SARS-CoV-2-positive swabs. This temporal association suggests that the manifestation of coagulopathic events is closely linked to the presence and detection of the SARS-CoV-2 virus. This observation highlights the dynamic nature of the relationship between viral infection and the onset of coagulation disorders, emphasizing the need for vigilant monitoring and timely interventions following a positive diagnosis to address and manage potential coagulopathic complications effectively. The understanding of this temporal sequence is crucial in refining clinical strategies and tailoring therapeutic approaches for individuals diagnosed with COVID-19, ensuring a comprehensive and timely response to mitigate the risk of coagulopathy-related complications. Biopsies from Alpha VOC SARS-CoV-2-positive swab patients were found positive for SARS-CoV-2 in situ presence, reporting both viral genome and NP protein expression mainly in thrombotic clots. The evaluation of the effect of different SARS-CoV-2 VOCs might be of extreme interest in understanding how they impact the infection outcome and persistence at the cardiovascular level.

The presence of SARS-CoV-2 in endothelial and thrombotic tissues is supported by an increased expression of both ACE2 and CD147 molecules. Interestingly, we reported a differential tissue expression of these two viral receptors in SARS-CoV-2-positive swab subjects, with a higher amount of ACE2 in the endothelial tissues, while CD147 was more expressed in thrombotic clots. ACE2 is known to be highly expressed on endothelial cells [34], where it represents the main receptor for virus entry [35]. Thus, ACE2 protein higher expression in endothelial tissues from SARS-CoV-2-positive swab patients could support the presence of both SARS-CoV-2 RBD RNA and NP protein at a vascular level. The increased CD147 expression at the thrombotic level might be due to the presence of platelets, that are known to express this receptor [36]. Interestingly, it has been shown that CD147 is able to induce ACE2 surface expression in infected cells [20,37], affecting virus entry into host cells (Figure 4).

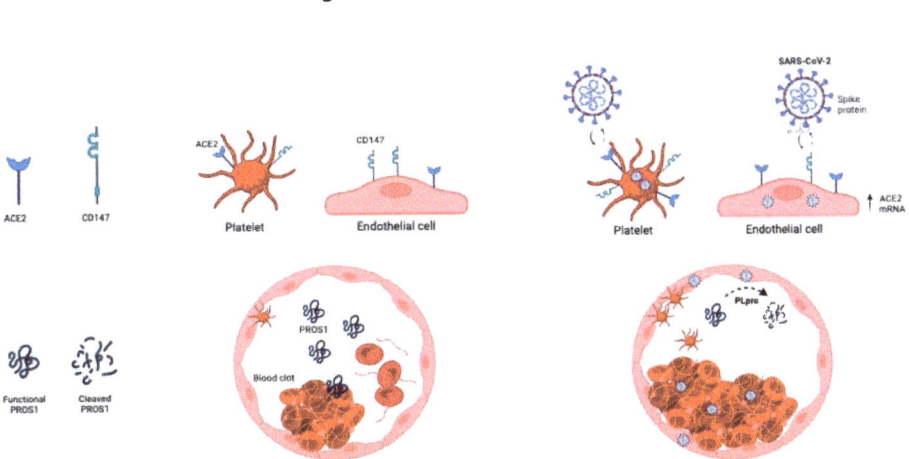

Figure 4. Schematic representation of blood clot formation in no COVID-19 and COVID-19 subjects.

The increased CD147 expression in SARS-CoV-2 positive thrombotic clots suggests a critical role in increasing SARS-CoV-2 in situ susceptibility, as already reported for gut viral tropism [11], possibly connected with a higher risk for developing thrombotic events (Figure 4).

This hypothesis is supported also by recent evidence suggesting a role for CD147 in both thrombosis and inflammation, establishing CD147+ platelets as a critical factor in SARS-CoV-2-dependent thrombotic events [36]. Indeed, the thrombotic events associated with COVID-19 are verified to exhibit an atypical state of hyperactivated platelets, linked to the surface expression of CD147 [38]. This reaffirms the involvement of platelets in the inflammatory and hemostatic aspects of the disease. Additionally, there is a proposed significance of the direct interplay between SARS-CoV-2-activated platelets and leukocytes in the formation of blood clots and the onset of a cytokine storm. This supports the consideration of antiplatelet therapies as a potential approach to counteract both thrombotic events and the spread of the infection [39]. These therapies emerge as a promising approach not only to mitigate the thrombotic events associated with COVID-19 but also to impede the spread of the infection. By targeting platelet activation, antiplatelet agents may not only address the hemostatic complications seen in COVID-19 patients, but also disrupt a crucial mechanism implicated in the inflammatory response and viral propagation. The exploration of antiplatelet therapies represents a multifaceted strategy in managing both the vascular complications and the infectious aspects of COVID-19, offering a comprehensive approach to enhance patient outcomes.

As a proof of concept of the possible implication of SARS-CoV-2 infection in coagulopathies, we evaluated the plasmatic levels of the anticoagulant factor PROS1 in correlation to infection status [22], showing lower levels in SARS-CoV-2 positive swab test patients in comparison with SARS-CoV-2 negative swab test patients, in line with previous results [11]. PROS1 is primarily synthesized in the liver, serving as a key site for its production. Additionally, its synthesis occurs locally in other crucial cellular components, such as the endothelium and megakaryocytes, which are the precursors of platelets. This diversified origin of PROS1 underscores its significance in various physiological processes, with contributions from both hepatic and non-hepatic sources, including the endothelial lining and megakaryocytic lineage, thereby emphasizing its multifaceted roles in hemostasis and thrombosis regulation. Furthermore, it has been documented that PROS1 undergoes proteolytic cleavage by the SARS-CoV-2 PLpro viral protease [40]. The observed decrease of PROS1 anticoagulant protein in SARS-CoV-2 positive biopsies strengthens the association between coagulopathies development and SARS-CoV-2 in situ presence, possibly through PROS1 impairment by proteolytic activity, carried out by SARS-CoV-2 PLpro viral protease [40] (Figure 4). The PLpro enzymatic modification of PROS1 raises significant clinical implications. The cleavage of PROS1 by PLpro may disrupt its anticoagulant and immunomodulatory functions, potentially contributing to the hypercoagulable state observed in COVID-19 patients. This molecular interaction highlights a potential mechanism by which SARS-CoV-2 may directly impact the intricate balance of hemostasis, providing valuable insights for understanding the pathophysiology of COVID-19-associated coagulopathies and suggesting new avenues for targeted therapeutic interventions aimed at restoring or mitigating PROS1 functionality. These therapeutic strategies may involve the development of specific inhibitors against the SARS-CoV-2 PLpro protease to prevent its cleavage of PROS1. Additionally, approaches that enhance PROS1 production or stability could be explored to counteract the detrimental effects of its cleavage. Investigating these novel therapeutic avenues holds promise for mitigating the hypercoagulable state associated with COVID-19, ultimately improving patient outcomes, and informing the development of tailored interventions in the evolving landscape of COVID-19 treatment strategies.

This hypothesis necessitates thorough validation through extensive investigations into the molecular mechanisms underlying the observed effects, aiming to offer additional insights into the intricate pathways involved. Specifically, future research endeavors should concentrate on elucidating the impact on the plasmatic levels of PROS1 in the presence of various SARS-CoV-2 VOCs. Focusing on these specific viral variants will allow a more nuanced understanding of how they potentially modulate PROS1 function, shedding light on any variant-specific effects on coagulation and hemostasis. This nuanced exploration is crucial for advancing our comprehension of the interplay between SARS-CoV-2 and PROS1, contributing to the refinement of targeted therapeutic strategies and informing public health measures tailored to the evolving landscape of viral variants and associated clinical manifestations.

Our study is constrained primarily by the limited number of participants included, the single center enrollment and the lack of quantification for the SARS-CoV-2 PLpro viral protease. Additionally, we did not assess inflammatory cytokine plasma levels or conduct coagulative assays. Specifically, a notable absence is the evaluation of plasma PROS1 activity, which could significantly enhance our comprehension of PROS1's physiological and pathological functionality in individuals with COVID-19. A more extensive enrollment of patients and the inclusion of quantitative measures for viral protease and other relevant factors would contribute to a more robust analysis. Furthermore, incorporating assessments of inflammatory markers and coagulation assays could provide a comprehensive understanding of the complex interplay between the virus and the host's hemostatic system, offering valuable insights into potential therapeutic interventions and improving the clinical relevance of our findings. The absence of long-term follow-up data in this study poses significant implications for understanding the persistence or resolution of coagulopathies over an extended period in individuals with SARS-CoV-2 infection. The dynamics of coagulation abnormalities in COVID-19 patients can vary over time, and a lack of prolonged observation hinders our ability to comprehensively assess the trajectory and outcomes of these complications. Long-term follow-up data and replication of this study in diverse settings are crucial to unravel the evolving nature of coagulopathies associated with SARS-CoV-2, shedding light on whether these abnormalities persist, resolve, or potentially reoccur after the acute phase of infection.

Nevertheless, the findings are noteworthy as they, for the first time, suggest a direct link between the in situ vascular presence of SARS-CoV-2 and the onset of coagulopathies, proposing an alteration in PROS1 expression as a potential key contributor to SARS-CoV-2-associated coagulation disorders. Identifying predisposing factors, such as the increased expression of CD147 and the reduction in plasmatic PROS1 levels, could be instrumental in proactively determining the risk of coagulopathies associated with SARS-CoV-2 infection and LCS. Monitoring altered plasmatic levels of PROS1 or incorporating its assessment during therapy could aid in identifying COVID-19 subjects at higher risk for PROS1-associated coagulopathies, which can significantly exacerbate the clinical course in COVID-19 patients. Screening for PROS1 mutations could be considered an additional preventive measure against coagulopathic events. Furthermore, recognizing the distinctive heterogeneity in clinical manifestations of COVID-19 is crucial in evaluating the onset of coagulopathic complications. Early assessment of PROS1 levels may contribute to reducing the incidence of COVID-19-associated cardiovascular events, particularly in LCS cases, by facilitating the early identification of the most susceptible patients.

5. Conclusions

In this study, we have unveiled, for the first time, a potential association between the in situ presence of SARS-CoV-2 at the cardiovascular level and thrombotic events involving PROS1. A discernible predisposing factor appears to be the distinctive expression patterns of ACE2 and CD147 receptors, with CD147 notably prevalent in thrombotic clots. This heightened presence potentially facilitates viral in situ replication, subsequently intensifying viral PLpro cleavage on PROS1. These findings underscore the pivotal role of SARS-CoV-2 infection in influencing PROS1 plasmatic levels, emerging as a significant risk factor for coagulopathies. Considering this, assessing PROS1 plasmatic levels and CD147 expression emerges as a potent diagnostic and therapeutic tool for COVID-19 patients, providing insights into the risk for SARS-CoV-2-associated coagulopathies. Furthermore, considering these revelations, the exploration of antiplatelet therapies becomes a valuable avenue for countering both thrombotic events and the propagation of infection in COVID-19 patients. To enhance the robustness of these findings, a replication of the data on a broader population is imperative, coupled with a comprehensive long-term follow-up investigation to elucidate the sustained impact of the PLpro viral protease on controlling PROS1 plasmatic levels.

Supplementary Materials: The following are available online at https://www.mdpi.com/article/10.3390/life14020237/s1, Figure S1: PROS1 ELISA sensitivity and specificity profile. (a) Increasing dilutions of pooled normal plasma (1/31.25—1/16,000, from 800 ng/mL to 1.56 ng/mL of PROS1) in PROS1 deficient plasma, were evaluated by ELISA sandwich, based on polyclonal antibodies. The very high reproducibility intra-assay is visible in the figure and the inter-assay variability is only 1.69%. Each point is the average of 3 measurements; (b) ELISA-PROS1 assay was conducted in pooled normal plasma by addition of C4BP protein (400 ng/mL, gray dashed line) or sample diluent (50 mM Tris, 150 mM NaCl, 5 mM CaCl2, pH 7.4, gray line) and no effect of this addition of this plasmatic physiological interactor of PROS1 was evaluable. This ELISA recognizes free and C4BP-bound PROS1 with identical affinity. Each point is the average of 2 evaluations.

Author Contributions: D.B. and R.R. conceptualization; D.B., R.R. and D.D.L. designed the experiments; M.B., S.B., G.S., S.R. and P.F. performed the experiments; M.B., S.B., D.B. and R.R. analyzed the data; A.P. and J.M.S.M. collected the samples and the clinical data; D.B., M.B. and R.R. wrote the manuscript; A.P. and D.D.L. edit the manuscript. All authors have read and agreed to the published version of the manuscript.

Funding: The study was financially supported by Grant from Italian Ministry of University and Research, University of Ferrara, Italy (FAR 2022), University of Ferrara crowdfunding, 5X1000 University of Ferrara grant and by "Bando FIRD 2023" University of Ferrara grant.

Institutional Review Board Statement: The study was conducted in accordance with the Declaration of Helsinki and approved by the Ethics Committee of Sant'Anna University Hospital in Ferrara (protocol code 540/2020/Oss/AOUFe—20 May 2020).

Informed Consent Statement: Informed consent was obtained from all subjects involved in the study.

Data Availability Statement: The data presented in this study are available on request from the corresponding author.

Acknowledgments: We thank Iva Pivanti and Giorgia Cianci for the experimental support, and Francesco Bernardi for the experimental counseling.

Conflicts of Interest: The authors declare no conflicts of interest.

References

1. Liu, J.; Li, Y.; Liu, Q.; Yao, Q.; Wang, X.; Zhang, H.; Chen, R.; Ren, L.; Min, J.; Deng, F.; et al. SARS-CoV-2 cell tropism and multiorgan infection. *Cell Discov.* **2021**, *7*, 17. [CrossRef] [PubMed]
2. Hoffmann, M.; Pohlmann, S. Novel SARS-CoV-2 receptors: ASGR1 and KREMEN1. *Cell Res.* **2022**, *32*, 1–2. [CrossRef] [PubMed]
3. Dong, M.; Zhang, J.; Ma, X.; Tan, J.; Chen, L.; Liu, S.; Xin, Y.; Zhuang, L. ACE2, TMPRSS2 distribution and extrapulmonary organ injury in patients with COVID-19. *Biomed. Pharmacother.* **2020**, *131*, 110678. [CrossRef] [PubMed]
4. Wang, K.; Chen, W.; Zhang, Z.; Deng, Y.; Lian, J.Q.; Du, P.; Wei, D.; Zhang, Y.; Sun, X.X.; Gong, L.; et al. CD147-spike protein is a novel route for SARS-CoV-2 infection to host cells. *Signal Transduct. Target Ther.* **2020**, *5*, 283. [CrossRef] [PubMed]
5. Park, M.B.; Park, E.Y.; Lee, T.S.; Lee, J. Effect of the Period From COVID-19 Symptom Onset to Confirmation on Disease Duration: Quantitative Analysis of Publicly Available Patient Data. *J. Med. Internet Res.* **2021**, *23*, e29576. [CrossRef] [PubMed]
6. Hartard, C.; Chaqroun, A.; Settembre, N.; Gauchotte, G.; Lefevre, B.; Marchand, E.; Mazeaud, C.; Nguyen, D.T.; Martrille, L.; Koscinski, I.; et al. Multiorgan and Vascular Tropism of SARS-CoV-2. *Viruses* **2022**, *14*, 515. [CrossRef]
7. Nalbandian, A.; Sehgal, K.; Gupta, A.; Madhavan, M.V.; McGroder, C.; Stevens, J.S.; Cook, J.R.; Nordvig, A.S.; Shalev, D.; Sehrawat, T.S.; et al. Post-acute COVID-19 syndrome. *Nat. Med.* **2021**, *27*, 601–615. [CrossRef] [PubMed]
8. Lechner-Scott, J.; Levy, M.; Hawkes, C.; Yeh, A.; Giovannoni, G. Long COVID or post COVID-19 syndrome. *Mult. Scler. Relat. Disord.* **2021**, *55*, 103268. [CrossRef]
9. López-León, S.; Wegman-Ostrosky, T.; Perelman, C.; Sepulveda, R.; Rebolledo, P.A.; Cuapio, A.; Villapol, S. More than 50 Long-Term Effects of COVID-19: A Systematic Review and Meta-Analysis. *SSRN Electron. J.* **2021**, *11*, 16144. [CrossRef]
10. Venkatesan, P. NICE guideline on long COVID. *Lancet Respir. Med.* **2021**, *9*, 129. [CrossRef]
11. Bortolotti, D.; Simioni, C.; Neri, L.M.; Rizzo, R.; Semprini, C.M.; Occhionorelli, S.; Laface, I.; Sanz, J.M.; Schiuma, G.; Rizzo, S.; et al. Relevance of VEGF and CD147 in different SARS-CoV-2 positive digestive tracts characterized by thrombotic damage. *FASEB J.* **2021**, *35*, e21969. [CrossRef]
12. Pretorius, E.; Vlok, M.; Venter, C.; Bezuidenhout, J.A.; Laubscher, G.J.; Steenkamp, J.; Kell, D.B. Persistent clotting protein pathology in Long COVID/Post-Acute Sequelae of COVID-19 (PASC) is accompanied by increased levels of antiplasmin. *Cardiovasc. Diabetol.* **2021**, *20*, 172. [CrossRef]
13. Iba, T.; Levy, J.H.; Levi, M.; Connors, J.M.; Thachil, J. Coagulopathy of Coronavirus Disease 2019. *Crit. Care Med.* **2020**, *48*, 1358–1364. [CrossRef]
14. Jose, R.J.; Manuel, A. COVID-19 cytokine storm: The interplay between inflammation and coagulation. *Lancet Respir. Med.* **2020**, *8*, e46–e47. [CrossRef]
15. Ganier, L.; Morelli, X.; Borg, J.P. CD147 (BSG) but not ACE2 expression is detectable in vascular endothelial cells within single cell RNA sequencing datasets derived from multiple tissues in healthy individuals. *Med. Sci.* **2020**, *36*, 42–46. [CrossRef]
16. Schimmel, L.; Chew, K.Y.; Stocks, C.J.; Yordanov, T.E.; Essebier, P.; Kulasinghe, A.; Monkman, J.; Dos Santos Miggiolaro, A.F.R.; Cooper, C.; de Noronha, L.; et al. Endothelial cells are not productively infected by SARS-CoV-2. *Clin. Transl. Immunol.* **2021**, *10*, e1350. [CrossRef] [PubMed]
17. Bortolotti, D.; Gentili, V.; Rizzo, S.; Schiuma, G.; Beltrami, S.; Spadaro, S.; Strazzabosco, G.; Campo, G.; Carosella, E.D.; Papi, A.; et al. Increased sHLA-G Is Associated with Improved COVID-19 Outcome and Reduced Neutrophil Adhesion. *Viruses* **2021**, *13*, 1855. [CrossRef]

18. Tang, N.; Li, D.; Wang, X.; Sun, Z. Abnormal coagulation parameters are associated with poor prognosis in patients with novel coronavirus pneumonia. *J. Thromb. Haemost.* **2020**, *18*, 844–847. [CrossRef] [PubMed]
19. Christensen, B.; Favaloro, E.J.; Lippi, G.; Van Cott, E.M. Hematology Laboratory Abnormalities in Patients with Coronavirus Disease 2019 (COVID-19). *Semin. Thromb. Hemost.* **2020**, *46*, 845–849. [CrossRef] [PubMed]
20. Zhang, S.; Liu, Y.; Wang, X.; Yang, L.; Li, H.; Wang, Y.; Liu, M.; Zhao, X.; Xie, Y.; Yang, Y.; et al. SARS-CoV-2 binds platelet ACE2 to enhance thrombosis in COVID-19. *J. Hematol. Oncol.* **2020**, *13*, 120. [CrossRef] [PubMed]
21. Pennings, G.J.; Yong, A.S.; Kritharides, L. Expression of EMMPRIN (CD147) on circulating platelets in vivo. *J. Thromb. Haemost.* **2010**, *8*, 472–481. [CrossRef]
22. Tutusaus, A.; Mari, M.; Ortiz-Perez, J.T.; Nicolaes, G.A.F.; Morales, A.; Garcia de Frutos, P. Role of Vitamin K-Dependent Factors Protein S and GAS6 and TAM Receptors in SARS-CoV-2 Infection and COVID-19-Associated Immunothrombosis. *Cells* **2020**, *9*, 2186. [CrossRef]
23. Castoldi, E.; Hackeng, T.M. Regulation of coagulation by protein S. *Curr. Opin. Hematol.* **2008**, *15*, 529–536. [CrossRef] [PubMed]
24. Ruzicka, J.A. Identification of the antithrombotic protein S as a potential target of the SARS-CoV-2 papain-like protease. *Thromb. Res.* **2020**, *196*, 257–259. [CrossRef] [PubMed]
25. Wypasek, E.; Karpinski, M.; Alhenc-Gelas, M.; Undas, A. Venous thromboembolism associated with protein S deficiency due to Arg451* mutation in PROS1 gene: A case report and a literature review. *J. Genet.* **2017**, *96*, 1047–1051. [CrossRef]
26. Baez-Santos, Y.M.; St John, S.E.; Mesecar, A.D. The SARS-coronavirus papain-like protease: Structure, function and inhibition by designed antiviral compounds. *Antivir. Res.* **2015**, *115*, 21–38. [CrossRef]
27. Pilli, V.S.; Plautz, W.; Majumder, R. The Journey of Protein S from an Anticoagulant to a Signaling Molecule. *JSM Biochem. Mol. Biol.* **2016**, *3*, 1014.
28. Ziebuhr, J. The coronavirus replicase. *Curr. Top Microbiol. Immunol.* **2005**, *287*, 57–94. [CrossRef]
29. Zaid, Y.; Puhm, F.; Allaeys, I.; Naya, A.; Oudghiri, M.; Khalki, L.; Limami, Y.; Zaid, N.; Sadki, K.; Ben El Haj, R.; et al. Platelets Can Associate with SARS-CoV-2 RNA and Are Hyperactivated in COVID-19. *Circ. Res.* **2020**, *127*, 1404–1418. [CrossRef]
30. Bortolotti, D.; Gentili, V.; Rizzo, S.; Schiuma, G.; Beltrami, S.; Strazzabosco, G.; Fernandez, M.; Caccuri, F.; Caruso, A.; Rizzo, R. TLR3 and TLR7 RNA Sensor Activation during SARS-CoV-2 Infection. *Microorganisms* **2021**, *9*, 1820. [CrossRef]
31. Baroni, M.; Pavani, G.; Marescotti, D.; Kaabache, T.; Borgel, D.; Gandrille, S.; Marchetti, G.; Legnani, C.; D'Angelo, A.; Pinotti, M.; et al. Membrane binding and anticoagulant properties of protein S natural variants. *Thromb. Res.* **2010**, *125*, e33–e39. [CrossRef]
32. Zhang, H.; Penninger, J.M.; Li, Y.; Zhong, N.; Slutsky, A.S. Angiotensin-converting enzyme 2 (ACE2) as a SARS-CoV-2 receptor: Molecular mechanisms and potential therapeutic target. *Intensive Care Med.* **2020**, *46*, 586–590. [CrossRef]
33. Zamboni, P.; Bortolotti, D.; Occhionorelli, S.; Traina, L.; Neri, L.M.; Rizzo, R.; Gafa, R.; Passaro, A. Bowel ischemia as onset of COVID-19 in otherwise asymptomatic patients with persistently negative swab. *J. Intern. Med.* **2022**, *291*, 224–231. [CrossRef]
34. Kumar, A.; Narayan, R.K.; Kumari, C.; Faiq, M.A.; Kulandhasamy, M.; Kant, K.; Pareek, V. SARS-CoV-2 cell entry receptor ACE2 mediated endothelial dysfunction leads to vascular thrombosis in COVID-19 patients. *Med. Hypotheses* **2020**, *145*, 110320. [CrossRef]
35. Beyerstedt, S.; Casaro, E.B.; Rangel, E.B. COVID-19: Angiotensin-converting enzyme 2 (ACE2) expression and tissue susceptibility to SARS-CoV-2 infection. *Eur. J. Clin. Microbiol. Infect. Dis.* **2021**, *40*, 905–919. [CrossRef] [PubMed]
36. Pennings, G.J.; Kritharides, L. CD147 in cardiovascular disease and thrombosis. *Semin. Thromb. Hemost.* **2014**, *40*, 747–755. [CrossRef] [PubMed]
37. Fenizia, C.; Galbiati, S.; Vanetti, C.; Vago, R.; Clerici, M.; Tacchetti, C.; Daniele, T. SARS-CoV-2 Entry: At the Crossroads of CD147 and ACE2. *Cells* **2021**, *10*, 1434. [CrossRef]
38. Maugeri, N.; De Lorenzo, R.; Clementi, N.; Antonia Diotti, R.; Criscuolo, E.; Godino, C.; Tresoldi, C.; Angels For COVID-Bio, B.S.G.B.; Bonini, C.; Clementi, M.; et al. Unconventional CD147-dependent platelet activation elicited by SARS-CoV-2 in COVID-19. *J. Thromb. Haemost.* **2022**, *20*, 434–448. [CrossRef] [PubMed]
39. Ghasemzadeh, M.; Ahmadi, J.; Hosseini, E. Platelet-leukocyte crosstalk in COVID-19: How might the reciprocal links between thrombotic events and inflammatory state affect treatment strategies and disease prognosis? *Thromb. Res.* **2022**, *213*, 179–194. [CrossRef] [PubMed]
40. Reynolds, N.D.; Aceves, N.M.; Liu, J.L.; Compton, J.R.; Leary, D.H.; Freitas, B.T.; Pegan, S.D.; Doctor, K.Z.; Wu, F.Y.; Hu, X.; et al. The SARS-CoV-2 SSHHPS Recognized by the Papain-like Protease. *ACS Infect. Dis.* **2021**, *7*, 1483–1502. [CrossRef] [PubMed]

Disclaimer/Publisher's Note: The statements, opinions and data contained in all publications are solely those of the individual author(s) and contributor(s) and not of MDPI and/or the editor(s). MDPI and/or the editor(s) disclaim responsibility for any injury to people or property resulting from any ideas, methods, instructions or products referred to in the content.

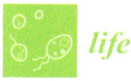

Review

Fibrin and Fibrinolytic Enzyme Cascade in Thrombosis: Unravelling the Role

Rajni Singh [1,*], Prerna Gautam [1], Chhavi Sharma [1] and Alexander Osmolovskiy [2,*]

[1] Amity Institute of Microbial Technology, Amity University Uttar Pradesh, Noida 201301, India; prerna.gautam.prerna@gmail.com (P.G.); sharmachhavi27@gmail.com (C.S.)
[2] Biological Faculty of Lomonosov, Moscow State University, 119234 Moscow, Russia
* Correspondence: rsingh3@amity.edu (R.S.); aosmol@mail.ru (A.O.); Tel.: +91-4392900 (R.S.)

Abstract: Blood clot formation in blood vessels (thrombosis) is a major cause of life-threatening cardiovascular diseases. These clots are formed by αA-, βB-, and Υ-peptide chains of fibrinogen joined together by isopeptide bonds with the help of blood coagulation factor XIIIa. These clot structures are altered by various factors such as thrombin, platelets, transglutaminase, DNA, histones, and red blood cells. Various factors are used to dissolve the blood clot, such as anticoagulant agents, antiplatelets drugs, fibrinolytic enzymes, and surgical operations. Fibrinolytic enzymes are produced by microorganisms (bacteria, fungi, etc.): streptokinase of *Streptococcus hemolyticus*, nattokinase of *Bacillus subtilis* YF 38, bafibrinase of *Bacillus* sp. AS-S20-I, longolytin of *Arthrobotrys longa*, versiase of *Aspergillus versicolor* ZLH-1, etc. They act as a thrombolytic agent by either enhancing the production of plasminogen activators (tissue or urokinase types), which convert inactive plasminogen to active plasmin, or acting as plasmin-like proteins themselves, forming fibrin degradation products which cause normal blood flow again in blood vessels. Fibrinolytic enzymes may be classified in two groups, as serine proteases and metalloproteases, based on their catalytic properties, consisting of a catalytic triad responsible for their fibrinolytic activity having different physiochemical properties (such as molecular weight, pH, and temperature). The analysis of fibrinolysis helps to detect hyperfibrinolysis (menorrhagia, renal failure, etc.) and hypofibrinolysis (diabetes, obesity, etc.) with the help of various fibrinolytic assays such as a fibrin plate assay, fibrin microplate assay, the viscoelastic method, etc. These fibrinolytic activities serve as a key aspect in the recognition of numerous cardiovascular diseases and can be easily produced on a large scale with a short generation time by microbes and are less expensive.

Keywords: fibrin; fibrinolysis; fibrinolytic assays; thrombosis; microbial fibrinolytic enzymes

1. Introduction

Cardiovascular diseases usually refer to conditions that involve the narrowing or blocking blood vessels, leading to stroke, heart attack, and angina [1]. The report provided by the World Health Organisation has shown that every year 17 million people die due to cardiovascular disorders. One of the main reasons for cardiovascular diseases is intravascular thrombosis (formation of blood clots in blood vessels) [2], which is caused due to the excessive activation of the blood coagulation cascade, wherein factor XII (the serine protease used to start the coagulation cascade) plays a role in thrombosis [3]. The high rates of mortality and morbidity are affiliated with venous and arterial thromboembolism (blockage of a blood vessel by a blood clot that has been dislodged from another site in the circulation) [4]. These blood clots are composed of fibrin fibres which provide a three-dimensional protein network and elasticity. These clots can be dissolved by the hydrolysis of fibrin by plasmin protein via the fibrinolysis process [2]. Fibrinolysis exhibits two kinds of activities: increased fibrinolysis that is seen in menorrhagia, renal failure, cirrhosis, malignancies, leukaemia, etc., and decreased fibrinolysis as seen in diabetes, obesity, hyperlipidaemia, and atherosclerosis [5].

Nowadays, various enzymes are used as anti-inflammatories, anticoagulants, oncolytics, thrombolytics, antimicrobials, digestive aids, and mucolytics [6]; among them, the enzymes responsible for clot dissolution are anticoagulant agents, antiplatelet drugs, and fibrinolytic enzymes (Figure 1) [7]. Fibrinolytic enzymes are extracted from microbes acting as potent biochemical catalysts with various biochemical applications. These fibrinolytic enzymes like streptokinase [8], nattokinase, longolytin, etc., show thrombolytic properties to treat cardiovascular diseases [9].

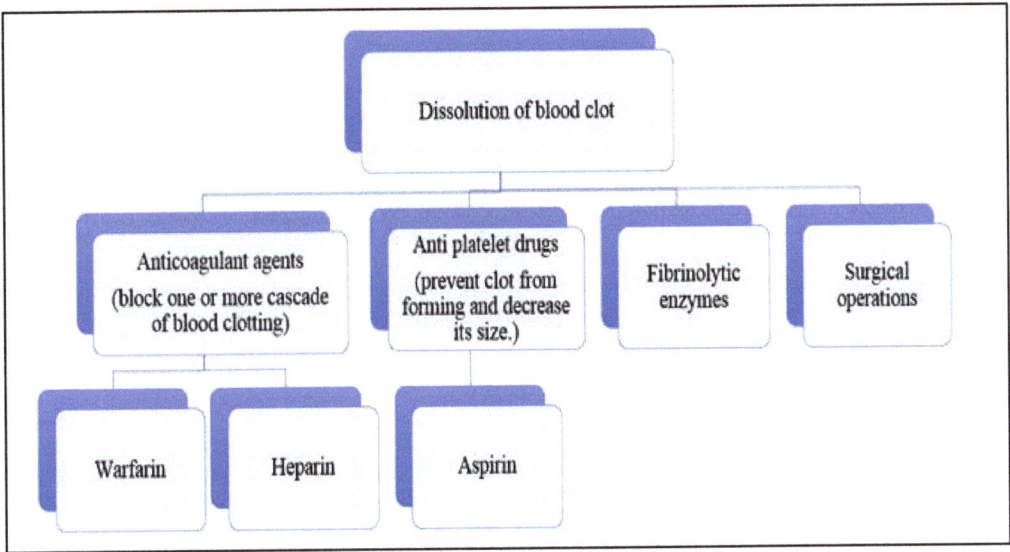

Figure 1. Different therapies for blood clot dissolution.

The fibrinolytic activity of these enzymes is estimated using various methods such as a fibrin plate assay, fibrin microplate assay, viscoelastic method, euglobulin clot lysis time, global fibrinolytic capacity, and rapid fibrin plate assay.

2. Materials and Methods

We performed an extensive literature search using scientific databases and commercial search engines like PubMed, Web of Science, ScienceDirect, ResearchGate, Google Scholar, etc., to search research papers, articles, and books for information related to mechanisms and applications. In total, 1896 different articles were scrutinized on the basis of availability; 53 elements of the latest data were finally selected with cross references, and information was compiled for the present study.

3. Results and Discussion

Worldwide cardiovascular diseases (CVDs) remain the biggest cause of death, accounting for about 31% of the total mortality rate (17.9 million deaths per year), which could exceed 23.6 million by 2030. A study from the Global Burden of Disease estimated a CVD death rate of 235 per 100,000 globally and estimated that 10.9 million people will be hospitalized for cardiovascular diseases by 2023, with 2.1 million deaths [2,3].

3.1. Cardiovascular Diseases and Thrombosis

Blood clotting and dissolution (i.e., fibrin formation and fibrinolysis) act in equilibrium. An imbalance in this equilibrium results in intravascular blood clotting, limiting the flow of blood through veins and arteries, resulting in thrombosis, leading to cardiac ailments. The leading cause of death worldwide is cardiovascular diseases which can be caused due to dysfunctional endothelial cells of the blood vessels. This leads to inflammation in the blood vessels and atherosclerotic lesions, resulting in myocardial infarction and stroke [10]. Cardiovascular diseases influenced by fibrinolytic activity occur in several other thrombotic disease states, such as acute myocardial infarction, coronary artery disease, venous thromboembolism, sepsis, and insulin-resistance syndrome. Such severe cases are associated with abnormalities such as obesity, overweight, diabetes mellitus, metabolic syndrome, hypertension, and lipid disorders (decreased HDL cholesterol and elevated triglyceride levels) [11–14]. Many studies have shown a strong relationship between plasma fibrinogen, incidence of stroke, and ischemic heart diseases. In the onset of ischemic heart diseases, factor VII (proconvertin, which causes blood to clot), and extrinsic pathway activity play a crucial role, whereas lipoproteins have a major impact on coagulability and atherogenesis [15,16].

Thrombosis is the development of blood clots inside the blood vessel, blocking the blood flow of the circulatory system. There can be two types: arterial thrombosis, which is concerned with high shear stress forming white thrombi (platelet-rich), and antiplatelet drugs like aspirin, triflusal, etc., are required for its treatment, and venous thrombosis, which concerns with low shear stress and blood flow forming red thrombi (red blood cell-rich) and anticoagulant drugs like heparin, warfarin, etc., are required for its treatment [11]. Three features that contribute to venous thrombosis (the Virchow Triad) are stasis, hypercoagulability, and endothelial injury [17]. A serious complication of thrombosis is seen in patients affected by myeloid and lymphoid leukaemia as leukemic cells activate procoagulants of platelets initiating thrombosis [18]. Procoagulant platelets facilitate the assembly of prothrombinase and tenase and thus result in thrombin burst, fibrin formation, and aggregation to create a fragile fibrin network [19] Deep venous thrombosis has a high risk for repeated venous thromboembolism that prevail for many years [20]. Oral anticoagulants are the standard treatment for deep vein thrombosis. It is also treated by drugs such as urokinase, streptokinase, tissue plasminogen activator, etc., which are injected into the foot/arm or directly at the site of the blood clot to dissolve the blood clot [21].

Ongoing clinical trials are determining the clinical efficiency of anti-inflammatory therapy in reducing the thrombus and defining the role of anti-platelet and anti-thrombotic therapy in inflammatory states [22].

3.2. Molecular Mechanism of Clot Formation

The basic unit of blood clots is fibrinogen, 340 kDa trinodular protein, present at a high concentration (2–4 mg/mL) in plasma and secreted by hepatocytes. It is composed of a dimer where an individual subunit consists of three polypeptide chains cross-linked by 29 disulfide linkages (αA-, βB- and Υ-chains) bound together as thread-like structures [23,24]. It participates in many biological processes like wound healing, haemostasis, inflammation, atherosclerosis, thrombosis, angiogenesis, etc. [25].

The six polypeptide chains form:
(1) The N terminal of the E nodule,
(2) The C terminal of the Υ- and βB-chains from the D nodule facing outwards,
(3) The C terminal of αA-chains is globular and situated near the E nodule (Figure 2a) [24,25].

Assembly of these fibrinogen to form fibrin fibres is a stepwise process in which prothrombin is transformed to thrombin by the action of activated factor X and factor V, with the formation of fibrin from fibrinogen ensuing [25–28]:
(1) Thrombin attaches to central E nodule cleaving N terminal peptides of Aα- and Bβ-chains (Figure 2b).
(2) Aα-chains are firstly cleaved by thrombin at a faster rate releasing fibrinopeptide A containing N terminal (16 residues), exposing the binding site containing Gly-Pro-Arg in E region (A knob) (Figure 2c).
(3) A knob has a complementary binding site of Υ-chain D region (a hole) creating (A: a) interaction mediating the formation of protofibrils, which are metastable peptide

assemblies observed during the growth of amyloid fibrils by a number of peptides (Figure 2d)

(4) Subsequently, removal of fibrinopeptide B containing N terminal (14 residues) causes a release, exposing the binding site containing Gly-His-Arg in E region (B knob) (Figure 2c).

(5) B knob also has a complementary binding site of β chain D region (b hole) creating (B: b) interaction, thus, mediating the lateral aggregation of fibrinogen (Figure 2d).

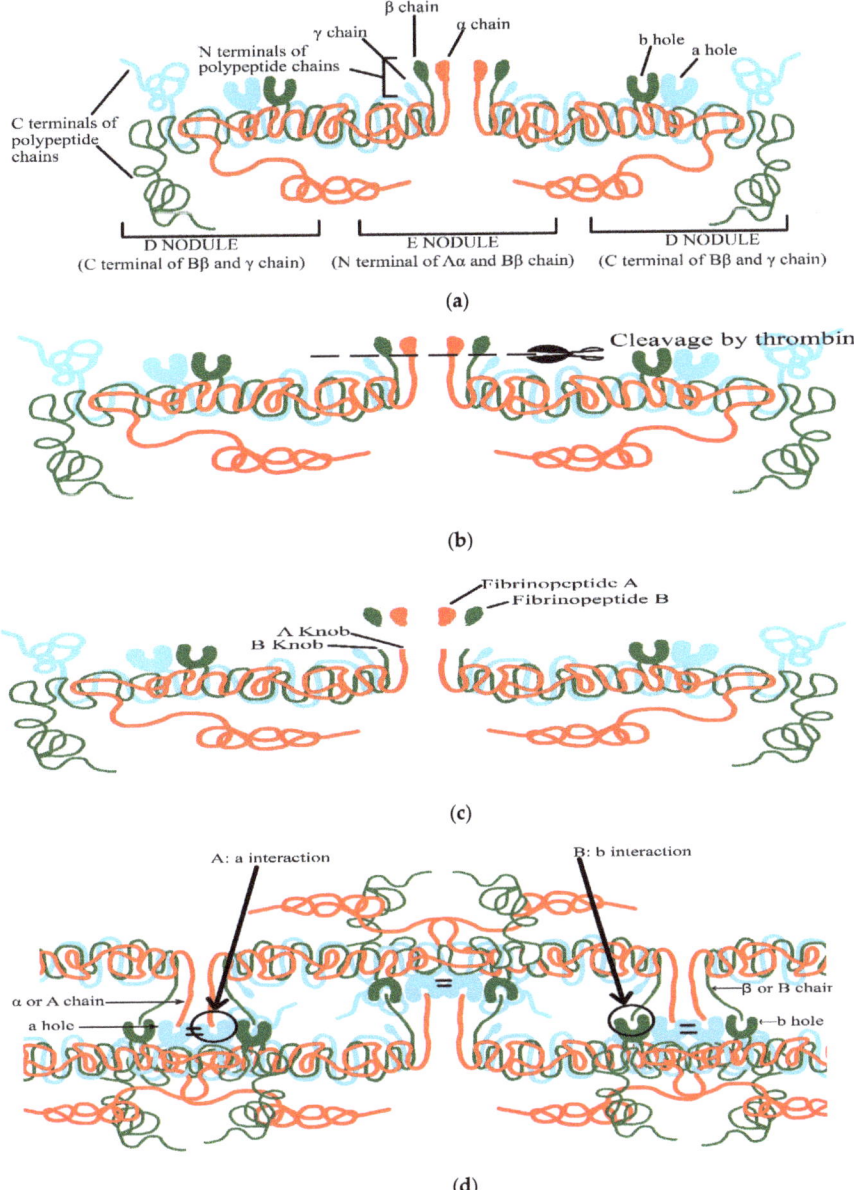

Figure 2. Cont.

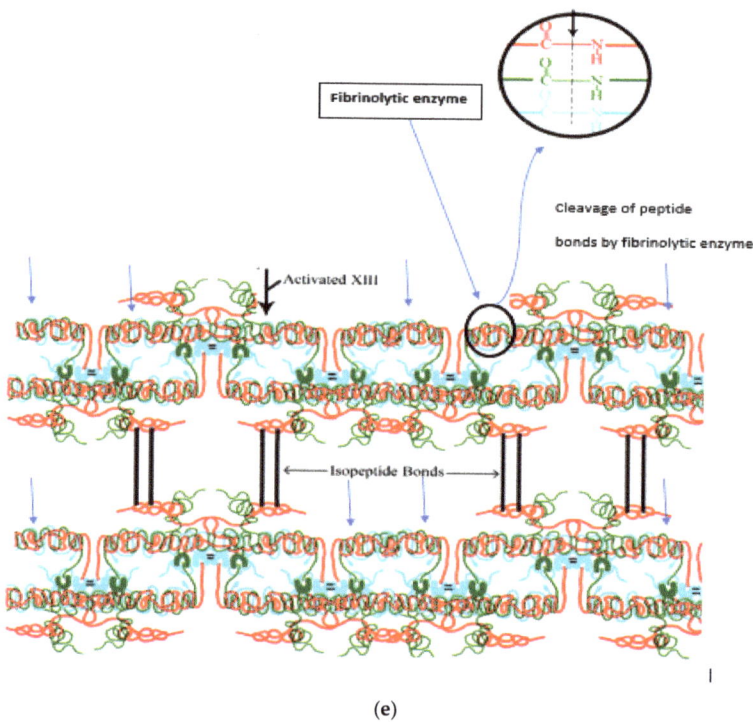

(e)

Figure 2. Mechanism of clot formation. (**a**) N terminal of the E nodule, C terminal of the ϒ- and βB-chains, C terminal of αA-chains situated near the E nodule. (**b**) Attachment of thrombin to central E nodule cleaving N terminal peptides of Aα- and Bβ-chains. (**c**) Cleavage of Aα-chains by thrombin. (**d**) Complementary binding sites of ϒ-chain and β-chain D region mediating protofibril formation and lateral aggregation of fibrinogen, respectively. (**e**) Formation of fibrin fibres.

This process results in the production of protofibrils which are then converted to fibrin fibres with the help of blood clotting factor XIII [29].

Factor XIII is a heterologous tetramer consisting of two catalytic A subunits (XIII A) produced by bone marrow and two inhibitory/carrier B subunits (XIII B) produced by hepatocytes. By the concentrated action of thrombin and calcium ions, inactive factor XIII is transformed into active factor XIII (active transglutaminase). Thrombin first cleaves off activation peptide XIII and in the presence of calcium ions, it dissociates XIII B. This cleaved XIII A dimer is presumed to be an enzymatic active configuration of factor XIII (XIIIa) [25]. XIIIa now forms an isopeptide bond between two adjacent monomers of αα-chains and αϒ-chains forming fibrin fibres, increasing the elasticity and stabilization of the individual protofibrils and the lateral aggregate structure (Figure 2e). Activated factor XIII also incorporates α2-antiplasmin into α-chains of fibrin to prevent lysis of the blood clot [30].

Elevated levels of fibrinogen increase the fibrin network concentration, blood clot rigorousness and resistance to the fibrinolytic process increasing the risk of venous thrombosis or venous thromboembolism [31]. Fibrin polymerization is an active process that is difficult to study and is monitored by available techniques like confocal microscopy, electron microscopy, and turbidity measurements [32].

3.3. Fibrin Architecture

Fibrin architecture is determined by fibrinogen and thrombin concentration. Within a certain range of thrombin concentration, the porosity, fibre dimension, and gel architecture of fibrin are formed in recalcified plasma. This concentration is determined by the initial rate of fibrinogen activation [33]. Many studies certify that denser clots (more tightly packed fibres, less porosity) lyse more slowly than clots with large pores (more loosely packed fibres) [34]. The size of the fibres and the arrangement of fibrinogen have a major impact on tissue plasminogen activator binding and rate of fibrinolysis [35].

Several factors that affect the fibrin architecture are as follows:

(1) Fibrin is formed in vivo at the site of blood vessel lesion where platelets are stimulated and bind to fibrin forming powerful adhesive forces. These fibres under tension regulate clot structure, constrain fibrin fibres, and increase their density in platelet-rich areas [36].

(2) Factor XIIIa (transglutaminase) proposes ϒ-glutamyllysine crosslinking between αC- and ϒC-domains of next fibrin monomers and tightens up the lateral (flanking) attachment of protofibrils. This covalent crosslinking results in a decrease in the fibrin diameter without any modification in the number of protofibrils in fibres. Thus, decreasing the vacant fluid space volume within the fibres causes a two-fold reduction in pore size [37,38].

(3) DNA and histones that are released by activated neutrophils form neutrophil extracellular traps. These have a major effect on clot lysis as they hold lysing fibrin (large fibrin degradative products) together resulting in a delay in the fibrinolytic process [39].

(4) The contractile force (induced by fibrin) of neighbouring fibres activates platelets which acts on red blood cells (RBCs) causing a change in their configuration from biconcave to polyhedral. This change induces gap-free compression of RBCs in unoccupied spaces between fibrin fibres forming a high lytic resistance structure and strong diffusion barrier [40]. These activities of RBCs increase blood viscosity, and express phosphatidylserine on their surface, which promotes fibrin deposition during venous thrombosis and reduces clot dissolution by suppressing plasmin [31].

3.4. Fibrinolysis

Fibrinolysis is the enzymatic breakdown of blood clots. The fibrinolytic system is composed of inactive proenzymes like plasminogen which is converted to plasmin (an active enzyme), degrading insoluble fibrin fibres into soluble FDPs (fibrin degradation products) [41].

Fibrinolysis activation is regulated by [42]:

(1) Tissue-type plasminogen activator (t-PA) which is enhanced in the presence of fibrin.
(2) Urokinase-type plasminogen activator (u-PA), which binds to specific u-PA receptors, enhancing the activation of cell-bound plasminogen (Figure 3).

In fibrinolysis, fibrin plays two major roles: it enhances the production of tissue plasminogen activator, and it also acts as a substrate for plasmin (Figure 4) [43].

Components of the Fibrinolytic System

(1) Plasminogen

Plasminogen (single polypeptide) is a glycoprotein of 92 kDa, consisting of 791 amino acids, 24 disulfide bridges and 5 homologous kringles (a triple loop structure having lysine binding sites for fibrin) [42].

Circulated plasminogen has amino terminal glutamic acid (glu-plasminogen), which upon proteolysis is modified to amino terminal lysine plasminogen (lys-plasminogen)—hydrolysis of the Lys-77—Lys-78 peptide bond forms modified zymogen that more readily binds to fibrin. Lys-plasminogen tends to be more readily activated by tissue plasminogen activator than Glu-plasminogen and its activation rate is increased by the addition of fibrinogen [44].

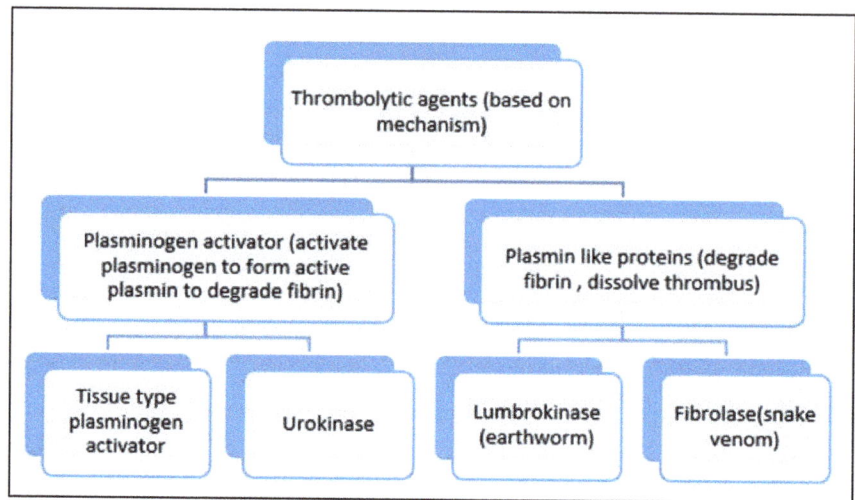

Figure 3. Categorization of thrombolytic agents on the basis of mechanism of action.

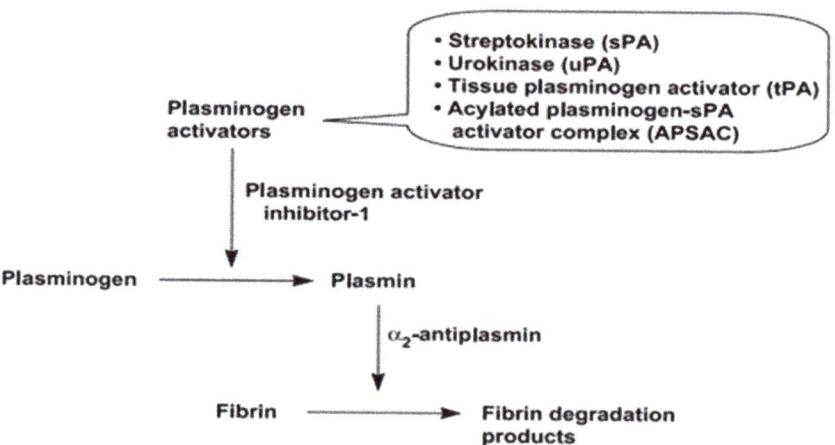

Figure 4. Schematic representation of fibrinolysis and proposed mode of action of fibrinolytic protease.

The peptide bond of plasminogen is cleaved by t-PA or u-PA between Arg-561 and Val-562, forming plasmin. This plasmin contains two polypeptide chains:
- Heavy chains have an N-terminal part of plasminogen including five kringles.
- Light chains having the C-terminal part of plasminogen containing serine peptidase (catalytic triad: His-603, Asp-646, Ser-741) [38].

(2) Tissue-type plasminogen activator (t-PA).

t-PA is a proteolytic enzyme that activates plasminogen to form plasmin and is found in blood (thrombolytic agent) and the brain (promoting neuronal synaptic plasticity) [45]. T-PA may be obtained as a single polypeptide chain of molecular weight of 72 kDa. Cleavage of the t-PA peptide bond Arg-275-Ile-276 by plasmin changes t-PA to disulphide-linked, double polypeptide chains of molecular weights of 30 to 40 kDa each [46].

Five discrete structural domains are present in t-PA, encompassing finger-growth factor–kringle 1–kringle 2–protease (F-G-K1-K2-P). It comprises several potential binding sites for cells and fibrin where F and K2 are the most important sites for fibrinolysis, but mutagenic analysis specifies that K2 is less concerned with fibrin binding than anticipated [47]. These domains are responsible for attachment to fibrin, cellular receptors, and fibrin-specific plasminogen activation [42]. It also has high mannose carbohydrate on Asn-11, an O-linked α-fucose residue on Thr-61, and complex oligosaccharide on Asn-448 which regulates its binding to cell surface receptors [48]. The discharge of t-PA is regulated through a diversity of interventions like bradykinin, adrenaline, thrombin, vasopressin, histamine, gonadotropins, exercise, acetylcholine, shear stress, and venous occlusion [49].

(3) Urokinase

Prourokinase (single chain urokinase-type plasminogen activator—pro-UK) is a pioneer of two active chains, urokinase plasminogen activator (u-PA). The prourokinase can be transformed to active u-PA by the hydrolysis of the Lys-158-Ile-159 peptide bond via plasmin, factor XII, trypsin, and plasma kallikrein [50]. u-PA consists of two chains with molecular weights of 20 and 30 k Da held together by a disulfide bridge. It is a serine protease that activates plasminogen to form plasmin. Less activity than u-PA and resistance to plasmin activation is seen in the case of thromb-UK (two-chain form) which is formed by the hydrolysis of the Arg-156-Phe-157 peptide bond of pro-UK by thrombin [51].

Urokinase plasminogen activator receptors (u-PAR) are specific membrane protein receptors and are assigned as CD 87 antigens. They are a highly glycosylated protein (50–65 kDa) linked to the plasma membrane by glycosylphosphatidylinositol [52]. They are encoded by 335 amino acids of which the initial 22 amino acids comprise the signal peptide. They contain a kringle module and a serine-binding domain. They are expressed in neutrophils, activated T-cells, mononuclear phagocytes, several types of tumour cells, and endothelial cells. They have a higher affinity for u-PA converting into active form on binding, thus gaining the capability to enzymatically digest plasminogen to plasmin [53]. Pro-UK as well as u-PA can both bind to u-PAR but thrombolysis by pro-UK is more effective and specific than u-PA. u-PA has a decreased affinity for fibrin fibres than t-PA and is a dynamic plasminogen activator mutually in the presence and absence of fibrin [54,55].

(4) Plasmin

The fibrinolytic enzyme plasmin is produced from plasminogen by activators such as t-PA and u-PA. Plasmin is a serine protease that cuts fibrin chains forming solvable FDPs exposing carboxyl-terminal lysine residues. This modification of the fibrin surface structure has major implications for plasmin, plasminogen, and t-PA-possessing kringle domains which mediate binding through lysine residues, affecting the regulation of fibrinolysis. The modification on the fibrin surface increases the rate of plasmin formation by three-fold when t-PA is a plasminogen activator [56].

Other roles of plasmin are:

- Plasmin deactivates and cleaves various clotting factors FV, FVIII, FIX, and FX in vitro which plays a major role in clot formation [57].
- The two catalytic A-subunits of active clotting factor XIII are degraded endogenously by plasmin during lysis of the blood clot [58].
- Plasmin is an important matrix metalloprotease activator, enhancing the lysis effect of plasmin on surrounding tissues [59].

(5) Plasminogen activator inhibitor

Plasminogen activator inhibitor 1 (PAI-1) consists of nine α-helices, three β-sheets, and an exposed loop containing the active site Arg-346-Met-347. Active PAI-1's overall structure is like the structure of other inhibitory serpins [60]. It is an important physiological inhibitor that inhibits the transformation of plasminogen to plasmin by t-PA and u-PA and plays a major part in the fibrinolytic process [61]. It also inhibits the endothelial cells present in plasma which react with single polypeptide t-PA, double polypeptide t-PA, and u-PA.

Strangely, it behaves as a competitive inhibitor of the binding of t-PA to fibrin. Since the inhibition constant of PAI-1 for t-PA is of the same order of magnitude as the dissociation constant of t-PA and fibrin interaction, the formation of t-PA PAI-1 complexes resulted in impaired fibrinolysis [62].

(6) α2-Antiplasmin

α2-antiplasmin (molecular weight 51 kDa) is a major inhibitor of plasmin and belongs to the Serpin family. Its synthesis takes place in the liver as an individual chain of glycoprotein comprising 464 amino acid residues (30% of circulating antiplasmin) and short chain polypeptide chain consisting of 452 amino acids (70% having higher proteolytic activity) [63]. It circulates in plasma at higher concentrations (0.9 nmol/L) with a plasma half-life of 2.4 days [49] and inhibits plasminogen activators like t-PA and u-PA [64].

α2-antiplasmin regulates fibrinolysis in three steps [60]:

- Inhibiting the adsorption of plasminogen to fibrin: the C-terminal end of α2-antiplasmin binds with a robust affinity towards the lysine binding site, where fibrin is bound non-covalently (competitive inhibition).
- Formation of a balanced inactive complex by plasmin: after the binding of α2-antiplasmin with the lysine binding site, it is quickly cleaved via plasmin at the active site releasing the peptides and forming a covalent plasmin—α2-antiplasmin complex.
- Cross-linkage via factor XIIIa: the portion of circulating α2-antiplasmin is tightly bound to fibrin via factor XIIIa, resulting in the amplified resistance of fibrin to fibrinolysis.

3.5. Why Measure Fibrinolysis?

Fibrinolysis under normal circumstances is a slow and natural process. Hyperfibrinolysis or enhanced fibrinolysis is life-threatening due to blood loss. Enhanced fibrinolysis has been seen in patients suffering from liver and lung disease, prostrate surgery or major trauma, cirrhosis, menorrhagia, renal failure, obstetric complications, and in some malignancies in leukaemia patients. This bleeding process starts when there is the absence of a fibrinolytic inhibitor. To combat this situation, anti-fibrinolytic lysine analogue, aprotinin, epsilon aminocaproic acid, and tranexamic acid are used.

In the case of hypofibrinolysis or impaired fibrinolysis, which may be due to environmental or heredity origin, these may be linked to thrombosis, associated with patients suffering from hyperlipidaemia, diabetes, obesity, and atherosclerosis. Various biomarkers are used that indicate reduced fibrinolysis such as elevated plasminogen activator inhibitor, α2-antiplasmin, changes in active t-PA level, and thrombin activatable fibrinolysis inhibitor. To combat this situation, anti-coagulant agents, anti-platelets drugs, and fibrinolytic enzymes are used [5].

The measurement of fibrinolytic activity is governed by various fibrinolytic assays determining hyperfibrinolysis or hypofibrinolysis conditions.

3.6. Fibrinolytic Activity Assay

Different methods are proposed to observe fibrinolytic action in blood and its elements [65].

(1) Fibrin plate assay

Fibrin plate assay determines fibrinolytic mediators present in the samples. It consists of two forms:

- Plasminogen-free fibrin plate (heated): This assay allows the direct activity of plasmin-like enzymes, formed from fibrinogen solution (5 mg human fibrinogen in 7 mL of 0.1 M Barbital buffer of 7.8 pH), 10 U thrombin solution and 7 mL of 10 g agarose/Liter) to be assessed in Petri plates. Then, for inactivating fibrinolytic enzymes, the plates were heated at 80 °C for 30 min. These plates were modified by means of bovine fibrinogen, calcium chloride, thrombin, and sodium chloride. The enzyme (10–30 µL) was dropped judiciously on a fibrin plate and incubated at 37 °C temperature for 3–18 h, and clear zones were obtained. A standard curve was plotted by using standard fibrinolytic enzyme (urokinase) to examine the fibrinolytic activity of an enzyme.

- Plasminogen-rich fibrin plate (non-heated): This consists of 5 U plasminogen in addition to the above fibrinolytic solution and is not heated. It is suitable for plasminogen activators [66].

The fibrin plate assay shows uncertainty in determining the accurate lysis zone and hence another method, the microtiter plate assay, was developed to overcome this problem.

(2) Fibrin microplate assay

This is a sensitive and quantitative assay to determine the fibrinolytic activity in the samples. In this assay, fibrin clots were adsorbed in 96-well microtiter plates with specific dye integration using fibrinogen. A mixture of para-nitroaniline and then thrombin were added to wells to form fibrin (overnight incubation at 37 °C). Inhibitors were removed from plasma using alcohol before being applied to the wells. Then, 20 µL of test mixture was applied in triplets with 5 µL plasminogen onto the fibrin gel. For positive reference, dilutions of urokinase (standard) were used. After 6 h incubation at 37 °C, the converted substrate (lysate) was removed with rinse buffer. A total of 20 µL plasmin (1 U/mL) was added to each of the remaining blood clots. After overnight incubation at 37 °C, complete lysis was obtained and then they were rinsed with buffer and mixed well. Fibrin was photometrically determined after dissolution by plasmin at 405 nm.

The fibrinolytic activity was observed by a difference in absorption value before and after lysis of the fibrin clot. The activity was determined by using a urokinase dose–response curve based on serial dilutions of standard urokinase.

This assay is highly reliable for the assessment of the degree of clot lysis by varying concentrations of urokinase and incubation time [67].

(3) Rapid fibrin plate assay

The long incubation period (16–20 h) is the key disadvantage of fibrin plate/microplate assay and is enhanced by plasminogen enrichment. The fibrin plates were enriched with 2 U of plasminogen to form opaque plates. The fibrin clots do not lyse spontaneously and yield prominent parallel lines for streptokinase and urokinase after 3 h of incubation. Urokinase assay is more precise as compared to streptokinase because of the shallow dose–response curve [7].

(4) Euglobulin clot lysis time (ECLT)

ECLT is used to evaluate fibrinolytic activity in plasma. It implies the interaction of the activity of t-PA with plasminogen-activating inhibitor [68]. The variation in the absorbance of recalcified euglobulin fraction at different time periods indicates the fibrinolytic activity [69].

In quantitative ECLT, turbidity is measured every 30 min using a microtiter plate reader where the midpoint between minimum and maximum turbidity determines the lysis time providing reliable and reproducive data. The mathematical examination determines critical points of lysis along with the kinetics analysis of fibrinolysis. Studies project that low ECLT values are linked with elevated plasmin–antiplasmin (PAP) complexes and free tissue plasminogen activator (tPA) levels in plasma [69,70]. It is highly recommended for surgeries like cardiovascular surgery, pharmacological surgery, and liver transplantation coagulation surgery to determine atherosclerosis, hyperlipidaemic conditions, and associated diseases [68].

(5) Global fibrinolytic capacity (GFC)

Global fibrinolytic capacity (GFC) is used to evaluate the fibrinolysis in a single sample by generating D-dimers (DD) from the fibrin clot prepared with fibrinogen and thrombin-free plasminogen [68]. Silicated fibrin tablets (25 µg) were added to plasma and t-PA and incubated at 37 °C for one-hour. The aprotinin accumulation and D-dimer production were assessed for the fibrinolytic process [65]. The method is quite costly due to the reagents used and the D-dimer evaluation to estimate fibrinolysis activity. This assay is useful for diabetes (type I and II), hypothyroidism, sepsis, chronic liver and mitral valve diseases, respiratory distress, and polycystic ovary syndromes [65].

(6) Viscoelastic method

The viscoelastic method is used to analyse the effect of blood cells and platelets on clotting and fibrinolytic processes in whole blood. This process is extremely fast and plays an important role during surgical procedures allied with blood loss, traumatic injury, liver transplant, and cardiothoracic surgery [5]. Viscoelastic changes in blood can be monitored by:

- Rotational thromboelastometry (ROTEM) computes different viscoelastic parameters like clotting time, clot growth kinetics, the pace of coagulation initiation, clot strength, and dissolution [66]. The five principal assays used with the ROTEM instrument are INTEM, HEPTEM, EXTEM, FIBTEM, and APTEM assays. The INTEM test initiates clotting via the intrinsic pathway using ellagic acid, while the HEPTEM assay uses heparinase in addition to ellagic acid. EXTEM uses tissue factor to initiate the extrinsic clotting cascade whereas FIBTEM uses cytochalasin D to inhibit platelet activity and provide clot tracing that indicates the presence of fibrinogen. This test is used extensively in cardiac and liver studies to monitor fibrinogen levels. APTEM is a modified EXTEM assay that incorporates aprotinin to stabilize the clot against hyperfibrinolysis. An electrical signal from an automatic electrical transducer leads to a graphical display supervised by a computer [71,72].
- Thromboelastography (TEG) is a non-invasive test that quickly determines coagulation rate (hypo/hyper) or solidification to fibrinolysis (involving prothrombin/thrombin/fibrin), the viscoelastic properties of blood samples during clotting under low shear stress. It uses reagents different from ROTEM and involves five different parameters: reaction time, kinetics, alpha angle, maximum amplitude, and lysis at 30 min (A30/LY30) [5,72].
- Sonoclot: This assesses the change in resistivity via a small disposable plastic probe spinning vertically on a coagulating blood sample in the cuvette. Fibrin components formed on the tip/ around the probe and on the internal wall of the cuvette increase the weight of the probe leading to an upsurge in the resistivity. This increase in resistivity is sensed via electronic circuits and transformed into an output signal. The output signal describes the viscoelastic properties of the blood coagulation initiated from fibrin development, aggregation of fibrin monomers, platelet interaction, clot retraction, and lysis [73].

Chromogenic assay. The chromogenic method is based on determining the target proteolytic activity with specific chromogenic peptide substrates of plasmin (H-D-Val-Leu-Lys-pNA or similar), tissue plasminogen activator (H-D-Ile-Pro-Arg-pNA or similar), and urokinase (pGlu-Gly-Arg-pNA or similar). As a rule, the sample is incubated with the substrate for 5 min at 37 °C. As a result of the reaction, a chromophore (para-nitroanaline) is split off from such substrates—para-nitroanilides—and absorption at 405 nm is measured in the mixture. The concentration of released para-nitroanaline is directly proportional to the activity of the proteolytic enzyme in the sample. The method is applicable to both mini-tubes and plates.

3.7. Microorganisms: Important Source of Fibrinolytic Enzymes

Numerous sources of fibrinolytic enzymes have been discovered such as microorganisms, snakes, earthworms, insects, plants, and fermented products. However, microorganisms have emerged as the most important sources, especially the genus *Bacillus* from traditional fermented foods [6]. A potent fibrinolytic enzyme (nattokinase) is used in thrombolytic therapy by cleaving the isopeptide bonds of fibrin (Figure 3) [74].

These fibrinolytic enzymes can be procured from different microbial sources such as bacterial species like *Streptococcus hemolyticus* (streptokinase) [75], *Bacillus subtilis* YF 38 (nattokinase) [8], *Staphylococcus aureus* (Staphylokinase) [76], *Bacillus* sp. DJ-4 (Subtilisin DJ4) [77], fungal species like *Arthrobotrys longa* [78], *Aspergillus oryzae* [79], *Aspergillus ochraceus* [80], *Aspergillus versicolor* [81], *Fusarium* sp. [82], *Penicillium* sp. [83], *Rhizopus chinensis* [84], *Sarocladium strictum* [85], or mushrooms such as *Cordyceps militaris* [86] and *Armillaria mella* [87].

Biochemical attributes of microbial fibrinolytic enzyme

The biochemical attributes of microbial fibrinolytic enzymes involve molecular weight, temperature optimum of activity, pH optimum of activity, substrate specificity, thermo- and pH-stability [2].

Based on catalytic properties, fibrinolytic enzymes are composed of different types of proteases. These proteases (synonyms: proteinases, peptidases, proteolytic enzymes) can hydrolyse peptide bonds in proteins. They can be found in less as well as in more complex organisms. These enzymes have excessive importance due to their major role in biochemical and cellular processes, and the life cycles of pathogens. Based on their catalytic mechanism, they are grouped as endopeptidase (cleavage takes place within the peptide backbone) and exopeptidase (cleavage takes place at the end of the peptide backbone) [88,89].

- Endopeptidase: Serine protease: trypsin, thrombin, chymotrypsin, subtilisin, etc. Cysteine protease: rhinovirus 3C, papain, etc. Metalloprotease: collagenase, thermolysin, etc. Aspartic protease: pepsin and cathepsin [83].

- Exopeptidase: Serine protease: carboxypeptidase Y. Cystine protease: cathepsin and DAPase. Metalloprotease: carboxypeptidase A, carboxypeptidase B [83]. Serine and metalloprotease have catalytic properties of fibrinolytic enzymes.

Serine protease. Most of the members are comprised of endopeptidase which varies extensively in their specificity. The cascades of consecutive activation of serine protease are required for the initiation of blood coagulation, complement fixation, and fibrinolysis process [90]. Enzymatic active members of the chymotrypsin family include His, Asp, and Ser whereas the enzymatic active members of the subtilisin family include different orders as Asp, His, and Ser. Therefore, we can say that serine protease represents different evolutionary lines [91]. Serine protease follows two-step reactions: acylation followed by deacylation occurring via a nucleophilic attack on intermediate by water, ensuing in the hydrolysis of a peptide.

These proteases are recognized by their irreversible inhibition by tosyl-L-lysine chloromethyl ketone (TLCK), L-3-carboxytrans 2,3-epoxypropyl-leucylamido (4-guanidine) butane, 3,4-dichloroisocoumarin (3,4-DCI), diisopropylfluorophosphate (DFP), and phenylmethylsulphonyl fluoride (PMSF) [92].

Fibrinolytic enzymes associated with the serine protease family belong to *Bacillus* sp. (subtilisin) and are active at alkaline to neutral pH (optimum pH 8–10), isoelectric points about 8 and molecular weights are between 27.7 and 44 KDa. The optimum temperature has a range between 30 and 70 °C, mostly 50 °C. It contains a catalytic triad containing Ser 221, His 64, and Asp 32 without any intramolecular disulphide linkage. Examples are Subtilisin DJ 4, CFR 15 protease, Subtilisin DFE, BAFFI, etc. (Table 1) [65].

Table 1. Microbial fibrinolytic enzymes and their properties.

Fibrinolytic Enzymes	Micro-Organisms Associated	Sources for Production	Physicochemical Properties	Functional Moiety	Mechanism of Action	References
Streptokinase	*Streptococcus hemolyticus*	Exudates of infected wounds	47 kDa pH 7.5 37 °C	Single polypeptide chain (414 amino acids) with multiple structural domains (α, β, γ)	plasminogen activation for the formation of β-domain SK plasminogen complex	[75,93]
Staphylokinase	*Staphylococcus aureus*	Human skin	15.5 kDa pH 8.5 37 °C	Single polypeptide chain (136 amino acids) without disulphide bridge	plasminogen activation due to higher affinity with plasmin	[76,94]
Serrapeptase	*Serratia marcescens* E 15	Intestine of silkworm	45–60 kDa pH 9.0 40 °C	Metalloprotease with one active site and three Zn atoms	Cleavage of peptide bond linkages	[95]
Nattokinase (wild Type)	*Bacillus subtilis* YF 38, natto	Fermented soybean Natto	27.7 kDa pH 8.6	Presence of catalytic triad (Asp-32, His-64 and Ser-221) and one oxyanion hole (Asn-155)	Resemblance with plasmin and enhanced production of plasmin and clot dissolving agents	[8,96]
Nattokinase	*Pseudomonas aeruginosa* CMSS (new strain)	Cow milk	21 kDa pH 7.0 25 °C	Like wild-type nattokinase with a two-fold increase in enzyme activation	Same as wild type nattokinase	[97]
CK fibrinolytic enzyme	*Bacillus* sp. CK	Chungkook-jang (Korea)	28.2 kDa pH 10.5 70 °C	Thermolytic alkaline serine protease (1882 protein atoms, 2 Ca^{2+} ions, and 44 water molecules)	Higher tissue plasminogen activator production.	[98,99]
Fibrinolytic enzyme	*Bacillus* sp. KA38	Jeot-gal (fermented fish, Korea)	41 kDa pH 7.0 40 °C	Metalloprotease	Degrade fibrin or form plasmin from plasminogen	[100]
CFR 15 protease	*Bacillus amyloliquefaciens* MCC2606 (strain CFR 15)	Dosa batter	32 kDa pH 10.5 45 °C	Serine protease with a catalytic triad (His-57, Ser-195, Asp-102)	Hydrolysis of αα-, ββ-, γ-chains of fibrin	[101]
B. amyloliquefaciens An6 fibrinase (BAF1)	*Bacillus amyloliquefaciens* An6	*Mirabilis jalapa* tuber powder (MJTP)	30 kDa pH 9.0 60 °C	Serine protease	Degrade fibrin or form plasmin from plasminogen	[102]
Subtilisin DJ-4	*Bacillus* sp. DJ-4	Doen-jang, Korea	29 kDa pH 10.0 40 °C	Plasmin-like serine protease	Rapid hydrolysis of αα-, ββ-, γ-chains of fibrin	[77]
Subtilisin QK02	*Bacillus* sp. QK02	Fermented soybean	28 kDa pH 8.5 55 °C	Serine protease with a catalytic triad (Asp-32, His-64 and Ser-221)	Cleaves peptide bond linkages	[103]

Table 1. Cont.

Fibrinolytic Enzymes	Micro-Organisms Associated	Sources for Production	Physicochemical Properties	Functional Moiety	Mechanism of Action	References
Subtilisin DFE	*Bacillus amyloliquefaciens* DC 4	Douchi (China)	28 kDa pH 9.0 48 °C	Serine protease	High specificity towards fibrin and hydrolyses thrombin	[104]
Fibrinolytic enzyme	*Bacillus tequilensis* CWD-67	Dumping soil	22 kDa pH 8.0 45 °C	Chymotrypsin-like serine metalloprotease containing hydrophobic S1 pocket	Hydrolysis of αα-, ββ-, γ-chains of fibrin	[105]
BacillokinaseII	*Bacillus subtilis* A1	Local soil (Korea)	31.4 kDa pH 7.0 50 °C	Chymotrypsin-like serine protease	Degrade fibrin and act as plasminogen activator	[106]
Fibrinolytic enzyme	*Bacillus* sp. KDO-13	Soybean paste (Korea)	45 kDa pH 7 60 °C	Metalloprotease with Catalytic domain with 170 amino acids, hinge region, and hemopexin domain of 200 amino acids	Degrade fibrin or form plasmin from plasminogen	[107,108]
Fibrinolytic enzyme	*Bacillus thuringiensis* IND 7	Cow dung	32 kDa pH 9.0	Serine protease	Degrade fibrin or form plasmin from plasminogen	[109]
Bafibrinase	*Bacillus* Sp. AS-S20-I	Soil (Assam)	32.3 kDa 7.4 pH 37 °C	Catalytic triad (Ser-221, His-64 and Asp-32) without intramolecular sulphide bond	Cleaves chains of fibrin (α, β) and fibrinogen	[110]
Subtilisin BK 17	*Bacillus subtilis* BK17	Decaying rice plant (Korea)	31 kDa	Serine protease	Degrade fibrin or form plasmin from plasminogen	[111]
Fibrinolytic enzyme	*Bacillus subtilis* KCK-7	Chungkookjang (fermented food)	45 kDa pH 7.0 60 °C	Serine protease requires hydroxyl group for activity	Degrade fibrin or form plasmin from plasminogen	[112]
Douchi fibrinolytic enzyme	*Bacillus subtilis* LD 8547	Soybean fermented food (China)	30 kDa	Serine protease	Activate t-PA	[113]
Fibrinolytic enzyme	*Paenibacillus* sp. IND8	Cooked Indian rice	-	-	Degrade fibrin or form plasmin from plasminogen	[114]
SW 1	*Streptomyces* sp. Y405	Soil isolate	30 kDa pH 8.0	Serine protease and metalloprotease	Degrade fibrin or form plasmin from plasminogen	[115]

Table 1. Cont.

Fibrinolytic Enzymes	Micro-Organisms Associated	Sources for Production	Physicochemical Properties	Functional Moiety	Mechanism of Action	References
Fibrinolytic enzyme	*Streptomyces rubiginosus*	Marine soil	45 kDa pH 7.2 32 °C	-	Degrade fibrin or form plasmin from plasminogen	[116]
Fibrinolytic enzyme	*Streptomyces* sp. MCMB-379	Seed culture	-	Serine endopeptidase type	Cleaves fibrin fibres by degradation of chains	[117]
β Haemolytic Streptokinase	*Streptococcus equinus*	Bovine milk	-	-	Degrade fibrin or form plasmin from plasminogen	[118]
Fibrinolytic enzyme	*Bacillus cereus* SRM-001	Chicken dump yard	28 kDa pH 7.0 37 °C	Serine protease	Plasmin catalysed hydrolysis of fibrin	[119]
Fibrinolytic enzyme	*Bacillus cereus* IND 5	Cuttle fish waste and cow dung	47 kDa pH 8.0 50 °C	Serine protease	Degrade fibrin or form plasmin from plasminogen	[120]
Fibrinolytic enzyme	*Bacillus pumilus*	Gembus (Indonesia fermented food)	20 kDa 50 °C	Serine protease	Degrade α- and β-chains of fibrinogen but not ϒ-chain	[121]
Fibrinolytic enzyme	*Serratia* sp. KG 2–1	Garbage dump yard	pH 8.0 40 °C	Metalloprotease	Degrade fibrin or form plasmin from plasminogen	[122]
Fibrinolytic enzyme	*Shewanella* sp. IND20	Fish *Sardinella longiceps*	55.5 kDa pH 8.0 50 °C	Serine protease	Direct clot lysis and plasminogen activation activity	[123]
Fibrinolytic enzyme	*Cordyceps militaris*	Mushroom	28 kDa pH 7.2 37 °C	Serine protease	Activate plasminogen to plasmin	[78]
Fibrinolytic enzyme	*Lasiodiplodia pseudotheobromae*	Aegle Marmelos (Golden apple)	80 kDa	-	Degrade fibrin or form plasmin from plasminogen	[124]
AMMP	*Armillaria mella*	Mushroom (Korea)	21 kDa pH 6.0 33 °C	Chymotrypsin like metalloprotease	Hydrolyse α-α fibrinogen	[79]
Fibrinolytic enzyme	*Mucor subtilissimus* UCP 1262	Soil (Brazil)	20 kDa pH 9.0 40 °C	Chymotrypsin like serine protease	Properties resemble to plasmin	[125]
Fibrinolytic enzyme	*Cochliobolus lunatus*	Surface culture	pH 6.8 40 °C	-	Degrade fibrin or form plasmin from plasminogen	[126]

Table 1. Cont.

Fibrinolytic Enzymes	Micro-Organisms Associated	Sources for Production	Physicochemical Properties	Functional Moiety	Mechanism of Action	References
Longolytin	*Arthrobotrys longa*	Soil, contains nematodes	28.6 kDa pH 6.0–9.0	Serine protease contains thiol groups	Hydrolyse fibrin and activate plasminogen like urokinase	[127,128]
Fibrinolytic enzyme	*Aspergillus ochraceus* L-1	Soil	36 kDa pH 10.0–11.0 45 °C	Serine protease	Hydrolyse fibrin and fibrinogen	[79]
Fibrinolytic enzyme	*Aspergillus oryzae* KSK-3	Commercial rice-koji for miso brewing	30 kDa pH 6.0 50 °C	Serine protease	Hydrolyse fibrin and fibrinogen	[80]
Versiase	*Aspergillus versicolor*	Marine sponge *Callyspongia* sp.	37.3 kDa pH 5.0 40 °C	Metalloprotease	Hydrolyse fibrin directly and indirectly via the activation of plasminogen, and it can hydrolyse α-, β- and γ-chains of fibrinogen.	[81]
Fu-P	*Fusarium* sp. CPCC480097	Shanghai Health Creation Center of Bio-pharmaceutical R&D	28 kDa pH 8.5 45 °C	Serine protease	Hydrolyse fibrin and fibrinogen	[82]
Fibrinolytic enzyme	*Paecilomyces tenuipes*	Culture Collection of DNA Bank of Mushrooms, Incheon, Republic of Korea.	14 kDa pH 5.0 35 °C	Serine protease	Hydrolyse the Aα chain of human fibrinogen, but do not hydrolyse the Bβ or γ chains	[83]
Fibrinolytic enzyme	*Rhizopus chinensis* 12	Brewing rice wine	18.0 kDa pH 10.5 45 °C	Serine protease. The first 12 amino acids of the N-terminal sequence of the enzyme were S-V-S-E-I-Q-L-M-H-N-L-G and had no homology with that of other fibrinolytic enzyme from other microorganism.	Hydrolyse fibrin and α-, β- and γ-chains of fibrinogen	[84]
Fibrinolytic enzyme	*Sarocladium strictum* 1	*Arhtrobotrys longa* co-culture	35.0 kDa pH 9.0 37 °C	Serine protease	Hydrolyse fibrin and activate plasminogen like urokinase	[85]

Metalloprotease. Metalloproteases are synthesized as inactive zymogens by heterotrophic bacteria [93]. All metalloproteases comprise one or two zinc ions and some enzymes contain one or two manganese or cobalt ions [94]. In the metalloprotease family, 13 members contain the HEXXH sequence providing two of three ligands for zinc atoms. This sequence occurs as a consensus of nine residues bXHEbbHbc (b: uncharged residue, X: any amino acid, and c: hydrophobic residue). The third ligand of the zinc atom is histidine in the case of autolysin, astacin, interstitial collagenase, and glutamic acid in the case of thermolysin, neprilysin, and alanyl aminopeptidase [91]. They can be deactivated by the addition of chelating mediators or dialysis [92].

Fibrinolytic enzymes associated with the metalloprotease family require divalent ions for their actions. They have an optimum pH between 6 and 7. Examples of metalloprotease are Ca^{2+} and Mg^{2+} for AMMP, Zn^{2+} for jeot gal and Co^{2+} Hg^{2+} for *Bacillus* sp. KDO 13 [65], as shown in Table 1.

From Table 1, common antithrombotic enzymes used for the treatment of various cardiovascular diseases are nattokinase, streptokinase, staphylokinase, serrapeptase and longolytin.

3.8. Nattokinase (NK)

A Japanese researcher, Hiroyuki Sumi (Chicago University Medical School) in 1980 invented natto which dissolves artificial fibrin. Sumi and his team members obtained an enzyme from natto that not only degrades fibrin clots but also degrades plasmin substrate. He termed this fibrinolytic enzyme "nattokinase". Natto is a fermented cheese-like food that has been used in Japan over thousands of years. It is made up of soybeans which are cooked and fermented with the action of bacterium *Bacillus subtilis* [129,130]. It degenerates fibrin directly during clot lysis with an action like plasmin and indirectly by affecting plasminogen activator activity (Figure 5A) [130,131].

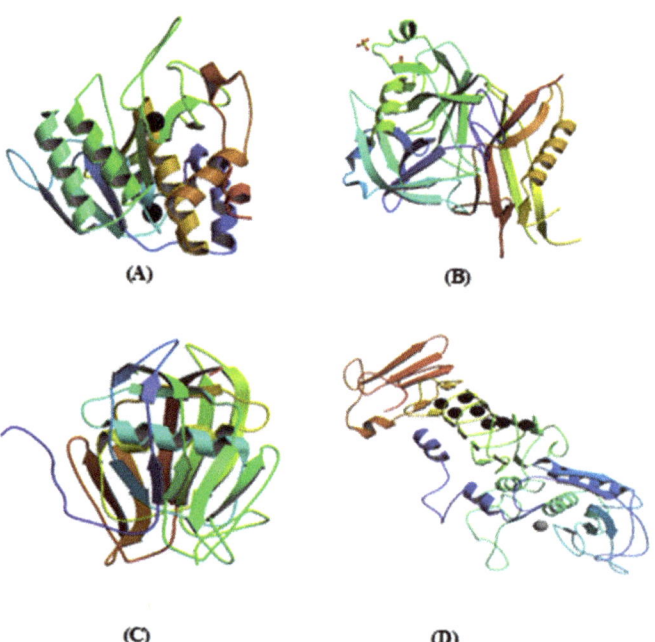

Figure 5. Three-dimensional structures of anti-thrombotics. (**A**) Structure of nattokinase. (**B**) Structure of streptokinase. (**C**) Structure of staphylokinase. (**D**) Structure of serrapeptase.

Nattokinase (NK) is a serine protease with 275 amino acid residues, and its molecular weight is 27.728 Da. It has immense homology with subtilisin, and DNA sequencing displays 99.5% homology with subtilisin E and 99.3% homology with *B. amylosaccharIticus*.

NK's effects are as well-known as aspirin (a well-known blood thinner) where NK improves blood flow with no side effects as compared to aspirin which often triggers gastric ulcers and bleeding. It is resistant to the acidic pH of the stomach (absorbed in the digestive tract), has a high pH (10), and resists high temperatures such as 50 °C [130]. It has various other applications such as a functional food additive, reduces blood viscosity and plasma II concentration, etc. [132].

In human trials, patients undergoing dialysis, patients with cardiovascular diseases, and healthy volunteers were administered orally with two capsules of (2000 FU/capsule) daily. After two months, it was observed that there was a decrease in factors VII and VIII due to which fibrinogen was observed in all three cases, causing no side effects with stable heart rate, uric acid production, and body weight. When dogs were administered orally with four NK capsules (2000 FU/capsule), the major leg vein containing chemically induced blot clot (thrombi) was dissolved completely in 5 h, restoring normal blood flow. Similarly, in the case of a rat's thrombosis in the carotid artery, this was treated with NK, and 62% of arterial blood flow was recovered. NK improves various diseases like atherosclerosis, Alzheimer's disease, hypertension, and stroke and is commercially used in the United States, Korea, Japan, Canada, China, and European Union Countries [129].

C. Yongjun et al. performed an experiment to improve the activity of nattokinase. Three homological genes from *B. natto* AS 1.107, *Bacillus licheniformis* CICC 10092, and *Bacillus amyloliquefaciens* CICC 20164 were intermixed properly to yield a mutant library. After the three cycles of DNA shuffling, one desired mutant of 16 amino acids was attained. For screening, the mutant library for improved activity, the plate-based method was used. The three-dimensional structure was obtained based on parental NK. The hydrophobic pocket present at the active site was broadened due to amino acid substitutions and this may lead to change in catalytic as well as enzymatic activity. The catalytic activity of mutant NK was found to be 2.3 times higher than the wild-type nattokinase [133].

3.9. Streptokinase (SK)

Dr. William Smith Tillet with Sol Sherry (scholar), in 1933, serendipitously laid the basis for the usage of streptokinase (SK) as a thrombolytic mediator in the treatment of acute myocardial infarction [134].

SK is an active plasminogen activator consisting of 414 amino acid residues. It forms a 1:1 stochiometric complex with plasmin (activating plasminogen to plasmin), thus resulting in clot lysis by the proteolytic cleavage of fibrin. It is also included in the World Health Organization's Model List of Essential Medicines and is clinically used an intravenous thrombolytic agent for preventing cardiovascular diseases [118].

Streptokinase N-terminal domain has low activation ability to complement plasminogen (60–414 amino acids) and C-terminal used in plasminogen substrate recognition and stimulation. Initially, 59 amino acid residues appear to have numerous binding domains for plasminogen. The important binding sites that are present in streptokinase are Asp41 and His48 and the coiled region of the Υ-domain plays an important role in plasminogen activation. Its mechanism is fibrin-dependent and independent (Figure 5B) [75,135]. As streptokinase is a non-human protein, its entry into the circulatory system may cause different anaphylactic reactions, including death, depending upon the concentration of anti-streptokinase antibodies existing in the blood circulation.

It is degraded by plasmin at proteolytic sites Lys59 and Lys386 due to which it has a shorter half-life; hence, modifications are performed to enhance its half-life by recombinant DNA technology, chemical or enzymatic alteration of indigenous streptokinase, and by genetic mutation. Recombinant streptokinase produced by yeast *Pichia pastoris* is resistant to proteolytic cleavage by plasmin [75].

3.10. Staphylokinase (SAK)

Staphylokinase is produced by lysogenic strains of *Staphylococcus aureus*, a subsidiary activator of plasminogen, and is a part of third-generation fibrinolytic enzymes [59,136]. It forms a 1:1 stochiometric complex with human plasmin catalysing further stimulation of plasminogen. This complex is sensitive to accelerated inhibition by α2-antiplasmin unless it is bound to fibrin by lysine-binding sites [137].

It is a 15.5 kDa protein consisting of 136 amino acids (single chain without disulfide linkage). Its 3D crystal structure involves five stand beta-sheets, a central alpha-helix (Lys-57-Thr-71) connected together by loops (Figure 5C) [55,138]. The main interaction between staphylokinase and plasminogen or staphylokinase and other staphylokinases (during the dimerization process) occurs at the region possessing alpha helix. The mutation in the active region (central alpha helix) results in a complete loss of activity of plasminogen. The N-terminal part (Lys 10) is responsible for proteolytic hydrolysis and protein interaction, whereas the C-terminal part (Lys-135-Lys-136) and its sterically positioned flexible loop (Lys-54) is responsible for dimerization and determinant of staphylokinase–plasminogen interaction [59].

Another role of SAK is its ability to nullify the activity of host antimicrobial peptides constituting various peptides secreted by mammals and other organisms. Hence, it plays its role against invading pathogens through a defence mechanism. SAK is able to bind with α2- antiplasmin that are secreted by human neutrophil proteins (HNPs) forming the SAK-HNP complex. This complex results in the mutual inhibition of protein bactericidal activities and thrombolytic activities [139].

3.11. Serrapeptase (SRP)

Serrapeptase is a proteolytic enzyme (metalloprotease with three zinc atoms and one active site) with molecular weight ranges from 45 to 60 kDa catalysing hydrolysis of peptide bonds in peptides. It is also known as serratiopeptidase, or serratia peptidase (SRP), due to its origin in *Serratia marcescens*. It has an affinity towards dead threads of proteins present in silkworms and dissolves them to make cocoons; it also dissolves non-living tissues present in mammals including plaques, mucous, and blood clots. It also degrades various protease inhibitors of the immune system and is the main reason for infection in mammalian epithelial cells [95].

It consists of 470 amino acids lacking sulphur-containing amino acids such as methionine and cysteine (Figure 5D) [90,140]. The activity of the serrapeptase enzyme is enhanced by zinc atoms [90]. It contains a zinc-binding consensus (HEXXHXXGXXH) where three histidine residues are zinc ligands, and the catalytic base is glutamic acid [140,141]. This enzyme belongs to the Serralysin group of enzymes which cleaves peptide bond linkage between Asn-Gln, Tyr-Tyr, Arg-Gly, CysSO$_3$H-Gly, Tyr-Tyr, His-Leu, Gly-Ala, Try-Thr, Gly-Gly, Phe-Tyr Ala-Leu, and Tyr-Leu; hence, it has broad substrate specificity [142].

Expression of SRP is available in the form of enteric-coated tablets (dry-coated with enteric polymer) as it undergoes gastric hydrolysis at a low pH decreasing the stability in the gastrointestinal tract. Hence, to maintain the stability of SRP, the recommended doses are 5–10 mg tablets three times a day. Orally given serratiopeptidase alters the viscoelasticity of sputum in patients (chronic airway disease), it also has various other side effects such as GI disturbance, nausea, and anorexia. Topical application of the SRP enzyme in the form of ointments and gels at the site of action increases the potential activity of the enzyme in the treatment of local inflammatory reactions. Non-steroidal anti-inflammatory drugs (NSAIDs), such as diclofenac sodium, ketoprofen, etc., which are used to treat chronic and acute arthritic conditions cause gastric irritation (causing ulcers) and other side effects. Hence, anti-inflammatory properties of SRP could be used as a suitable alternative to NSAIDs. It also enhances the efficiency of some antibiotics such as ampicillin, cefotiam, ciclacillin, cephalexin, and minocycline. A team of Italian researchers suggested that SRP enhances the effectiveness against microbial biofilms and inhibits its formation [143].

3.12. Longolytin

Longolytin is the preparation of extracellular proteolytic enzymes obtained from the culture fluid of the strain *Arthrobortys longa* Mecht. No. 1. The drug has fibrinolytic, thrombolytic, esterase, small proteolytic, and plasminogen activator activities. When separating longolitin, six protein fractions were identified, among which only one was fibrinolytically active. The enzyme had a pI of 3.7 and a molecular weight of 28.6 kDa. The optimal activity was at pH 6.0–9.0 and a temperature of 37 °C. Based on the action of inhibitors, the enzyme was tentatively assigned to serine-type proteinases containing thiol groups. The effectiveness of longolytin has been proven in in vitro and in vivo experiments. A pronounced affinity of the drug for fibrin was shown, and its intravenous administration to animals increased the fibrinolytic and activator properties of plasma and proved its local effect on the structure of blood clots. An increase in the amount of plasmin in the blood of animals that received high doses of the drug showed the ability of the drug to activate plasminogen. Longolytin was first proposed as a thrombolytic drug for the treatment of thrombophlebitis and phlebothrombosis, due to its ability to penetrate the epidermis and underlying soft tissues into the microcirculation system and systemic circulation and cause adequate physiological and biochemical reactions.

A model of venous thrombosis on the rabbit marginal ear vein was developed by Podorol'skaya et al., 2007 [127]. The thrombolytic activity of longolytin applied externally onto the thrombotic venous segment was evaluated. When applied externally, longolytin (both individually and in combination with heparin) causes a significant acceleration of thrombolysis, acting locally on the thrombus structure, and does not affect haemostasis. Heparin significantly accelerated the process of dissolution of blood clots only when it was used together with longolytin. Thus, longolytin reduced the time of thrombus dissolution by 2 times and increased the rate of thrombolysis by 4.5 times. The combined use of longolytin and heparin increased jugular vein thrombolysis by 30 times compared with the control group. Biochemical indicators of haemostasis (fibrinogen content, fibrinolytic activity, recalcification time) remained unchanged during thrombolysis both in the experiment and in the control, which indicates the specificity and selectivity of longolytin. The introduction of longolytin into the stomach cavity and into the oral cavity of rats also demonstrated the effect of a significant increase in the fibrinolytic and anticoagulant activity of the blood of animals. Sharkova and Podorolskaya, 2017 [128] have used longolytin by per os administration in rats to reveal the influence on haemostasis and fibrinolysis. In their experiments, 120 white rats were introduced to a 0.1 mL 3% solution of longolytin in glycerol (activity 30–40 C.U.) orally every day for 7 days and observed an increase in anticoagulant and fibrinolytic activities in experimental rats. The resulting effects turned out to be prolonged, remaining for another week after the drug was discontinued and creating a favourable antithrombotic background in the animal body, in contrast to the inhibition of fibrinolysis characteristic of intravenous administration at the end of the course of use. So, longolytin can be used orally for both therapeutic and prophylactic purposes [144].

3.13. Clinical Significance of Fibrinolytic Enzymes

Fibrinolytic enzymes are clinically administered for the treatment of myocardial infarctions, strokes, cardiac and respiratory failure. Therefore, in this section, we intend to discuss some of the clinical trials of fibrinolytic enzymes stating their significance and importance.

The efficacy of a single dose of nattokinase (2000 FU) was evaluated in a double-blind, placebo-controlled cross-over nattokinase intervention human trial. The results showed that after the administration of nattokinase, D-dimer concentrations at 6 and 8 h and fibrin/fibrinogen degradation at 4 h elevated significantly with respective p-values of < 0.05. Also, antithrombin concentration in the blood was also higher at 2 and 4 h, and thus the outcomes suggest that fibrinolysis and anti-coagulation are enhanced using nattokinase via numerous pathways [145]. In addition, treatment with streptokinase in a controlled clinical trial revealed that angiographic evidence of thrombolysis was significantly greater ($p < 0.01$) in patients treated with streptokinase when compared to heparin. However, aftereffects such as bleeding were more common with streptokinase than with heparin but was not a critical concern [146]. Another clinical trial by Gusev EI et al. performed a multicentre, open-label, randomized, parallel-group, and non-inferiority trial and studied the effect of non-immunogenic recombinant staphylokinase versus alteplase for patients with acute ischaemic stroke 4–5 h after symptom onset. The difference in the rate of favourable response at day 90 was 9.5% (95% CI −1.7 to 20.7) and the lower limit did not cross the margin of non-inferiority (p non-inferiority <0.0001). After-effects such as symptomatic intracranial haemorrhage affected 8% and 3% of patients ($p = 0.087$) in the non-immunogenic staphylokinase group and alteplase group, respectively. Also, on the follow-up day 90, 14% and 10% of patients ($p = 0.32$) died in the non-immunogenic staphylokinase group and alteplase group, respectively [147]. These brief data from clinical trials indicate that fibrinolytic enzymes might serve as an efficient alternative to synthetic antithrombotic agents. However, treatments with these drugs are associated with an increased risk of complications such as haemorrhage, and therefore, the search for safer and more efficient methods is evident.

3.14. Other Potential Applications of Fibrinolytic Enzymes

Fibrinolytic enzymes along with blood clot dissolution, exhibit numerous other potential applications in food, industrial, and clinical sectors. They have been reported as aiding in blood pressure regulation and proteolysis in addition to fibrin. Fibrinolytic enzymes have also found their applicability as antimicrobials, detergent additives, anti-inflammatory agents, etc. [2]. A randomized clinical trial reported the positive effects of nattokinase on blood pressure/hypertension and confirmed that nattokinase results in a reduction in systolic and diastolic blood pressure [148]. Another study detailed that oral administration of nattokinase and serrapeptase is effective against Alzheimer's disease [149]. Serrapeptase exhibits significant anti-inflammatory and other essential applications along with anti-thrombotic activity [6,66,150,151]. In addition, serrapeptase has shown a potent effect with respect to venous inflammatory diseases and chronic airway diseases such as decreased neutrophil count, sputum output and viscosity, and chronic sinusitis [152–155]. Scientific studies also provide insight into the significant role of fibrinolytic enzymes in food fortification and nutraceutical applications [156,157]. Fibrinolytic protease from *Lactobacillus plantarum* KSK-II was found to inhibit the growth of *S. aureus* (29%), *B. cereus* (21%), *P. aeruginosa* (13%), *P. vulgaris* (10%), and *E. coli* (7%) and thus exhibit anti-microbial activity [6].

Fibrinolytic enzymes also aid in proteolysis in addition to fibrin and are considered as an apt detergent additive. The enzyme from *L. plantarum* was found to hydrolyse plasma proteins along with collagen and fibrin and was also compatible/stable with the detergent formulations of Persil (112%), X-tra® (98%), Ariel® (92%), Tide® (86%), Lang® (81%), Dac® (80%), Isis® (77%), Bonux® (75%), Dixan® (67%), and Oxi® (64%) [6]. A detergent-resistant nattokinase from *B. subtilis* showed an increase of 141% with non-ionic detergents (Tween-20, Tween-80, and Triton X-100) [158]. Furthermore, an enzyme from *Bacillus* sp. IND12 bovine serum albumin, chicken skin, hydrolysed egg white, and goat blood clots was recommended for use in both wastewater treatment and clinical practices [159].

4. Conclusions

In the present review, we have discussed in detail the mechanism of blood clotting, different microbial sources used as anti-thrombotic agents, and their mechanism of action. We have summarized the mechanism of blood clot formation, and clot lysis (fibrinolysis) with the help of plasminogen activators or plasmin-like molecules involving fibrinolytic enzymes. Different methods are proposed to observe fibrinolytic action in blood and its elements. Fibrinolytic activities can be linked with the patient's cardiovascular disease status which can be taken care of well in advance to avoid serious cardiac arrest. Fibrinolytic enzymes have the capability to dissolve blood clots. These enzymes obtained from microorganisms cleave fibrin fibres and clot peptide bonds of chains ($\alpha\alpha$-, $\beta\beta$-, Υ-) forming fibrin degradative products, dissolving the blood clots present in blood vessels for normal blood flow. Several types of reported/ commercially available fibrinolytic enzymes have also been described along with their clinical trials and applications. Human trials suggest microbial fibrinolytic enzymes as efficient substitutes to other antithrombotic agents, but after-effects such as hemorrhage leave an urgent urge to search for more safer and potent therapies. Lastly, other potential applications of fibrinolytic enzymes such as detergent additives, blood pressure regulators, anti-microbial/anti-inflammatory agents, etc., pave the way for their diverse use. However, the mechanisms behind the above-mentioned uses are uncertain so far.

Author Contributions: Writing—original draft preparation, P.G., C.S. and R.S.; writing—review and editing, R.S. and A.O.; supervision, R.S., and A.O. All authors have read and agreed to the published version of the manuscript.

Funding: This research received no external funding.

Institutional Review Board Statement: Not Applicable.

Informed Consent Statement: Not Applicable.

Data Availability Statement: Not Applicable.

Conflicts of Interest: The authors declare no conflict of interest.

References

1. MFMER: Rochester, MN, USA. Available online: https://www.mayoclinic.org/diseases-conditions/heart-disease/symptoms-causes/syc-20353118 (accessed on 15 September 2023).
2. Sharma, C.; Osmolovskiy, A.; Singh, R. Microbial Fibrinolytic Enzymes as Anti-Thrombotics: Production, Characterisation and Prodigious Biopharmaceutical Applications. *Pharmaceutics* **2021**, *13*, 1880. [CrossRef] [PubMed]
3. Geddings, J.E.; Mackamn, N. Recently identified factors that regulate hemostatsis and thrombosis. *Thromb. Haemost.* **2014**, *111*, 570–574. [CrossRef] [PubMed]
4. Available online: https://www.merriam-webster.com/dictionary/thromboembolism (accessed on 15 September 2023).
5. Longstaff, C. Measuring fibrinolysis: From research to routine diagnostic assays. *J. Thromb. Haemost.* **2018**, *16*, 652–662. [CrossRef] [PubMed]
6. Kotb, E. The Biotechnological Potential of Fibrinolytic Enzymes in the Dissolution of Endogenous Blood Thrombi. *Biotechnol. Prog.* **2014**, *30*, 656–672. [CrossRef]
7. Marsh, N.A.; Gaffney, P.J. A rapid fibrin plate: A method for plasminogen activator assay. *Thromb. Haemost.* **1977**, *38*, 545–551. [CrossRef]
8. Hmidet, N.; Nawani, N.; Ghorbel, S. Recent Development in Production and Biotechnological Application of Microbial Enzymes. *Biomed. Res. Int.* **2014**, *2015*, 2. [CrossRef]
9. Liang, X.; Jia, S.; Sun, Y.; Chen, M.; Chen, X.; Zhong, J.; Huan, L. Secretory Expression of Nattokinase from *Bacillus subtilis* YF38 in *Escherichia coli*. *Mol. Biotechnol.* **2007**, *37*, 187–194. [CrossRef]
10. Dimmeler, S. Cardiovascular diseases review series. *EMBO Mol. Med.* **2011**, *3*, 697. [CrossRef]
11. Lijfering, W.; Flinterman, L.; Vandenbroucke, J.; Rosendaal, F.; Cannegieter, S. Relationship between Venous and Arterial Thrombosis: A Review of the Literature from a Causal Perspective. *Semin. Thromb. Hemost.* **2011**, *37*, 885–896. [CrossRef]
12. Lijnen, H.R.; Collen, D. Impaired fibrinolysis and the risk for coronary heart disease. *Circulation* **1996**, *94*, 2052–2054. [CrossRef]
13. Unar, A.; Bertolino, L.; Patauner, F.; Gallo, R.; Durante-Mangoni, E. Pathophysiology of Disseminated Intravascular Coagulation in Sepsis: A Clinically Focused Overview. *Cells* **2023**, *12*, 2120. [CrossRef]
14. Unar, A.; Bertolino, L.; Patauner, F.; Gallo, R.; Durante-Mangoni, E. Decoding Sepsis-Induced Disseminated Intravascular Coagulation: A Comprehensive Review of Existing and Emerging Therapies. *J. Clin. Med.* **2023**, *12*, 6128. [CrossRef] [PubMed]
15. Thomas, W.; Meade, D.M. Thrombosis and cardiovascular disease. *Med. Clin. N. Am.* **1992**, *82*, 511–525.
16. Nabel, E.G. Cardiovascular disease. *N. Engl. J. Med.* **2003**, *349*, 60–72. [CrossRef]
17. Bagot, C.N.; Arya, R. Virchow and his triad: A question of attribution. *Br. J. Haematol.* **2008**, *143*, 180–190. [CrossRef] [PubMed]
18. Del Principe, M.I.; Del Principe, D.; Venditti, A. Thrombosis in adult patients with acute leukemia. *Curr. Opin. Oncol.* **2017**, *29*, 448–454. [CrossRef] [PubMed]
19. Chu, Y.; Guo, H.; Zhang, Y.; Qiao, R. Procoagulant platelets: Generation, characteristics, and therapeutic target. *J. Clin. Lab. Anal.* **2021**, *35*, e23750. [CrossRef] [PubMed]

20. Sharma, C.; Salem, G.E.M.; Sharma, N.; Gautam, P.; Singh, R. Thrombolytic Potential of Novel Thiol-Dependent Fibrinolytic Protease from *Bacillus cereus* RSA1. *Biomolecules* **2020**, *10*, 3. [CrossRef]
21. Watson, L.; Broderick, C.; Armon, M.P. Thrombolysis for acute deep vein thrombosis. *Cochrane Database Syst. Rev.* **2016**, *11*, CD002783. [CrossRef]
22. Nagareddy, P.; Smyth, S.S. Inflammation and thrombosis in cardiovascular disease. *Curr. Opin. Hematol.* **2013**, *20*, 457–463. [CrossRef]
23. Chapin, J.C.; Hajjar, K.A. Fibrinolysis and the control of blood coagulation. *Blood Rev.* **2015**, *29*, 17–24. [CrossRef]
24. La Corte, A.L.C.; Philippou, H.; Ariens, R.A.S. Role of fibrin structure in thrombosis and vascular disease. *Adv. Protein Chem. Struct. Biol.* **2011**, *83*, 75–127.
25. Lord, S.T. Fibrinogen and fibrin: Scaffold proteins in haemostasis. *Curr. Opin. Hematol.* **2007**, *14*, 236–241. [CrossRef]
26. Schuligaa, M.; Graingeb, C.; Westall, G.; Knigh, D. The fibrogenic actions of the coagulant and plasminogen activation systems in pulmonary fibrosis. *Int. J. Biochem. Cell Biol.* **2018**, *97*, 108–117. [CrossRef]
27. Wolberg, A.S. Thrombin generation and fibrin clot structure. *Blood Rev.* **2007**, *21*, 131–142. [CrossRef] [PubMed]
28. Cooper, A.V.; Standeven, K.F.; Arie, R.A.S. Fibrinogen gamma-chain splice variant alters fibrin formation and structure. *Blood* **2003**, *102*, 535–540. [CrossRef] [PubMed]
29. Bagoly, Z.; Koncz, Z.; Hársfalvi, J.; Muszbek, L. Factor XIII, clot structure, thrombosis. *Thromb. Res.* **2011**, *129*, 382–387. [CrossRef] [PubMed]
30. Ariens, R.A.S. Fibrin (ogen) and Thrombotic disease. *J. Thromb. Haemost.* **2013**, *11*, 294–305. [CrossRef]
31. Aleman, M.M.; Walton, B.L.; Byrnes, J.R.; Wolberg, A.S. Fibrinogen and red blood cells in venous thrombosis. *Thromb. Res.* **2014**, *133*, S38–S40. [CrossRef] [PubMed]
32. Chernysh, I.N.; Nagaswami, C.; Weisel, J.W. Visualization and identification of the structures formed during early stages of fibrin polymerization. *Blood* **2016**, *117*, 4609–4614. [CrossRef]
33. Blombäck, B.; Carlsson, K.; Fatah, K.; Hessel, B.; Procyk, R. Fibrin in human plasma: Gel architectures governed by rate and nature of fibrinogen activation. *Thromb. Res.* **1994**, *75*, 521–538. [CrossRef]
34. Bridge, K.I.; Philippou, H.; Ariëns, R.A.S. Clot properties and cardiovascular disease. *Thromb. Haemost.* **2014**, *112*, 901–908. [CrossRef] [PubMed]
35. Collet, J.P.; Lesty, C.; Montalescot, G.; Weisel, J.W. Dynamic Changes of Fibrin Architecture during Fibrin Formation and Intrinsic Fibrinolysis of Fibrin-rich Clots. *J. Biol. Chem.* **2013**, *278*, 21331–21335. [CrossRef] [PubMed]
36. Lam, W.A.; Chaudhuri, O.; Crow, A.; Webster, K.D.; Li, T.-D.; Kita, A.; Huang, J.; Fletcher, D.A. Mechanics and contraction dynamics of single platelets and implications for clot stiffening. *Nat. Mater.* **2011**, *10*, 61–66. [CrossRef] [PubMed]
37. Ryan, E.A.; Mockros, L.F.; Weisel, J.W.; Lorand, L. Structural Origins of Fibrin Clot Rheology. *Biophys. J.* **1999**, *77*, 2813–2826. [CrossRef]
38. Hethershaw, E.L.; La Corte, A.C.; Duval, C.; Ali, M.; Grant, P.J.; Ariëns, R.A.; Philippou, H. The effect of blood coagulation factor XIII on fibrin clot structure and fibrinolysis. *J. Thromb. Haemost.* **2014**, *12*, 197–205. [CrossRef]
39. Longstaff, C.; Varjú, I.; Sótonyi, P.; Szabó, L.; Krumrey, M.; Hoell, A.; Bóta, A.; Varga, Z.; Komorowicz, E.; Kolev, K. Mechanical Stability and Fibrinolytic Resistance of Clots Containing Fibrin, DNA, and Histones. *J. Biol. Chem.* **2013**, *288*, 6946–6956. [CrossRef]
40. Longstaff, C.; Kolev, K. Basic mechanisms and regulation of fibrinolysis. *J. Thromb. Haemost.* **2015**, *13*, S98–S105. [CrossRef]
41. Sharma, C.; Nigam, A.; Singh, R. Computational-approach understanding the structure-function prophecy of Fibrinolytic Protease RFEA1 from *Bacillus cereus* RSA1. *PeerJ* **2021**, *9*, e11570. [CrossRef]
42. Rijken, D.J.; Lijnen, H.R. New insights into the molecular mechanisms of the fibrinolytic system. *J. Thromb. Haemost.* **2009**, *7*, 4–13. [CrossRef]
43. Gabriel, D.A.; Muga, K.; Boothroyd, E.M. The Effect of Fibrin Structure on Fibrinolysis. *J. Biol. Chem.* **1992**, *267*, 24259–24263. [CrossRef] [PubMed]
44. Hoylaerts, M.; Rijken, D.C.; Lijnen, H.R.; Collen, D. Kinetics of the Activation of Plasminogen by Human Tissue Plasminogen Activator. Role of Fibrin. *J. Biol. Chem.* **1982**, *257*, 2912–2919. [CrossRef] [PubMed]
45. Tsai, S.J. Role of tissue-type plasminogen activator and plasminogen activator inhibitor-1 in psychological stress and depression. *Oncotarget* **2017**, *8*, 113258–113268. [CrossRef] [PubMed]
46. Rijken, D.C.; Hoylaerts, M.; Collen, D. Fibrinolytic Properties of One-chain and Two-chain Human Extrinsic (Tissue-type) Plasminogen Activator. *J. Biol. Chem.* **1982**, *257*, 2920–2925. [CrossRef] [PubMed]
47. Longstaff, C.; Thelwell, C.; Williams, S.C.; Silva, M.M.; Szabó, L.; Kolev, K. The interaction between tissue plasminogen activator domains and fibrin structure studies in the regulation of fibrinolysis: Kinetic and microscopic structure. *Blood* **2010**, *117*, 661–668. [CrossRef] [PubMed]
48. Harris, R.J.; Leonard, C.K.; Guzzetta, A.W.; Spellman, M.W. Tissue plasminogen activator has an O-linked fucose attached to threonine-61 in the epidermal growth factor domain. *Biochem. J.* **1991**, *30*, 2311–2314. [CrossRef]
49. Cesarman-Maus, G.; Hajjar, K.A. Molecular mechanisms of fibrinolysis. *Br. J. Haematol.* **2005**, *129*, 307–321. [CrossRef] [PubMed]
50. Munk, G.A.W.; Groeneveld, E.; Rijken, D.C. Acceleration of the Thrombin Inactivation of Single Chain Urokinase-type Plasminogen Activator (Pro-urokinase) by Thrombomodulin. *J. Clin. Investig.* **1991**, *88*, 1680–1684. [CrossRef]
51. Liu, J.N.; Gurewich, V. The kinetics of plasminogen activation by thrombin-cleaved pro-urokinase and promotion of its activity by fibrin fragment E-2 and by tissue plasminogen activator. *Blood* **1993**, *81*, 980–987. [CrossRef]

52. Ploug, M.; Ellis, V. Structure-function relationships in the receptor for urokinase-type plasminogen activator. Comparison to other members of the Ly-6 family and snake venom a-neurotoxins. *FEBS Lett.* **1994**, *349*, 163–168. [CrossRef]
53. Bohuslav, J.; Horejsí, V.; Hansmann, C.; Stöckl, J.; Weidle, U.H.; Majdic, O.; Bartke, I.; Knapp, W.; Stockinger, H. Urokinase Plasminogen Activator Receptor, 2-Integrins, and Src-kinases within a Single Receptor Complex of Human Monocytes. *J. Exp. Med.* **1995**, *181*, 1381–1390. [CrossRef]
54. Gurewich, V.; Pannell, R.; Louie, S.; Kelley, P.; Suddith, R.L.; Greenlee, R. Effective and Fibrin-specific Clot Lysis by a Zymogen Precursor Form of Urokinase (Pro-urokinase) A Study In Vitro and in Two Animal Species. *J. Clin. Investig.* **1984**, *73*, 1731–1739. [CrossRef]
55. Lijnen, H.R.; Zamarron, C.; Blaber, M.; Winkler, M.E.; Collen, D. Activation of Plasminogen by Pro-urokinase. *J. Biol. Chem.* **1985**, *261*, 1253–1258. [CrossRef]
56. Schneider, M.; Brufatto, N.; Neill, E.; Nesheim, M. Activated Thrombin-activatable Fibrinolysis Inhibitor Reduces the Ability of High Molecular Weight Fibrin Degradation Products to Protect Plasmin from Antiplasmin. *J. Biol. Chem.* **2004**, *279*, 13340–13345. [CrossRef] [PubMed]
57. Hoover-Plow, J. Does plasmin have anticoagulant activity? *Vasc. Health Risk Manag.* **2010**, *6*, 199–205. [CrossRef] [PubMed]
58. Hur, W.S.; Mazinani, N.; Lu, X.J.D.; Britton, H.M.; Byrnes, J.R.; Wolberg, A.S.; Kastrup, C.J. Coagulation factor XIIIa is inactivated by plasmin. *Blood* **2015**, *126*, 2329–2337. [CrossRef] [PubMed]
59. Bokarewa, M.I.; Jin, T.; Tarkowski, A. *Staphylococcus aureus*: Staphylokinase. *Int. J. Biochem. Cell Biol.* **2005**, *38*, 504–509. [CrossRef]
60. Nar, H.; Bauer, M.; Stassen, J.-M.; Lang, D.; Gils, A.; Declerck, P.J. Plasminogen Activator Inhibitor 1. Structure of the Native Serpin, Comparison to its Other Conformers and Implications for Serpin Inactivation. *J. Mol. Biol.* **2000**, *297*, 683–695. [CrossRef]
61. Pant, A.; Kopec, A.K.; Baker, K.S.; Cline-Fedewa, H.; Lawrence, D.A.; Luyendyk, J.P. Plasminogen Activator Inhibitor-1 Reduces tPA-Dependent Fibrinolysis and Intrahepatic Hemorrhage in Experimental Acetaminophen Overdose. *Am. J. Pathol.* **2018**, *188*, 1204–1212. [CrossRef]
62. Masson, C.; Angles-Cano, E. Kinetic analysis of the interaction between plasminogen activator inhibitor-1 and tissue-type plasminogen activator. *Biochem. J.* **1988**, *256*, 237–244. [CrossRef]
63. Zakrzewski, M.; Zakrzewska, E.; Kiciński, P.; Przybylska-Kuć, S.; Dybała, A.; Myśliński, W.; Pastryk, J.; Tomaszewski, T.; Mosiewicz, J. Evaluation of Fibrinolytic Inhibitors: Alpha-2 Antiplasmin and Plasminogen Activator Inhibitor 1 in Patients with Obstructive Sleep Apnoea. *PLoS ONE* **2016**, *11*, e0166725. [CrossRef] [PubMed]
64. Carpenter, S.L.; Mathew, P. α2-Antiplasmin and its deficiency: Fibrinolysis out of balance. *Haemophilia* **2008**, *16*, 1250–1254. [CrossRef]
65. Ilich, A.; Bokarev, I.; Key, N.S. Global assays of fibrinolysis. *Int. J. Lab. Hematol.* **2017**, *39*, 441–447. [CrossRef] [PubMed]
66. Kotb, E. Activity assessment of microbial fibrinolytic enzymes. *Appl. Microbiol. Biotechnol.* **2013**, *97*, 6647–6665. [CrossRef] [PubMed]
67. Fossum, S.; Hoem, N.O. Urokinase and non-urokinase fibrinolytic activity in protease-inhibitor-deprived plasma, assayed by a fibrin micro-plate method. *Immunopharmacology* **1996**, *32*, 119–121. [CrossRef]
68. Boudjeltia, K.Z.; Cauchie, P.; Remacle, C.; Guillaume, M.; Brohée, D.; Hubert, J.L.; Vanhaeverbeek, M. A new device for measurement of fibrin clot lysis: Application to the Euglobulin Clot Lysis Time. *BMC Biotechnol.* **2002**, *2*, 8. [CrossRef] [PubMed]
69. Ilich, A.; Kumar, V.; Ferrara, M.J.; Henderson, M.W.; Noubouossie, D.F.; Jenkins, D.H.; Kozar, R.A.; Park, M.S.; Key, N.S. Euglobulin clot lysis time reveals a high frequency of fibrinolytic activation in trauma. *Thromb. Res.* **2021**, *204*, 22–28. [CrossRef]
70. Smith, A.A.; Jacobson, L.J.; Miller, B.I.; Hathaway, W.E.; Manco-Johnson, M.J. A new euglobulin clot lysis assay for global fibrinolysis. *Thromb. Res.* **2004**, *112*, 329–337. [CrossRef]
71. Schöchl, H.; Nienaber, U.; Hofer, G.; Voelckel, W.; Jambor, C.; Scharbert, G.; Kozek-Langenecker, S.; Solomon, C. Goal-directed coagulation management of major trauma patients using thromboestatometry (ROTEM)-guided administration of fibrinogen concentration and prothrombin complex concentrate. *Crit. Care* **2010**, *14*, R55. [CrossRef]
72. Mou, Q.; Zhou, Q.; Liu, S. Blood clot parameters: Prejudgment of fibrinolysis in thromboelastography. *Clin. Chim. Acta* **2018**, *479*, 94–97. [CrossRef]
73. Hett, D.A.; Walker, D.; Pilkington, S.N.; Smith, D.C. Sonoclot analysis. *Br. J. Anaesth.* **1995**, *75*, 771–776. [CrossRef]
74. Singh, R.; Kumar, M.; Mittal, A.; Mehta, P.K. Microbial enzymes: Industrial progress in 21st century. *3 Biotech* **2016**, *6*, 174. [CrossRef]
75. Banerjee, A.; Chisti, Y.; Banerjee, U.C. Streptokinase—A clinically useful thrombolytic agent. *Biotechnol. Adv.* **2003**, *22*, 287–307. [CrossRef] [PubMed]
76. Collen, D.; Lijnen, H.R.; Vanderschueren, S. Staphylokinase: Fibrinolytic properties and current experience in patients with occlusive arterial thrombosis. *Verh.-K. Acad. Voor Geneeskd. Van Belg.* **1995**, *57*, 183–196.
77. Choi, N.S.; Chang, K.T.; Jae Maeng, P.; Kim, S.H. Cloning, expression and fibrin(ogen)olytic properties of a Subtilisn DJ-4 Gene from *Bacillus* sp. DJ 4. *FEMS Microbiol. Lett.* **2004**, *236*, 325–331. [CrossRef]
78. Sharkova, T.S.; Kornienko, E.I.; Osmolovskii, A.A.; Kreier, V.G.; Baranova, N.A.; Egorov, N.S. Morphological and physiological properties of the micromycete *Arthrobotrys longa*, a producer of longolytin, a proteolytic complex with a thrombolytic effect. *Microbiology* **2016**, *85*, 180–184. [CrossRef]
79. Shirasaka, N.; Naitou, M.; Okamura, K.; Kusuda, M.; Fukuta, Y.; Terashita, T. Purification and characterization of a fibrinolytic protease from *Aspergillus oryzae* KSK-3. *Mycoscience* **2012**, *53*, 354–364. [CrossRef]

80. Osmolovskiy, A.A.; Rukavitsyna, E.D.; Kreier, V.G.; Baranova, N.A.; Egorov, N.S. Production of proteinases with fibrinolytic and fibrinogenolytic activity by a micromycete *Aspergillus ochraceus*. *Microbiology* **2017**, *86*, 512–516. [CrossRef]
81. Zhao, L.; Lin, X.; Fu, J.; Zhang, J.; Tang, W.; He, Z. A Novel Bi-Functional Fibrinolytic Enzyme with Anticoagulant and Thrombolytic Activities from a Marine-Derived Fungus *Aspergillus versicolor* ZLH-1. *Mar. Drugs* **2022**, *20*, 356. [CrossRef]
82. Wu, B.; Wu, L.; Chen, D.; Yang, Z.; Luo, M. Purification and characterization of a novel fibrinolytic protease from *Fusarium* sp. CPCC 480097. *J. Ind. Microbiol. Biotechnol.* **2009**, *36*, 451–459. [CrossRef]
83. Baggio, L.M.; Panagio, L.A.; Gasparin, F.G.M.; Sartori, D.; Celligoi, M.A.P.C.; Baldo, C. Production of fibrinogenolytic and fibrinolytic enzymes by a strain of *Penicillium* sp. Isolated from contaminated soil with industrial effluent. *Acta Scientiarum. Health Sci.* **2019**, *41*, e40606. [CrossRef]
84. Liu, X.-L.; Du, L.-X.; Lu, F.-P.; Zheng, X.Q.; Xiao, J. Purification and characterization of a novel fibrinolytic enzyme from *Rhizopus chinensis* 12. *Appl. Microbiol. Biotechnol.* **2005**, *67*, 209–214.
85. Kornienko, E.I.; Osmolovskiy, A.A.; Kreyer, V.G.; Baranova, N.A.; Kotova, I.B.; Egorov, N.S. Characteristics and Properties of the Complex of Proteolytic Enzymes of the Thrombolytic Action of the Micromycete *Sarocladium strictum*. *Appl. Biochem. Microbiol.* **2021**, *57*, 57–64. [CrossRef]
86. Liu, X.; Kopparapu, N.K.; Li, Y.; Deng, Y.; Zheng, X. Biochemical characterization of a novel fibrinolytic enzyme from *Cordeceps militaris*. *Int. J. Biol. Macromol.* **2016**, *94*, 793–801. [CrossRef] [PubMed]
87. Lee, S.Y.; Kim, J.S.; Kim, J.E.; Sapkota, K.; Shen, M.H.; Kim, S.; Chun, H.S.; Yoo, J.C.; Choi, H.S.; Kim, M.K.; et al. Purification and characterisation of fibrinolytic enzyme from cultured mycelia of *Armillaria mella*. *Protein Expr. Purif.* **2005**, *43*, 10–17. [CrossRef] [PubMed]
88. Mótyán, J.A.; Tóth, F.; Tőzsér, J. Research application in proteolytic enzymes in molecular microbiology. *Biomolecules* **2013**, *3*, 923–942. [CrossRef]
89. Ryan, B.J.; Henehan, G.T. Overview of Approaches to Preventing and Avoiding Proteolysis During Expression and Purification of Proteins. *Curr. Protoc. Protein Sci.* **2013**, *71*, 5–25. [CrossRef]
90. Hedstrom, L. Serine Protease mechanism and specificity. *Chem. Rev.* **2002**, *102*, 4501–4523. [CrossRef]
91. Rawlings, N.D.; Barrett, A.J. Evolutionary families of peptidases. *Biochem. J.* **1993**, *290*, 205–218. [CrossRef]
92. Rao, M.B.; Tanksale, A.M.; Ghatge, M.S.; Deshpande, V.V. Molecular and Biotechnological Aspects of Microbial Proteases. *Microbiol. Mol. Biol. Rev.* **1998**, *62*, 597–635. [CrossRef]
93. Wu, J.W.; Chen, X.L. Extracellular metalloprotease from bacteria. *Appl. Microbiol. Biotechnol.* **2011**, *92*, 253–262. [CrossRef]
94. Fukasawa, K.M.; Hata, T.; Ono, Y.; Hirose, J. Metal Preferences of Zinc-Binding Motif on Metalloproteases. *J. Amino Acids* **2011**, *2011*, 574816. [CrossRef]
95. Ethiraj, S.; Gopinat, S. Production, purification, characterization, immobilization, and application of Serrapeptase: A review. *Front. Biol.* **2017**, *12*, 333–348. [CrossRef]
96. Wu, S.; Feng, C.; Zhong, J.; Huan, L. Roles of S3 Site Residues of Nattokinase on Its Activity and Substrate Specificity. *Biochem. J.* **2007**, *142*, 357–364. [CrossRef] [PubMed]
97. Chandrasekaran, S.D.; Vaithilingam, M.; Shanker, R.; Kumar, S.; Thiyur, S.; Babu, V.; Selvakumar, J.N.; Prakash, S. Exploring the In Vitro Thrombolytic Activity of Nattokinase from a New Strain *Pseudomonas aeruginosa* CMSS. *Jundishapur J. Microbiol.* **2015**, *8*, e23567. [CrossRef]
98. Kim, W.; Choi, K.; Kim, Y.; Park, H.; Choi, J.; Lee, Y.; Oh, H.; Kwon, I.; Lee, S. Purification and Characterization of a Fibrinolytic Enzyme Produced from *Bacillus* sp. Strain CK 11-4 Screened from Chungkook-Jang. *Appl. Environ. Microbiol.* **1996**, *62*, 2482–2488. [CrossRef] [PubMed]
99. Yamane, T.A.; Kani, T.A.; Hatanaka, T.A.; Suzuki, A.T.; Ashida, T.A.; Kobayashi, T.; Ito, S.; Yamashita, O. Structure of a New Alkaline Serine Protease (M-Protease) from *Bacillus* sp. KSM-KI6. *Acta Crystallogr. Sect. D Biol. Crystallogr.* **1994**, *51*, 199–206. [CrossRef]
100. Kim, H.K.; Kim, G.T.; Kim, D.K.; Choi, W.A.; Park, S.H.; Jeong, Y.K.; Kong, I.S. Purification and characterisation of a novel fibrinolytic enzyme from *Bacillus* sp. KA 38 originated from fermented fish. *J. Ferment. Bioeng.* **1997**, *84*, 307–312.
101. Devaraj, Y.; Rajender, S.K.; Halami, P.M. Purification, characterization of fibrinolytic protease from *Bacillus amyloliquefaciens* MCC2606 and analysis of fibrin degradation product by MS/MS. *Prep. Biochem. Biotechnol.* **2018**, *48*, 172–180. [CrossRef] [PubMed]
102. Agrebi, R.; Hmidet, N.; Hajji, M.; Ktari, N.; Haddar, A.; Fakhfakh-Zouari, N.; Nasri, M. Fibrinolytic Serine Protease Isolation from *Bacillus amyloliquefaciens* An6 Grown on *Mirabilis jalapa* Tuber Powders. *Appl. Biochem. Biotechnol.* **2010**, *162*, 75–88. [CrossRef]
103. Ko, J.H.; Yan, J.P.; Zhu, L.; Qi, Y.P. Identification of two novel fibrinolytic enzymes from *Bacillus subtilis* QK02. *Comp. Biochem. Physiol. C Toxicol. Pharmacol.* **2003**, *137*, 65–74. [CrossRef] [PubMed]
104. Xiao, L.; Zhang, R.-H.; Peng, Y.; Zhang, Y.-Z. Highly efficient gene expression of a fibrinolytic enzyme (subtilisin DFE) in Bacillus subtilis mediated by the promoter of α-amylase gene from *Bacillus amyloliquefaciens*. *Biotechnol. Lett.* **2004**, *26*, 1365–1369. [CrossRef]
105. Velusamy, P.; Pachaiappan, R.; Christopher, M.; Vaseeharan, B.; Anbu, P.; So, J.-S. Isolation and identification of a novel fibrinolytic *Bacillus tequilensis* CWD-67 from dumping soils enriched with poultry wastes. *J. Gen. Appl. Microbiol.* **2015**, *61*, 241–247. [CrossRef] [PubMed]

106. Yeo, W.S.; Seo, M.J.; Kim, M.J.; Lee, H.H.; Kang, B.W.; Park, J.U.; Choi, Y.H.; Jeong, Y.K. Biochemical analysis of fibrinolytic enzyme purified from *Bacillus subtilis* strain A1. *J. Microbiol.* **2011**, *49*, 376–380. [CrossRef] [PubMed]
107. Lee, S.K.; Bae, D.H.; Kwon, T.J.; Lee, S.B.; Lee, H.H.; Park, J.H.; Heo, S.; Johnson, M.G. Purification and Characterization of a fibrinolytic enzyme from *Bacillus* sp. KDO-13 Isolated from Soyabean Paste. *J. Microbiol. Biotechnol.* **2001**, *11*, 845–852.
108. Nagase, H.; Visse, R.; Murphy, G. Structure and function of matrix metalloproteinases and TIMPS. *Cardiovasc. Res.* **2006**, *69*, 562–573. [CrossRef]
109. Vijayaraghavan, P.; Arun, A.; Vincent, S.G.P.; Arasu, M.V.; Al-Dhabi, N.A. Cow Dung Is a Novel Feedstock for Fibrinolytic Enzyme Production from Newly Isolated *Bacillus* sp. IND 7 and Its Application in In Vitro Clot Lysis. *Front. Microbiol.* **2016**, *7*, 361. [CrossRef] [PubMed]
110. Mukherjee, A.K.; Rai, S.K.; Thakur, R.; Chattopadhyay, P.; Kar, S.K. Bafibrinase: A non-toxic, non-hemorrhagic, direct-acting fibrinolytic serine protease from *Bacillus* sp. Strain AS-S20-I exhibits in vivo anticoagulant activity and thrombolytic potency. *Biochimie* **2012**, *94*, 1300–1308. [CrossRef]
111. Jeong, Y.K.; Park, J.U.; Baek, H.; Park, S.H.; Kong, I.S.; Kim, D.W.; Joo, W.H. Purification and biochemical characterization of a fibrinolytic enzyme from *Bacillus subtilis* BK-17. *World J. Microbiol. Biotechnol.* **2001**, *17*, 89–92. [CrossRef]
112. Paik, H.D.; Lee, S.K.; Heo, S.; Kim, S.Y.; Lee, H.H.; Kwon, T.J. Purification and Characterization of the Fibrinolytic Enzyme Produced by *Bacillus subtilis* KCK-7 from Chungkookjang. *J. Microbiol. Biotechnol.* **2004**, *14*, 829–835.
113. Yuan, J.; Yang, J.; Zhuang, Z.; Yang, Y.; Lin, L.; Wang, S. Thrombolytic effects of Douchi Fibrinolytic enzyme from *Bacillus subtilis* LD-8547 in vitro and in vivo. *BMC Biotechnol.* **2012**, *12*, 36. [CrossRef]
114. Vijayaraghavan, P.; Prakash Vincent, S.G. Medium Optimization for the Production of Fibrinolytic Enzyme by *Paenibacillus* sp. IND8 Using Response Surface Methodology. *Sci. World J.* **2014**, *2014*, 276942. [CrossRef]
115. Wang, J.; Wang, M.; Wang, Y. Purification and characterization of a novel fibrinolytic enzymes from *Streptomyces* sp. *Clin. J. Biotechnol.* **1999**, *15*, 83–89.
116. Verma, P.; Chatterjee, S.; Keziah, M.S.; Devi, S.C. Fibrinolytic protease from marine *Streptomyces rubiginosus* VITPSSM. *Cardiovasc. Hematol. Agents Med. Chem.* **2018**, *16*, 44–55. [CrossRef] [PubMed]
117. Chitte, R.R.; Deshmukh, S.V.; Kanekar, P.P. Production, Purification, and Biochemical Characterization of a Fibrinolytic Enzyme from Thermophilic *Streptomyces* sp. MCMB-379. *Appl. Biochem. Biotechnol.* **2011**, *165*, 1406–1413. [CrossRef] [PubMed]
118. Babu, V.; Devi, C.S. Exploring the in vitro thrombolytic potential of streptokinase-producing β-hemolytic *Streptococci* isolated from bovine milk. *J. Gen. Appl. Microbiol.* **2015**, *61*, 139–146. [CrossRef]
119. Narasimhan, M.K.; Ethiraj, S.; Krishnamurthi, T.; Rajesh, M. Purification, biochemical and thermal properties of fibrinolytic enzyme secreted by *Bacillus cereus* SRM-001. *Prep. Biochem. Biotechnol.* **2017**, *48*, 34–42. [CrossRef]
120. Biji, G.D.; Arun, A.; Muthulakshmi, E.; Vijayaraghavan, P.; Arasu, M.V.; Al-Dhabi, N.A. Bio-prospecting of cuttle fish waste and cow dung for the production of fibrinolytic enzyme from *Bacillus cereus* IND5 in solid state fermentation. *3 Biotech* **2016**, *6*, 231. [CrossRef]
121. Afifah, D.N.; Sulchan, M.; Syah, D.; Yanti, Y.; Suhartono, M.T.; Kim, J.H. Purification and Characterization of a Fibrinolytic Enzyme from *Bacillus pumilus* 2.g Isolated from Gembus, an Indonesian Fermented Food. *Prev. Nutr. Food Sci.* **2014**, *19*, 213–219. [CrossRef]
122. Taneja, K.; Bajaj, B.K.; Kumar, N.; Dilbaghi, N. Production, purification and characterization of fibrinolytic enzyme from *Serratia* sp. KG-2-1 using optimized media. *3 Biotech* **2017**, *7*, 184. [CrossRef]
123. Vijayaraghavan, P.; Prakash Vincent, S.G. A low-cost fermentation medium for potential fibrinolytic enzyme production by a newly isolated marine bacterium *Shewanella* sp. IND 20. *Biotechnol. Rep.* **2015**, *7*, 135–142. [CrossRef] [PubMed]
124. Meshram, V.; Saxena, S. Potential fibrinolytic activity of an endophytic *Lasiodiplodia pseudotheobromae* species. *3 Biotech* **2016**, *6*, 114. [CrossRef] [PubMed]
125. Nascimento, T.P.; Sales, A.E.; Porto, T.S.; Costa, R.M.P.B.; Breydo, L.; Uversky, V.N.; Porto, A.L.F.; Converti, A. Purification, biochemical, and structural characterization of a novel fibrinolytic enzyme from *Mucor subtilissimus* UCP 1262. *Bioprocess Biosyst. Eng.* **2017**, *40*, 1209–1219. [CrossRef]
126. Abdel-Fattah, A.F.; Ismail, A.M.S. Preparation and Properties of Fibrinolytic Enzymes Produced by *Cochliobolus lunatus*. *Biotechnol. Bioeng.* **1983**, *26*, 37–40. [CrossRef] [PubMed]
127. Weng, Y.; Yao, J.; Sparks, S.; Wang, K.Y. Nattokinase: An Oral Antithrombotic Agent for the Prevention of Cardiovascular Disease. *Int. J. Mol. Sci.* **2017**, *18*, 523. [CrossRef]
128. Meruvu, H.; Vangalapati, M. Nattokinase: A Review on Fibrinolytic Enzyme. *Int. J. Chem. Environ. Pharm. Res.* **2011**, *2*, 61–66.
129. RCSB PDB. Available online: http://www.rcsb.org/structure/4DWW (accessed on 15 September 2023).
130. Cal, D.; Zhu, C.; Chen, S. Microbial production of nattokinase: Current, challenge and prospect. *World J. Microbiol. Biotechnol.* **2017**, *33*, 84.
131. Yongjun, C.; Wei, B.; Shujun, J.; Meizhi, W.; Yan, J.; Yan, Y.; Zhongliang, Z.; Goulin, Z. Directed evolution improves the fibrinolytic activity of nattokinase from *Bacillus natto*. *FEMS Microbiol. Lett.* **2011**, *325*, 155–161. [CrossRef]
132. Sikri, N.; Bardia, A. A History of Streptokinase use in Acute Myocardial Infarction. *Tex. Heart Inst. J.* **2007**, *34*, 318–327.
133. RCSB PDB. Available online: https://www.rcsb.org/structure/1L4D (accessed on 15 September 2023).
134. Vakili, B.; Nezafat, N.; Negahdaripour, M.; Yari, M.; Zare, B.; Ghasemi, Y. Staphylokinase Enzyme: An Overview of Structure, Function and Engineered Forms. *Curr. Pharm. Biotechnol.* **2017**, *18*, 1026–1037. [CrossRef]

135. Peetermans, M.; Vanassche, T.; Liesenborghs, L.; Claes, J.; Velde, G.V.; Kwiecinksi, J.; Jin, T.; De Geest, B.; Hoylaerts, M.F.; Lijnen, R.H.; et al. Plasminogen activation by staphylokinase enhances local spreading of *S. aureus* in skin infections. *BMC Microbiol.* **2014**, *14*, 310. [CrossRef]
136. RCSB PDB. Available online: http://www.rcsb.org/structure/1C78 (accessed on 15 September 2023).
137. Nguyen, L.T.; Vogel, H.J. Staphylokinase has distinct modes of interaction with antimicrobial peptides, modulating its plasminogen-activation properties. *Sci. Rep.* **2016**, *6*, 31817. [CrossRef]
138. RCSB PDB. Available online: https://www.rcsb.org/structure/1SRP (accessed on 15 September 2023).
139. Selan, L.; Papa, R.; Tilotta, M.; Vrenna, G.; Carpentieri, A.; Amoresano, A.; Pucci, P.; Artini, M. Serratiopeptidase: A well-known metalloprotease with a new non-proteolytic activity against *S. aureus* biofilm. *BMC Microbiol.* **2015**, *15*, 207. [CrossRef]
140. Gupte, V.; Luthra, U. Analytical techniques for Serratiopeptidase: A review. *J. Pharm. Anal.* **2017**, *7*, 203–207. [CrossRef] [PubMed]
141. Nirale, N.M.; Menon, M.D. Topical Formulations of Serratiopeptidase: Development and Pharmacodynamic Evaluation. *Indian J. Pharm. Sci.* **2010**, *72*, 65–71. [PubMed]
142. Podorol'skaya, L.V.; Serebryakova, T.N.; Sharkova, T.S.; Neumyvakin, L.V.; Khromov, I.S.; Khokhlov, N.V.; Tarantul, V.Z. Tarantul Experimental thrombosis in rabbit marginal ear vein and evaluation of the thrombolytic action of longolytin. *Bull. Exp. Biol. Med.* **2007**, *143*, 577–580. [CrossRef]
143. Sharkova, T.; Podorolskaya, L. Increase of Fibrinilytic and Anticoagulant Activity by per os Administrating of Proteinase Complex Longolytin in Rats. *J. Thromb. Haemost.* **2017**, *16*, 355.
144. Osmolovskiy, A.A.; Kreyer, V.G.; Baranova, N.A.; Egorov, N.S. Proteolytic Enzymes of Mycelial Fungi with Plasmin-like and Plasminogen-Activator Activity. *Usp. Sovr. Biol.* **2021**, *141*, 467–482.
145. Kurosawa, Y.; Nirengi, S.; Homma, T.; Esaki, K.; Ohta, M.; Clark, J.F.; Hamaoka, T. A single-dose of oral nattokinase potentiates thrombolysis and anti-coagulation profiles. *Sci. Rep.* **2015**, *5*, 11601. [CrossRef] [PubMed]
146. Ly, B.; Arnesen, H.; Eie, H.; Hol, R. A controlled clinical trial of streptokinase and heparin in the treatment of major pulmonary embolism. *Acta Med. Scand.* **1978**, *203*, 465–470. [CrossRef]
147. Gusev, E.I.; Martynov, M.Y.; Nikonov, A.A.; Shamalov, N.A.; Semenov, M.P.; Gerasimets, E.A.; Yarovaya, E.B.; Semenov, A.M.; Archakov, A.I.; Markin, S.S.; et al. Non-immunogenic recombinant staphylokinase versus alteplase for patients with acute ischaemic stroke 4.5 h after symptom onset in Russia (FRIDA): A randomised, open label, multicentre, parallel-group, non-inferiority trial. *Lancet Neurol.* **2021**, *20*, 721–728. [CrossRef]
148. Kim, J.Y.; Gum, S.N.; Paik, J.K.; Lim, H.H.; Kim, K.C.; Ogasawara, K.; Inoue, K.; Park, S.; Jang, Y.; Lee, J.H. Effects of nattokinase on blood pressure: A randomized, controlled trial. *Hypertens. Res.* **2008**, *31*, 1583–1588. [CrossRef]
149. Fadl, N.N.; Ahmed, H.H.; Booles, H.F.; Sayed, A.H. Serrapeptase and nattokinase intervention for relieving Alzheimer's disease pathophysiology in rat model. *Hum. Exp. Toxicol.* **2013**, *32*, 721–735. [CrossRef]
150. Moriya, N.; Nakata, M.; Nakamura, M.; Takaoka, M.; Iwasa, S.; Kato, K.; Kakinuma, A. Intestinal absorption of serrapeptase (TSP) in rats. *Biotechnol. Appl. Biochem.* **1994**, *20*, 101–108. [CrossRef]
151. Kotb, E. Fibrinolytic bacterial enzymes with thrombolytic activity. In *Fibrinolytic Bacterial Enzymes with Thrombolytic Activity*; Springer: Berlin/Heidelberg, Germany, 2012.
152. Majima, Y.; Inagaki, M.; Hirata, K.; Takeuchi, K.; Morishita, A.; Sakakura, Y. The effect of an orally administered proteolytic enzyme on the elasticity and viscosity of nasal mucus. *Arch. Otorhinolaryngol.* **1988**, *44*, 355–359. [CrossRef]
153. Bracale, G.; Selvetella, L. Clinical study of the efficacy of and tolerance to seaprose S in inflammatory venous disease. Controlled study versus serratio-peptidase. *Minerva Cardioangiol.* **1996**, *44*, 515–524. [PubMed]
154. Esch, P.M.; Gerngross, H.; Fabian, A. Reduction of postoperative swelling. Objective measurement of swelling of the upper ankle joint in treatment with serrapeptase: A prospective study. *Fortschritte Der Med.* **1989**, *107*, 67–68.
155. Mazzone, A.; Catalani, M.; Costanzo, M.; Drusian, A.; Mandoli, A.; Russo, S.; Guarini, E.; Vesperini, G. Evaluation of *Serratia* peptidase in acute or chronic inflammation of otorhinolaryngology pathology: A multicentre, double blind, randomized trial versus placebo. *J. Int. Med. Res.* **1990**, *18*, 379–388. [CrossRef]
156. Mine, Y.; Wong, A.H.K.; Jiang, B. Fibrinolytic enzymes in Asian traditional fermented foods. *Food Res. Int.* **2005**, *38*, 243–250. [CrossRef]
157. Wong, A.H.; Mine, Y. Novel fibrinolytic enzyme in fermented shrimp paste, a traditional Asian fermented seasoning. *J. Agric. Food Chem.* **2004**, *52*, 980–986. [CrossRef] [PubMed]
158. Nguyen, T.T.; Quyen, T.D.; Le, H.T. Cloning and enhancing production of a detergent- and organic-solvent-resistant nattokinase from *Bacillus subtilis* VTCC-DVN-12-01 by using an eight-protease-gene-deficient *Bacillus subtilis* WB800. *Microb. Cell Factories* **2013**, *12*, 79. [CrossRef] [PubMed]
159. Vijayaraghavan, P.; Rajendran, P.; Prakash Vincent, S.G.; Arun, A.; Abdullah Al-Dhabi, N.; Valan Arasu, M.; Young Kwon, O.; Kim, Y.O. Novel sequential screening and enhanced production of fibrinolytic enzyme by *Bacillus* sp. IND12 using response surface methodology in solid-state fermentation. *BioMed Res. Int.* **2017**, *2017*, 3909657. [CrossRef] [PubMed]

Disclaimer/Publisher's Note: The statements, opinions and data contained in all publications are solely those of the individual author(s) and contributor(s) and not of MDPI and/or the editor(s). MDPI and/or the editor(s) disclaim responsibility for any injury to people or property resulting from any ideas, methods, instructions or products referred to in the content.

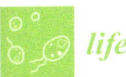

Article

Long-Term Clinical Impact of Patients with Multi-Vessel Non-Obstructive Coronary Artery Disease

Jin Jung, Su-Nam Lee *, Sung-Ho Her, Ki-Dong Yoo, Keon-Woong Moon, Donggyu Moon and Won-Young Jang

Department of Cardiology, St. Vincent's Hospital, College of Medicine, The Catholic University of Korea, Seoul 16247, Republic of Korea; colaking@naver.com (J.J.); hhhsungho@naver.com (S.-H.H.); yookd@catholic.ac.kr (K.-D.Y.); cardiomoon@gmail.com (K.-W.M.); babaheesu@gmail.com (D.M.); raph83@naver.com (W.-Y.J.)
* Correspondence: sunam1220@gmail.com

Abstract: Background: Non-obstructive coronary artery disease (CAD) is a disease commonly diagnosed in patients undergoing coronary angiography. However, little is known regarding the long-term clinical impact of multi-vessel non-obstructive CAD. Therefore, the object of this study was to investigate the long-term clinical impact of multi-vessel non-obstructive CAD. Method: A total of 2083 patients without revascularization history and obstructive CAD were enrolled between January 2010 and December 2015. They were classified into four groups according to number of vessels involved in non-obstructive CAD (25% ≤ luminal stenosis < 70%): zero, one, two, or three diseased vessels (DVs). We monitored the patients for 5 years. The primary outcome was major cardiovascular and cerebrovascular events (MACCEs), defined as a composite of cardiac death, stroke, and myocardial infarction (MI). Result: The occurrence of MACCEs increased as the number of non-obstructive DVs increased, and was especially high in patients with three DVs. After adjustment, patients with three DVs still showed significantly poorer clinical outcomes of MACCEs, stroke, and MI compared those with zero DVs. Conclusion: Multi-vessel non-obstructive CAD, especially in patients with non-obstructive three DVs, is strongly associated with poor long-term clinical outcomes. This finding suggests that more intensive treatment may be required in this subset of patients.

Keywords: non-obstructive coronary artery disease; multi-vessel; stroke; long-term clinical outcome; major cardiovascular and cerebrovascular event; myocardial infarction; cardiac death

1. Introduction

In the past few decades, the prevalence of coronary artery disease (CAD) has been increasing continuously due to population growth and aging. Therefore, CAD remains the leading cause of morbidity and mortality worldwide, and the importance of the early diagnosis of CAD is increasing [1,2]. Consistent with this trend, coronary angiography (CAG) is actively used as a gold standard diagnostic tool. In addition, the use of coronary computerized tomography angiography (CCTA), instead of the use of the electrocardiogram test [3,4], allows the identification of many patients with mild to moderate stenosis.

Although non-obstructive CAD, including mild to moderate stenosis, is a relatively common finding in patients undergoing CAG and CCTA [5–7], non-obstructive CAD has been characterized as "insignificant CAD" in previous studies because of the low incidence of adverse outcomes [7,8]. Therefore, because most previous studies on CAD focused on patients with obstructive CAD, the risks associated with non-obstructive CAD were underestimated [9,10]. For this reason, management is well established for patients who have undergone percutaneous coronary intervention (PCI) or patients with obstructive CAD [3]. In particular, for statin treatment, different obvious target values are presented depending on the risk level, and for antiplatelet treatment, the combination, intensity, and duration are also obviously presented [11,12]. On the other hand, management for primary prevention in patients with non-obstructive CAD has not yet been established.

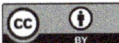

However, a prior study suggested that myocardial infarction (MI) occurred frequently in patients with non-obstructive lesions [13], and subsequent studies have supported an association between non-obstructive CAD and poor clinical outcomes [14,15]. Therefore, there is a growing awareness of the importance of non-obstructive CAD, and many studies are being conducted. However, the long-term clinical impact of multi-vessel non-obstructive CAD is still poorly understood. Therefore, the object of this study was to investigate the long-term clinical effect of multi-vessel non-obstructive CAD.

2. Materials and Methods

2.1. Study Design and Population

This was a non-randomized, retrospective, single-center study. We reviewed the medical records of 4287 patients who underwent CAG in St. Vincent Hospital, Suwon, Republic of Korea between January 2010 and December 2015. The angiographic findings, including degree of stenosis and extent of CAD, were evaluated visually by the attending interventional cardiologist. Referring to the standard definition used in a previous study and guidelines [14,16], obstructive CAD was defined as 50% or greater stenosis in the left main (LM) coronary artery or 70% or greater in other coronary arteries. Non-obstructive CAD was defined as CAD with mild (25–49%) to moderate (50–69%) stenosis, but LM CAD was defined as 20% or greater but less than 50% stenosis. Of the total patients, 2204 were excluded, including patients undergoing initial PCI, patients with previous PCI/coronary artery bypass graft history, and those with follow-up loss or obstructive CAD (Figure 1). The remaining 2083 patients were classified into 4 groups according to number of epicardial coronary arteries with non-obstructive CAD at the time of initial CAG: zero diseased vessels (DV) (0 DV), one diseased vessel (1 DV), two diseased vessels (2 DV), and three diseased vessels (3 DV). Patients with isolated non-obstructive LM disease were classified as 2 DV.

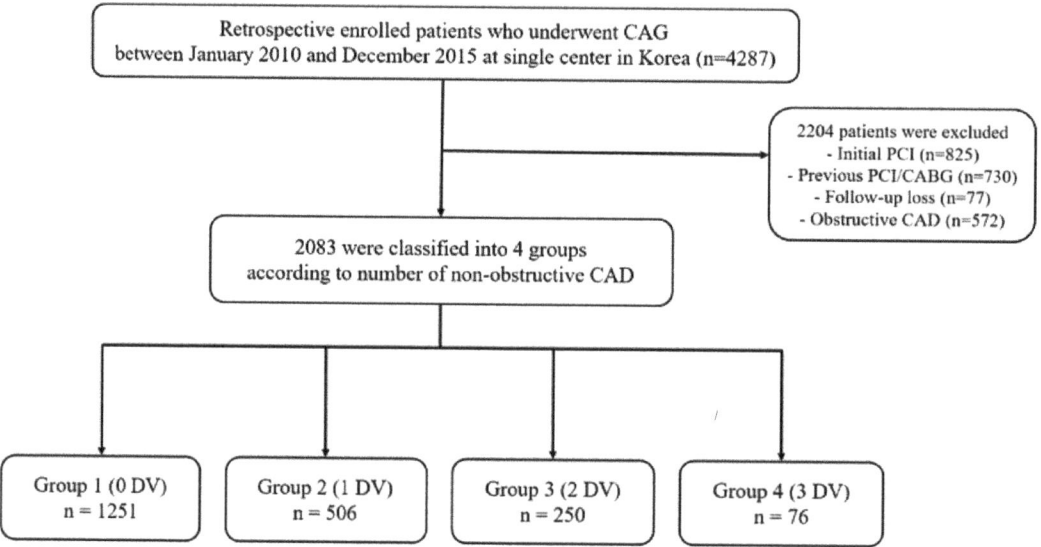

Figure 1. Study population flow chart. DV, diseased vessel; CAG, coronary angiography; CAD, coronary artery disease; PCI, percutaneous coronary intervention; CABG, coronary artery bypass grafting.

This study was approved by Institutional Review Board (IRB) of St. Vincent hospital (IRB VC20RISI0087) and complied with 1975 Declaration of Helsinki. The need for individual patient consent was waived.

2.2. Study Endpoint and Definition

The primary outcome of the study was major cardiovascular and cerebrovascular events (MACCEs), defined as a composite of cardiac death, stroke, and MI. The secondary outcomes were all-cause death, cardiac death, MI, and stroke. Because patients who initially underwent PCI were excluded from the study, MI referred to only spontaneous MI, defined as any troponin or creatine kinase-myocardial band increase above the upper limit of the normal range with ischemic signs or symptoms during the follow-up period after discharge, and periprocedural MI was excluded. Stroke was defined as neurological symptoms associated with radiologic evidence based on magnetic resonance imaging or computed tomography. The time-to-event duration was determined as that between study enrollment and the first event. Smoking was defined as having smoked cigarettes within 3 months of admission [17]. Chronic kidney disease (CKD) was defined as an estimated glomerular filtration rate <60 mL/min/1.73 m^2, as calculated using the Modification of Renal Diet equation from baseline serum creatinine [18]. All clinical events were confirmed by source documentation collected at each hospital and centrally adjudicated by an independent group of clinicians unaware of the revascularization type.

2.3. Statistical Analyses

Continuous variables were presented as median and interquartile range or mean ± standard deviation and analyzed using Student's t-test or Mann–Whitney test. Categorical variables were summarized as counts (percentages) and compared using the chi-square test or Fisher's exact test, as appropriate. Event rates were calculated based on the Kaplan–Meier estimates in time-to-first event analysis and compared using the log-rank test. Univariable and multivariable Cox regression analyses were performed to analyze the clinical outcomes. The hazard ratio (HR) and 95% confidence interval (CI) were also calculated. Multivariable Cox regression models were adjusted for age, sex, hypertension (HTN), diabetes mellitus (DM), cerebrovascular accident (CVA), intravascular ultrasonography (IVUS), fractional flow reserve (FFR), aspirin, P2Y12 inhibitor, cilostazol, statin, vasodilator, left ventricular ejection fraction (LV EF), and creatinine.

All statistical analyses were conducted using Statistical Analysis Software (SAS, version 9.2, SAS Institute, Cary, NC, USA) and p-value < 0.05 was considered statistically significant.

3. Results

During the study period, 2083 patients with non-obstructive CAD or 0 DV were analyzed. Of those, 1251 (60%) were classified as 0 DV, and the remaining patients were divided into three groups according to number of non-obstructive DVs (1 DV: 506 [24% of total patients], 2 DV: 250 [12%], 3 DV: 76 [4.0%]).

3.1. Baseline Characteristics

Baseline characteristics are displayed in Table 1. Compared to patients with low burden of atherosclerotic disease (non-obstructive 0 DV and 1 DV), older age and prevalence of HTN and DM were higher in patients with multi-vessel non-obstructive CAD (age, 0 DV: 59.2 ± 11.9, 1 DV: 64.1 ± 10.7, 2 DV: 65.8 ± 11.1, 3 DV: 65.1 ± 12.9, $p < 0.001$; HTN, 0 DV: 561 [44.8%], 1 DV: 274 [54.2%], 2 DV: 162 [64.8%], 3 DV: 53 [69.7%], $p < 0.001$; DM, 0 DV: 231 [18.5%], 1 DV: 126 [24.9%], 2 DV: 81 [32.4%], 3 DV: 23 [30.3%], $p < 0.001$). Moreover, previous CVA was most frequent in patients with 3VD (Previous CVA, 0 DV: 83 [6.6%], 1 DV: 33 [6.5%], 2 DV: 26 [10.4%], 3 DV: 15 [19.7%], $p < 0.001$). The rates of aspirin, P2Y12 inhibitor, and statin medication use related to these underlying diseases showed the same tendency (aspirin, 0 DV: 385 [30.8%], 1 DV: 278 [54.9%], 2 DV: 177 [70.8%], 3 DV: 51 [67.1%], $p < 0.001$; P2Y12 inhibitor, 0 DV:46 [3.7%], 1 DV: 45 [8.9%], 2 DV: 29 [11.6%], 3 DV: 10 [13.2%], $p < 0.001$; Statin, 0 DV: 276 [22.1%], 1 DV: 184 [36.4%], 2 DV: 104 [41.6%], 3 DV: 31 [40.8%], $p < 0.001$). Laboratory and procedural characteristics showed no difference in groups except creatinine and FFR usage (creatinine, 0.9 ± 0.9, 1 DV: 1.4 ± 1.7, 2 DV:

1.0 ± 0.8, 3 DV: 1.5 ± 1.7, p = 0.046; FFR, 0 DV: 0 [0.0%], 1 DV: 7 [1.4%], 2 DV: 4 [1.6%], 3 DV: 0 [0.0%], p < 0.001).

Table 1. Baseline demographic and clinical characteristics.

	0 DV n = 1251	1 DV n = 506	2 DV n = 250	3 DV n = 76	p-Value
Age (years)	59.2 ± 11.9	64.1 ± 10.7	65.8 ± 11.1	65.1 ± 12.9	<0.001
Male	629 (50.3)	241 (47.6)	101 (40.4)	32 (42.1)	0.024
BMI	24.4 ± 3.6	24.6 ± 3.4	24.2 ± 3.1	24.3 ± 4.1	0.544
Smoking	353 (28.2)	158 (31.2)	78 (31.2)	24 (31.6)	0.529
HTN	561 (44.8)	274 (54.2)	162 (64.8)	53 (69.7)	<0.001
DM	231 (18.5)	126 (24.9)	81 (32.4)	23 (30.3)	<0.001
Dyslipidemia	229 (18.3)	109 (21.5)	57 (22.8)	17 (22.4)	0.216
CKD	23 (1.8)	14 (2.8)	7 (2.8)	2 (2.6)	0.574
Previous CVA	83 (6.6)	33 (6.5)	26 (10.4)	15 (19.7)	<0.001
LV EF (%)	59.3 ± 10.6	60.9 ± 8.9	61.6 ± 7.7	58.0 ± 11.8	0.013
Aspirin	385 (30.8)	278 (54.9)	177 (70.8)	51 (67.1)	<0.001
P2Y12 inhibitor	46 (3.7)	45 (8.9)	29 (11.6)	10 (13.2)	<0.001
Cilostazol	19 (1.5)	13 (2.6)	14 (5.6)	3 (4.0)	0.001
Statin	276 (22.1)	184 (36.4)	104 (41.6)	31 (40.8)	<0.001
Beta blocker	185 (14.8)	87 (17.2)	42 (16.8)	17 (22.4)	0.229
ACEi/ARB	242 (19.3)	105 (20.8)	67 (26.8)	15 (19.7)	0.068
Vasodilator	333 (26.6)	201 (39.7)	111 (44.4)	38 (50.0)	<0.001
IVUS	1 (0.1)	4 (0.8)	2 (0.8)	1 (1.3)	0.045
FFR	0 (0.0)	7 (1.4)	4 (1.6)	0 (0.0)	<0.001
HbA1c (%)	6.4 ± 1.2	6.6 ± 1.3	7.1 ± 1.7	6.3 ± 1.0	0.058
Proximal LAD	0 (0.0)	83 (16.4)	50 (20.0)	28 (36.8)	<0.001
LAD (lesion)	0 (0.0)	260 (51.4)	155 (62.0)	52 (68.4)	<0.001
Mild stenosis (lesion)	0 (0.0)	164 (32.4)	86 (34.4)	27 (35.5)	
Moderate stenosis (lesion)	0 (0.0)	96 (19.0)	69 (27.6)	25 (32.9)	
LCx (lesion)	0 (0.0)	65 (12.9)	109 (43.6)	67 (88.2)	<0.001
Mild stenosis (lesion)	0 (0.0)	42 (8.3)	56 (22.4)	30 (39.5)	
Moderate stenosis (lesion)	0 (0.0)	23 (4.6)	53 (21.2)	37 (48.7)	
RCA (lesion)	0 (0.0)	114 (22.5)	166 (66.4)	76 (100.0)	<0.001
Mild stenosis (lesion)	0 (0.0)	75 (14.8)	116 (46.4)	39 (51.3)	
Moderate stenosis (lesion)	0 (0.0)	39 (7.7)	50 (20.0)	37 (48.7)	
Creatinine (mg/dL)	0.9 ± 0.9	1.4 ± 1.7	1.0 ± 0.8	1.5 ± 1.7	0.046
Hemoglobin (g/dL)	13.6 ± 1.8	13.6 ± 1.9	13.6 ± 1.8	13.1 ± 2.2	0.738
Hematocrit (%)	39.6 ± 5.0	39.7 ± 4.6	39.8 ± 5.0	37.9 ± 5.8	0.876
Platelet ($\times 10^9$/L)	238.9 ± 68.2	238.7 ± 63.5	236.3 ± 71.6	232.6 ± 76.5	0.853
White blood cell ($\times 10^9$/L)	7.9 ± 10.6	7.8 ± 6.2	8.3 ± 4.3	7.3 ± 2.6	0.939
Total cholesterol (mg/dL)	181.1 ± 43.1	183.5 ± 41.8	186.9 ± 53.3	169.4 ± 38.0	0.649
Triglyceride (mg/dL)	129.7 ± 113.4	131.0 ± 81.0	142.7 ± 105.2	105.9 ± 59.2	0.485
HDL cholesterol (mg/dL)	43.2 ± 11.6	43.0 ± 11.8	40.8 ± 11.7	43.7 ± 12.1	0.346
LDL cholesterol (mg/dL)	107.8 ± 33.5	109.5 ± 35.6	106.5 ± 41.6	102.1 ± 29.6	0.240
C-Reactive protein (mg/dL)	1.1 ± 3.1	1.0 ± 5.1	1.8 ± 3.5	0.5 ± 0.6	0.116
Albumin	4.3 ± 1.2	4.4 ± 4.7	4.2 ± 0.6	4.2 ± 0.3	0.114

Data are expressed as mean ± standard deviation or number (%); DV, diseased vessel; BMI, body mass index; HTN, hypertension; DM, diabetic mellitus; CKD, chronic kidney disease; CVA, cerebrovascular accident; LV EF, left ventricular ejection fraction; ACEi, angiotensin-converting–enzyme inhibitor; ARB, angiotensin II receptor blocker; IVUS, intravascular ultrasonography; FFR, fractional flow reserve; HbA1c, glycated hemoglobin; LAD, left anterior descending artery; LCx, left circumflex artery; RCA, right coronary artery.

3.2. Long-Term Clinical Outcomes

All-cause death and cardiac death did not show statistically significant differences in the groups (All-cause death, 0 DV: 118 [9.4%], 1 DV: 45 [8.9%], 2 DV: 28 [11.2%], 3 DV: 14 [18.4%], p = 0.680; Cardiac death, 0 DV: 31 [2.5%], 1 DV: 11 [2.2%], 2 DV: 3 [1.2%], 3 DV: 1 [1.3%], p = 0.597), but they were significantly different in patients with MACCEs, MI, or stroke (MACCEs, 0 DV: 78 [6.2%], 1 DV: 33 [6.5%], 2 DV: 17 [6.8%], 3 DV: 14 [18.4%], $p < 0.001$; MI, 0 DV: 3 [0.2%], 1 DV: 5 [1.0%], 2 DV: 1 [0.4%], 3 DV: 3 [4.0%], $p < 0.001$; Stroke, 0 DV: 43 [3.9%], 1 DV: 18 [3.6%], 2 DV: 13 [5.2%], 3 DV: 10 [13.2%], $p = 0.001$). The occurrence of MACCEs increased as the number of non-obstructive DVs increased and, in particular, with a nearly 3 times higher occurrence rate in the 3 DVs compared to the 2 DVs group. In addition, the occurrence of MACCEs was mainly due to stroke rather than cardiac events (Table 2) (Figure 2).

Table 2. Five-year clinical outcomes.

	0 DV n = 1251	1 DV n = 506	2 DV n = 250	3 DV n = 76	*p*-Value
MACCEs	78 (6.2)	33 (6.5)	17 (6.8)	14 (18.4)	<0.001
All-cause death	118 (9.4)	45 (8.9)	28 (11.2)	9 (11.8)	0.680
Cardiac death	31 (2.5)	11 (2.2)	3 (1.2)	1 (1.3)	0.597
Myocardial infarction	3 (0.2)	5 (1.0)	1 (0.4)	3 (4.0)	<0.001
Stroke	49 (3.9)	18 (3.6)	13 (5.2)	10 (13.2)	0.001

Data are shown as n (%); DV, diseased vessel; MACCEs, major adverse cardiovascular and cerebrovascular events.

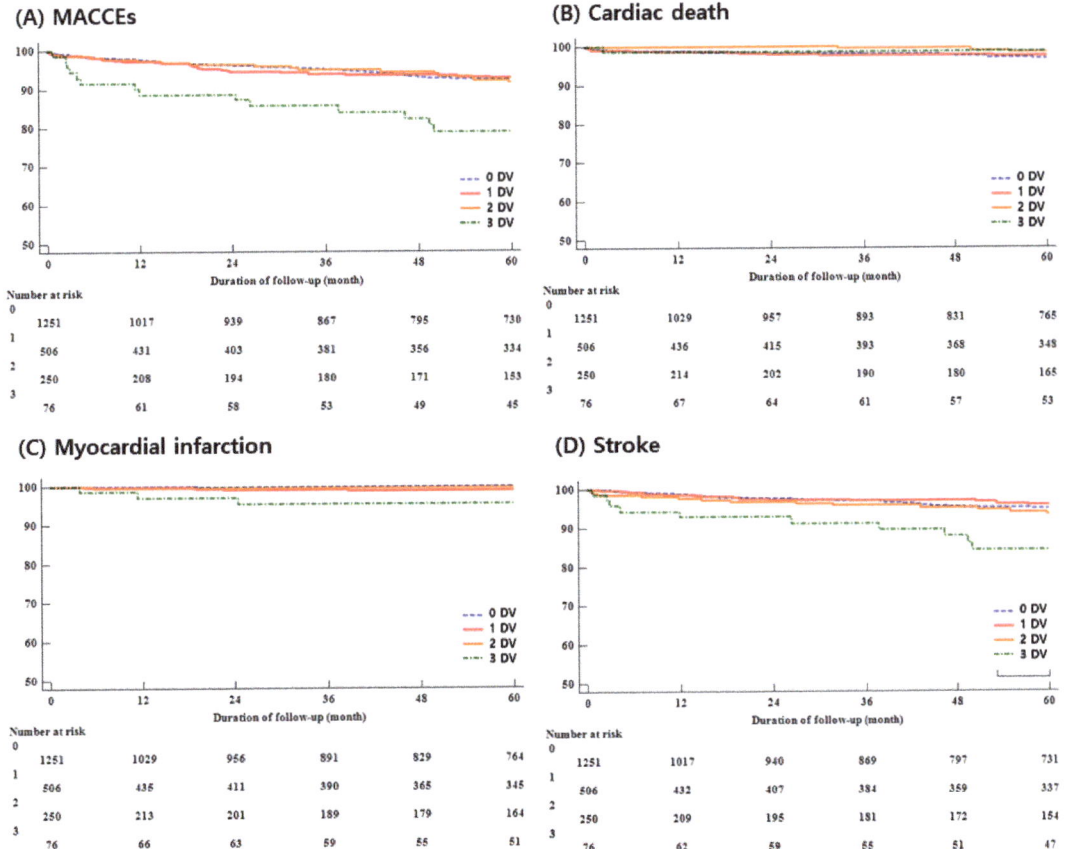

Figure 2. (**A**) Major cardiovascular and cerebrovascular events; (**B**) Cardiac death; (**C**) Myocardial infarction; (**D**) Stroke.

In multivariable analysis, patients with non-obstructive 3 DVs showed significantly worse long-term clinical outcomes than those with 0 DVs in terms of MACCEs, stroke, and MI (MACCEs: hazard ratio [HR] 2.09, 95% confidence interval [CI] 1.15–3.79, $p = 0.016$; Stroke: HR 2.04, 95% CI 1.01–4.16, $p = 0.049$, MI: HR 15.17, 95% CI 2.37–97.25, $p = 0.004$) (Table 3).

Table 3. Five-year hazard ratio of MACCEs, all-cause death, cardiac death, myocardial infarction, and stroke.

	Univariate HR (95% CI)	p-Value	Multivariate HR [a] (95% CI)	p-Value
MACCEs				
0 DVs (reference)	1.00	-	1.00	-
1 DV	0.98 (0.65–1.48)	0.928	0.83 (0.54–1.27)	0.386
2 DVs	1.05 (0.62–1.78)	0.854	0.70 (0.40–1.23)	0.212
3 DVs	2.97 (1.68–5.24)	<0.001	2.09 (1.15–3.79)	0.016
All-cause death				
0 DVs (reference)	1.00	-	1.00	-
1 DV	0.87 (0.62–1.12)	0.434	0.77 (0.54–1.10)	0.148
2 DVs	1.11 (0.74–1.68)	0.612	0.85 (0.55–1.32)	0.466
3 DVs	1.13 (0.57–2.22)	0.734	0.77 (0.39–1.55)	0.469
Cardiac death				
0 DVs (reference)	1.00	-	1.00	-
1 DV	0.83 (0.42–1.65)	0.595	0.80 (0.39–1.65)	0.548
2 DVs	0.46 (0.14–1.51)	0.201	0.37 (1.11–1.29)	0.118
3 DVs	0.49 (0.07–3.60)	0.485	0.45 (0.06–3.35)	0.433
Myocardial infarction				
0 DVs (reference)	1.00	-	1.00	-
1 DV	3.92 (0.94–16.42)	0.061	3.31 (0.73–14.99)	0.120
2 DVs	1.60 (0.17–15.40)	0.683	1.44 (0.13–15.77)	0.765
3 DVs	15.65 (3.16–77.56)	<0.001	15.17 (2.37–97.25)	0.004
Stroke				
0 DVs (reference)	1.00	-	1.00	-
1 DV	0.85 (0.49–1.45)	0.540	0.67 (0.38–1.16)	0.152
2 DVs	1.27 (0.69–2.34)	0.441	0.74 (0.39–1.42)	0.362
3 DVs	3.30 (1.67–6.52)	<0.001	2.04 (1.01–4.16)	0.049

[a] adjusted by age, sex, hypertension, diabetic mellitus, cerebrovascular accident, intravascular ultrasonography, fractional flow reserve, aspirin, P2Y12 inhibitor, cilostazol, statin, vasodilator, left ventricular ejection fraction, and creatinine. HR, hazard ratio; CI, confidence interval; DV, diseased vessel; MACCEs, major adverse cardiovascular and cerebrovascular events.

4. Discussion

The main findings of the study were as follows: (1) Non-obstructive CAD was associated with adverse long-term clinical outcomes, especially in patients with non-obstructive three DVs; as the number of non-obstructive DVs increased, the frequency of 5-year MACCE increased; (2) Compared to patients without non-obstructive DV, patients with three DVs showed twice the risk of MACCE and stroke and 15 times the risk of MI; (3) The occurrence of MACCE was primarily due to stroke and not cardiac events.

The population in the present study had no previous history of revascularization and were diagnosed with non-obstructive CAD after initial CAG and did not undergo PCI. These patients are often encountered in clinical practice, while clinical relevance may be underestimated as they are considered low risk for adverse events and clear guidelines for the management of these patients have not been established. Currently, FFR is used in addition to angiography for therapeutic decisions in these patients. However, in many cardiac laboratories, it is still common to base a clinical decision on coronary angiography findings alone due to equipment availability, financial considerations, and insurance issues. In that respect, our study was similar to real-world clinical practice.

Our results show that non-obstructive CAD is associated with poor clinical outcomes, consistent with several previous studies showing such a negative impact [14,15,19,20] and with prior studies indicating that a majority of plaque ruptures and MIs are related to non-obstructive rather than obstructive lesions [9,13,21]. In addition, as the number of obstructive vessels increases, the clinical outcomes worsen, especially in patients with obstructive three DVs [6,9,14]. Through this study, the same trend was confirmed in non-obstructive CAD. These results are also consistent with the results of previous studies that evaluated CAD with CCTA [22,23]. In a previous study [22] of patients with no history of PCI, patients with a small number of segments with disease did not differ from patients without non-obstructive CAD when comparing survival free from cardiovascular death or MI. However, among patients with non-obstructive CAD, those with extensive segments with disease experienced a higher rate of cardiovascular death or myocardial infarction, comparable with those who have a small number of segments with disease and showed similar clinical outcomes to patients with obstructive CAD. In another study [23] of a similar patient group, patients with non-obstructive CAD had a 6% higher risk of death for each additional segment with non-obstructive plaque. These studies have shown the importance of not only the presence of non-obstructive CAD but also its extent. This conclusion is in line with our study, where the number of adverse events increased as the number of non-obstructive DVs increased.

Patients with multi-vessel non-obstructive CAD were older, had a higher female proportion, and had a higher co-morbid incidence including DM, HTN, and CVA. These baseline characteristic differences were more evident between one DV and two DVs than between two DVs and three DVs, and have shown the same trend in a previous major study [14]. In particular, the female ratio of two DVs was similar to three DVs, but higher than one DV. Gender may have influenced these differences because female patients show higher HTN, DM incidence than their male counterparts [24]. Age was known to be a strong predictor of adverse events in non-obstructive CAD patients, and so was the DM [25]. In the presence of DM, both non-obstructive CAD and obstructive CAD patients had poorer clinical outcomes than patients without DM, and diabetic patients with non-obstructive CAD had the worse outcome, which was comparable to patients with obstructive CAD alone [26]. Hypertension was well known as a cardiovascular risk factor and was associated with the extent of non-obstructive CAD and triple vessel disease [27]. Prior CVA was also independently associated with a higher risk of MACCEs [28]. Therefore, these factors may have affected the present study results. However, after adjusting for these factors, non-obstructive three DVs remained an independent predictor of MACCEs, unlike one DV and two DVs. These results were the same as those of Maddox et al. [14], who presented short-term (1-year) outcomes of similar patients using similar definitions of non-obstructive CAD. Our study confirmed that this trend was maintained in the long term (5 years).

Contrary to age, gender, and co-morbidity, there were no differences between groups in terms of laboratory characteristics. In particular, CPR, a representative inflammation marker, was well known as a marker that can predict cardiovascular events in previous studies [29,30], but no difference was found in this study. Previous studies targeted a selective population such as patients with typical chest pain and evidence of ischemia [29] or patients with a high risk of atherosclerotic disease [30]. On the other hand, this study was a retrospective study that excluded patients with a history of previous revascularization and consisted of a less selective population. Therefore, the study population may have had an influence. Additionally, the association between CRP and cardiovascular events demonstrated statistical significance, but the association with stroke did not [31]. In our study, MACCEs occurred more frequently in stroke than in cardiac events, so this may also have had an impact.

There was a statistically significant difference in coronary involvement in all groups. In particular, the location of the lesion is important in patients with non-obstructive CAD, and it is well known that proximal coronary involvement was associated with increased adverse event risk in patients with non-obstructive CAD [32]. Our study results also showed that proximal left anterior descending (LAD) involvement increased as DV increased and showed poor outcomes.

Even in non-obstructive CAD, multi-vessel non-obstructive CAD, reflecting a greater atherosclerotic burden, affected the poor clinical impact, suggesting that not only the degree of stenosis, but also the total atherosclerotic burden, are important factors in prognosis. Previous studies have reported that the burden of atherosclerotic disease is a strong predictor of prognosis [33–35]. A study using CCTA, another diagnostic modality, also showed poor clinical outcomes, as calcified plaque burden and non-calcified plaque burden increased independently of CAD severity [36]. Maddox et al. [14], mentioned above, showed that, as CAD extent increased, the clinical outcome, defined as a composite of MI and mortality, worsened. In obstructive CAD, HR progressively increased as the number of involved vessels increased. The same trend was seen in non-obstructive CAD, but it was statistically significant only in three DVs. A similar result was also demonstrated in a study evaluating CAD extent with CCTA [37]. Mortensen et al. [15] demonstrated that patients with comparable total atherosclerotic burden had a similar risk for cardiovascular events regardless of non-obstructive or obstructive CAD. This indicates that the main predictor of clinical outcome is not the degree of stenosis, but the total atherosclerotic burden, which would have had a significant impact on the derivation of our findings.

Endothelial dysfunction may also have influenced the result that patients with multi-vessel non-obstructive CAD showed a poorer clinical outcome. The vascular endothelium plays an important role in vascular tone and flow, as well as permeability and thrombosis homeostasis. Therefore, endothelial dysfunction causes a decline in these functions, resulting in a decrease in anti-atherosclerotic and anti-thrombotic properties [38]. In other words, endothelial dysfunction is a marker of atherosclerosis and itself contributes to the progression of atherosclerosis [39]. A large cohort study with 5 years of follow-up has already shown that endothelial dysfunction was a major predictor of MACCE, defined identically to our study [40], and, as in our study, the presence of endothelial dysfunction increased cardiac events even in patients with non-obstructive CAD [41]. Such endothelial dysfunction worsened as the number of DVs increased [41,42], which is consistent with the present study, showing that patients with multi-vessel non-obstructive CAD had worse clinical outcomes. The presence of endothelial dysfunction in patients with non-obstructive CAD predicts adverse cardiovascular outcomes, but careful interpretation is necessary because endothelial dysfunction is not always present in non-obstructive CAD.

Gender difference may also have contributed to poor prognosis with multi-vessel non-obstructive CAD. Contrary to obstructive CAD, the prevalence of non-obstructive CAD is higher in women, but, paradoxically, women show higher rates of myocardial ischemia and mortality than men [43,44]. Our study also showed a higher female ratio, especially in multi-vessel CAD, which is the same result as the previous study [24]. The reason why females have a worse outcome is not yet fully explained, but it is thought that the higher frequency of inflammatory disease and microvascular dysfunction, adverse pregnancy outcome, and hormonal and menopause effects may have had an effect [44,45].

Many cardiologists focus only on significant CAD in patients who have undergone CAG. However, given that atherosclerosis is a systemic process and the prevalence of polyvascular atherosclerosis is common [46,47], the potential risk of other atherosclerosis should be considered. In particular, CAD often coexists with stroke because they share risk factors and pathogenesis [48,49] and the extent of CAD is associated with an incremental risk of stroke. In our study, the overall CVA prevalence among patients with non-obstructive CAD including one DV, two DVs, and three DVs was 8.9% (74/832), which is much higher than the prevalence of 3.72% for general Koreans of a similar age group [50]. This figure is similarly confirmed in the CVA prevalence (9.8%) in another study targeting Koreans with non-obstructive CAD [51]. In the present study, the occurrence of stroke but not a cardiac event contributed most to the occurrence of MACCE. These results have important implications for East Asian countries such as Korea, because stroke has a higher mortality than CAD in East Asia, opposed to findings in Western and other Asian countries [49].

Our results suggest that the total atherosclerotic burden is a more important factor in long-term prognosis than the dichotomous definition of CAD as obstructive or non-obstructive. That is, even non-obstructive CAD is associated with a worse prognosis if it is multi-vessel, especially non-obstructive three DVs. However, there are no clear guidelines for the management of patients with non-obstructive CAD, and there is lack of awareness that intensive treatment should be provided. Recently, management for the primary prevention of non-obstructive CAD patients has been studied [23,52]. In particular, a large-scale study [23] showed that aspirin had no benefit in patients with non-obstructive CAD, whereas statin was associated with a significant reduction in mortality for individuals with non-obstructive CAD. However, further research is still needed on the statin intensity or target level. In addition, non-obstructive CAD patients also have different effects across subgroups [51], requiring research on which patient groups are effective. Considering the results of our study, clinicians should consider intensive medical care when treating patients with multi-vessel non-obstructive CAD.

5. Limitations

The present study had several limitations. First, as a retrospective and observational study, selection bias could have contributed to the results. Second, since the degree of CAD stenosis and distribution were evaluated subjectively, there was a possibility of misclassification. However, this would have been offset by the performance in a single center. Third, plaque location such as proximal or distal and characteristics could affect MACCEs, but only the proximal LAD was analyzed, and the proximal left circumflex artery and right coronary artery involvement were not analyzed. Fourth, in patients with non-obstructive CAD, coronary artery spasm may have been one of the causes leading to sudden cardiac death and myocardial infarction, which may have influenced the results showing poor prognosis. However, coronary artery spasm was not investigated. Finally, despite a follow-up of 5 years, the occurrence of cardiac events was relatively small, so there was a limit to the interpretation. Therefore, data for a longer period are needed.

6. Conclusions

Multi-vessel non-obstructive CAD, reflecting higher atherosclerotic burden, is associated with poor long-term (5 years) clinical outcomes, mainly stroke. These findings suggest that more intensive treatment may be required in this subset of patients, and the risk of stroke, as well as of cardiovascular events, should be considered. Further large-scale prospective studies are needed to determine proper management to prevent future events in these patients.

Author Contributions: Conceptualization, J.J. and S.-N.L.; Methodology, S.-H.H.; Data curation, S.-N.L., S.-H.H., K.-D.Y., K.-W.M. and D.M.; Writing—original draft preparation, J.J.; Writing—review and editing, S.-N.L., W.-Y.J. and S.-H.H., Supervision, S.-N.L. All authors have read and agreed to the published version of the manuscript.

Funding: This study was supported by a grant from the Yuhan Corporation, Seoul, Republic of Korea (grant number: 5-2020-D0166-00004).

Institutional Review Board Statement: This study was approved by the Institutional Review Board (IRB) of St. Vincent hospital (IRB VC20RISI0087) and complied with the 1975 Declaration of Helsinki. The need for individual patient consent was waived.

Informed Consent Statement: The need for individual patient consent was waived.

Data Availability Statement: The data presented in this study are available on request from the corresponding author.

Conflicts of Interest: The authors declare that they have no known competing financial interests or personal relationships that could have appeared to influence the work reported in this paper.

References

1. Roth, G.A.; Mensah, G.A.; Johnson, C.O.; Addolorato, G.; Ammirati, E.; Baddour, L.M.; Barengo, N.C.; Beaton, A.Z.; Benjamin, E.J.; Benziger, C.P.; et al. Global Burden of Cardiovascular Diseases and Risk Factors, 1990–2019: Update From the GBD 2019 Study. *J. Am. Coll. Cardiol.* **2020**, *76*, 2982–3021. [CrossRef]
2. Yusuf, S.; Reddy, S.; Ounpuu, S.; Anand, S. Global burden of cardiovascular diseases: Part II: Variations in cardiovascular disease by specific ethnic groups and geographic regions and prevention strategies. *Circulation* **2001**, *104*, 2855–2864. [CrossRef]
3. Knuuti, J.; Wijns, W.; Saraste, A.; Capodanno, D.; Barbato, E.; Funck-Brentano, C.; Prescott, E.; Storey, R.F.; Deaton, C.; Cuisset, T.; et al. 2019 ESC Guidelines for the diagnosis and management of chronic coronary syndromes. *Eur. Heart J.* **2020**, *41*, 407–477. [CrossRef]
4. Gulati, M.; Levy, P.D.; Mukherjee, D.; Amsterdam, E.; Bhatt, D.L.; Birtcher, K.K.; Blankstein, R.; Boyd, J.; Bullock-Palmer, R.P.; Conejo, T.; et al. 2021 AHA/ACC/ASE/CHEST/SAEM/SCCT/SCMR Guideline for the Evaluation and Diagnosis of Chest Pain: A Report of the American College of Cardiology/American Heart Association Joint Committee on Clinical Practice Guidelines. *Circulation* **2021**, *144*, e368–e454.
5. Kim, Y.K.; Jang, C.W.; Kwon, S.H.; Kim, J.H.; Lerman, A.; Bae, J.H. Ten-year clinical outcomes in patients with intermediate coronary stenosis according to the combined culprit lesion. *Clin. Cardiol.* **2021**, *44*, 1161–1168. [CrossRef]
6. Olesen, K.K.W.; Madsen, M.; Lip, G.Y.H.; Egholm, G.; Thim, T.; Jensen, L.O.; Raungaard, B.; Nielsen, J.C.; Botker, H.E.; Sorensen, H.T.; et al. Coronary artery disease and risk of adverse cardiac events and stroke. *Eur. J. Clin. Investig.* **2017**, *47*, 819–828. [CrossRef]
7. Kemp, H.G.; Kronmal, R.A.; Vlietstra, R.E.; Frye, R.L. Seven year survival of patients with normal or near normal coronary arteriograms: A CASS registry study. *J. Am. Coll. Cardiol.* **1986**, *7*, 479–483. [CrossRef]
8. Patel, M.R.; Chen, A.Y.; Peterson, E.D.; Newby, L.K.; Pollack, C.V., Jr.; Brindis, R.G.; Gibson, C.M.; Kleiman, N.S.; Saucedo, J.F.; Bhatt, D.L.; et al. Prevalence, predictors, and outcomes of patients with non-ST-segment elevation myocardial infarction and insignificant coronary artery disease: Results from the Can Rapid risk stratification of Unstable angina patients Suppress ADverse outcomes with Early implementation of the ACC/AHA Guidelines (CRUSADE) initiative. *Am. Heart J.* **2006**, *152*, 641–647.
9. Stergiopoulos, K.; Boden, W.E.; Hartigan, P.; Mobius-Winkler, S.; Hambrecht, R.; Hueb, W.; Hardison, R.M.; Abbott, J.D.; Brown, D.L. Percutaneous coronary intervention outcomes in patients with stable obstructive coronary artery disease and myocardial ischemia: A collaborative meta-analysis of contemporary randomized clinical trials. *JAMA Intern. Med.* **2014**, *174*, 232–240. [CrossRef]
10. Sorajja, P.; Gersh, B.J.; Cox, D.A.; McLaughlin, M.G.; Zimetbaum, P.; Costantini, C.; Stuckey, T.; Tcheng, J.E.; Mehran, R.; Lansky, A.J.; et al. Impact of multivessel disease on reperfusion success and clinical outcomes in patients undergoing primary percutaneous coronary intervention for acute myocardial infarction. *Eur. Heart J.* **2007**, *28*, 1709–1716. [CrossRef]
11. Mach, F.; Baigent, C.; Catapano, A.L.; Koskinas, K.C.; Casula, M.; Badimon, L.; Chapman, M.J.; De Backer, G.G.; Delgado, V.; Ference, B.A.; et al. 2019 ESC/EAS Guidelines for the management of dyslipidaemias: Lipid modification to reduce cardiovascular risk. *Eur. Heart J.* **2020**, *41*, 111–188. [CrossRef]
12. Valgimigli, M.; Bueno, H.; Byrne, R.A.; Collet, J.P.; Costa, F.; Jeppsson, A.; Juni, P.; Kastrati, A.; Kolh, P.; Mauri, L.; et al. 2017 ESC focused update on dual antiplatelet therapy in coronary artery disease developed in collaboration with EACTS: The Task Force for dual antiplatelet therapy in coronary artery disease of the European Society of Cardiology (ESC) and of the European Association for Cardio-Thoracic Surgery (EACTS). *Eur. Heart J.* **2018**, *39*, 213–260.
13. Ambrose, J.A.; Tannenbaum, M.A.; Alexopoulos, D.; Hjemdahl-Monsen, C.E.; Leavy, J.; Weiss, M.; Borrico, S.; Gorlin, R.; Fuster, V. Angiographic progression of coronary artery disease and the development of myocardial infarction. *J. Am. Coll. Cardiol.* **1988**, *12*, 56–62. [CrossRef]
14. Maddox, T.M.; Stanislawski, M.A.; Grunwald, G.K.; Bradley, S.M.; Ho, P.M.; Tsai, T.T.; Patel, M.R.; Sandhu, A.; Valle, J.; Magid, D.J.; et al. Nonobstructive coronary artery disease and risk of myocardial infarction. *JAMA* **2014**, *312*, 1754–1763. [CrossRef]
15. Mortensen, M.B.; Dzaye, O.; Steffensen, F.H.; Botker, H.E.; Jensen, J.M.; Ronnow Sand, N.P.; Kragholm, K.H.; Sorensen, H.T.; Leipsic, J.; Maeng, M.; et al. Impact of Plaque Burden Versus Stenosis on Ischemic Events in Patients With Coronary Atherosclerosis. *J. Am. Coll. Cardiol.* **2020**, *76*, 2803–2813. [CrossRef]
16. Levine, G.N.; Bates, E.R.; Blankenship, J.C.; Bailey, S.R.; Bittl, J.A.; Cercek, B.; Chambers, C.E.; Ellis, S.G.; Guyton, R.A.; Hollenberg, S.M.; et al. 2011 ACCF/AHA/SCAI Guideline for Percutaneous Coronary Intervention. A report of the American College of Cardiology Foundation/American Heart Association Task Force on Practice Guidelines and the Society for Cardiovascular Angiography and Interventions. *J. Am. Coll. Cardiol.* **2011**, *58*, e44–e122. [CrossRef]
17. Redfors, B.; Furer, A.; Selker, H.P.; Thiele, H.; Patel, M.R.; Chen, S.; Udelson, J.E.; Ohman, E.M.; Eitel, I.; Granger, C.B.; et al. Effect of Smoking on Outcomes of Primary PCI in Patients With STEMI. *J. Am. Coll. Cardiol.* **2020**, *75*, 1743–1754. [CrossRef]
18. Matsuo, S.; Imai, E.; Horio, M.; Yasuda, Y.; Tomita, K.; Nitta, K.; Yamagata, K.; Tomino, Y.; Yokoyama, H.; Hishida, A.; et al. Revised equations for estimated GFR from serum creatinine in Japan. *Am. J. Kidney Dis.* **2009**, *53*, 982–992. [CrossRef]
19. Nakazato, R.; Arsanjani, R.; Achenbach, S.; Gransar, H.; Cheng, V.Y.; Dunning, A.; Lin, F.Y.; Al-Mallah, M.; Budoff, M.J.; Callister, T.Q.; et al. Age-related risk of major adverse cardiac event risk and coronary artery disease extent and severity by coronary CT angiography: Results from 15 187 patients from the International Multisite CONFIRM Study. *Eur. Heart J. Cardiovasc. Imaging* **2014**, *15*, 586–594. [CrossRef]

20. Rodriguez-Capitan, J.; Sanchez-Perez, A.; Ballesteros-Pradas, S.; Millan-Gomez, M.; Cardenal-Piris, R.; Oneto-Fernandez, M.; Gutierrez-Alonso, L.; Rivera-Lopez, R.; Guisado-Rasco, A.; Cano-Garcia, M.; et al. Prognostic Implication of Non-Obstructive Coronary Lesions: A New Classification in Different Settings. *J. Clin. Med.* **2021**, *10*, 1863. [CrossRef]
21. Little, W.C.; Constantinescu, M.; Applegate, R.J.; Kutcher, M.A.; Burrows, M.T.; Kahl, F.R.; Santamore, W.P. Can coronary angiography predict the site of a subsequent myocardial infarction in patients with mild-to-moderate coronary artery disease? *Circulation* **1988**, *78*, 1157–1166. [CrossRef] [PubMed]
22. Bittencourt, M.S.; Hulten, E.; Ghoshhajra, B.; O'Leary, D.; Christman, M.P.; Montana, P.; Truong, Q.A.; Steigner, M.; Murthy, V.L.; Rybicki, F.J.; et al. Prognostic value of nonobstructive and obstructive coronary artery disease detected by coronary computed tomography angiography to identify cardiovascular events. *Circ. Cardiovasc. Imaging* **2014**, *7*, 282–291. [CrossRef] [PubMed]
23. Chow, B.J.; Small, G.; Yam, Y.; Chen, L.; McPherson, R.; Achenbach, S.; Al-Mallah, M.; Berman, D.S.; Budoff, M.J.; Cademartiri, F.; et al. Prognostic and therapeutic implications of statin and aspirin therapy in individuals with nonobstructive coronary artery disease: Results from the CONFIRM (COronary CT Angiography EvaluatioN For Clinical Outcomes: An InteRnational Multicenter registry) registry. *Arterioscler. Thromb. Vasc. Biol.* **2015**, *35*, 981–989. [PubMed]
24. Jamee, A.; Abed, Y.; Jalambo, M.O. Gender difference and characteristics attributed to coronary artery disease in Gaza-Palestine. *Glob. J. Health Sci.* **2013**, *5*, 51–56. [CrossRef]
25. Kissel, C.K.; Chen, G.; Southern, D.A.; Galbraith, P.D.; Anderson, T.J.; For the APPROACH investigators. Impact of clinical presentation and presence of coronary sclerosis on long-term outcome of patients with non-obstructive coronary artery disease. *BMC Cardiovasc. Disord.* **2018**, *18*, 173. [CrossRef]
26. Zhang, H.W.; Jin, J.L.; Cao, Y.X.; Guo, Y.L.; Wu, N.Q.; Zhu, C.G.; Xu, R.X.; Dong, Q.; Li, J.J. Association of diabetes mellitus with clinical outcomes in patients with different coronary artery stenosis. *Cardiovasc. Diabetol.* **2021**, *20*, 214. [CrossRef]
27. Berge, C.A.; Eskerud, I.; Almeland, E.B.; Larsen, T.H.; Pedersen, E.R.; Rotevatn, S.; Lonnebakken, M.T. Relationship between hypertension and non-obstructive coronary artery disease in chronic coronary syndrome (the NORIC registry). *PLoS ONE* **2022**, *17*, e0262290. [CrossRef]
28. Wang, H.; Ning, X.; Zhu, C.; Yin, D.; Feng, L.; Xu, B.; Guan, C.; Dou, K. Prognostic significance of prior ischemic stroke in patients with coronary artery disease undergoing percutaneous coronary intervention. *Catheter. Cardiovasc. Interv.* **2019**, *93*, 787–792. [CrossRef]
29. Cosin-Sales, J.; Pizzi, C.; Brown, S.; Kaski, J.C. C-reactive protein, clinical presentation, and ischemic activity in patients with chest pain and normal coronary angiograms. *J. Am. Coll. Cardiol.* **2003**, *41*, 1468–1474. [CrossRef]
30. Ridker, P.M.; Bhatt, D.L.; Pradhan, A.D.; Glynn, R.J.; MacFadyen, J.G.; Nissen, S.E.; Prominent, R.-I.; Investigators, S. Inflammation and cholesterol as predictors of cardiovascular events among patients receiving statin therapy: A collaborative analysis of three randomised trials. *Lancet* **2023**, *401*, 1293–1301. [CrossRef]
31. McCabe, J.J.; Walsh, C.; Gorey, S.; Harris, K.; Hervella, P.; Iglesias-Rey, R.; Jern, C.; Li, L.; Miyamoto, N.; Montaner, J.; et al. C-Reactive Protein, Interleukin-6, and Vascular Recurrence After Stroke: An Individual Participant Data Meta-Analysis. *Stroke* **2023**, *54*, 1289–1299. [CrossRef] [PubMed]
32. Han, D.; Chen, B.; Gransar, H.; Achenbach, S.; Al-Mallah, M.H.; Budoff, M.J.; Cademartiri, F.; Maffei, E.; Callister, T.Q.; Chinnaiyan, K.; et al. Prognostic significance of plaque location in non-obstructive coronary artery disease: From the CONFIRM registry. *Eur. Heart J. Cardiovasc. Imaging* **2022**, *23*, 1240–1247. [CrossRef] [PubMed]
33. Eskerud, I.; Gerdts, E.; Larsen, T.H.; Simon, J.; Maurovich-Horvat, P.; Lonnebakken, M.T. Total coronary atherosclerotic plaque burden is associated with myocardial ischemia in non-obstructive coronary artery disease. *Int. J. Cardiol. Heart Vasc.* **2021**, *35*, 100831. [CrossRef] [PubMed]
34. Mushtaq, S.; De Araujo Goncalves, P.; Garcia-Garcia, H.M.; Pontone, G.; Bartorelli, A.L.; Bertella, E.; Campos, C.M.; Pepi, M.; Serruys, P.W.; Andreini, D. Long-term prognostic effect of coronary atherosclerotic burden: Validation of the computed tomography-Leaman score. *Circ. Cardiovasc. Imaging* **2015**, *8*, e002332. [CrossRef] [PubMed]
35. Arbab-Zadeh, A.; Fuster, V. The Risk Continuum of Atherosclerosis and its Implications for Defining CHD by Coronary Angiography. *J. Am. Coll. Cardiol.* **2016**, *68*, 2467–2478. [CrossRef] [PubMed]
36. Yamaura, H.; Otsuka, K.; Ishikawa, H.; Shirasawa, K.; Fukuda, D.; Kasayuki, N. Determinants of Non-calcified Low-Attenuation Coronary Plaque Burden in Patients Without Known Coronary Artery Disease: A Coronary CT Angiography Study. *Front. Cardiovasc. Med.* **2022**, *9*, 824470. [CrossRef]
37. Otsuka, K.; Fukuda, S.; Tanaka, A.; Nakanishi, K.; Taguchi, H.; Yoshiyama, M.; Shimada, K.; Yoshikawa, J. Prognosis of vulnerable plaque on computed tomographic coronary angiography with normal myocardial perfusion image. *Eur. Heart J. Cardiovasc. Imaging* **2014**, *15*, 332–340. [CrossRef]
38. Gutierrez, E.; Flammer, A.J.; Lerman, L.O.; Elizaga, J.; Lerman, A.; Fernandez-Aviles, F. Endothelial dysfunction over the course of coronary artery disease. *Eur. Heart J.* **2013**, *34*, 3175–3181. [CrossRef]
39. Lerman, A.; Cannan, C.R.; Higano, S.H.; Nishimura, R.A.; Holmes, D.R., Jr. Coronary vascular remodeling in association with endothelial dysfunction. *Am. J. Cardiol.* **1998**, *81*, 1105–1109. [CrossRef]
40. Yeboah, J.; Crouse, J.R.; Hsu, F.C.; Burke, G.L.; Herrington, D.M. Brachial flow-mediated dilation predicts incident cardiovascular events in older adults: The Cardiovascular Health Study. *Circulation* **2007**, *115*, 2390–2397. [CrossRef]
41. Suwaidi, J.A.; Hamasaki, S.; Higano, S.T.; Nishimura, R.A.; Holmes, D.R., Jr.; Lerman, A. Long-term follow-up of patients with mild coronary artery disease and endothelial dysfunction. *Circulation* **2000**, *101*, 948–954. [CrossRef]

42. Manganaro, A.; Ciraci, L.; Andre, L.; Trio, O.; Manganaro, R.; Saporito, F.; Oreto, G.; Ando, G. Endothelial dysfunction in patients with coronary artery disease: Insights from a flow-mediated dilation study. *Clin. Appl. Thromb. Hemost.* **2014**, *20*, 583–588. [CrossRef]
43. Vaccarino, V.; Parsons, L.; Every, N.R.; Barron, H.V.; Krumholz, H.M. Sex-based differences in early mortality after myocardial infarction. National Registry of Myocardial Infarction 2 Participants. *N. Engl. J. Med.* **1999**, *341*, 217–225. [CrossRef]
44. Waheed, N.; Elias-Smale, S.; Malas, W.; Maas, A.H.; Sedlak, T.L.; Tremmel, J.; Mehta, P.K. Sex differences in non-obstructive coronary artery disease. *Cardiovasc. Res.* **2020**, *116*, 829–840. [CrossRef]
45. Schamroth Pravda, N.; Karny-Rahkovich, O.; Shiyovich, A.; Schamroth Pravda, M.; Rapeport, N.; Vaknin-Assa, H.; Eisen, A.; Kornowski, R.; Porter, A. Coronary Artery Disease in Women: A Comprehensive Appraisal. *J. Clin. Med.* **2021**, *10*, 4664. [CrossRef]
46. Fernandez-Friera, L.; Penalvo, J.L.; Fernandez-Ortiz, A.; Ibanez, B.; Lopez-Melgar, B.; Laclaustra, M.; Oliva, B.; Mocoroa, A.; Mendiguren, J.; Martinez de Vega, V.; et al. Prevalence, Vascular Distribution, and Multiterritorial Extent of Subclinical Atherosclerosis in a Middle-Aged Cohort: The PESA (Progression of Early Subclinical Atherosclerosis) Study. *Circulation* **2015**, *131*, 2104–2113. [CrossRef]
47. Baber, U.; Mehran, R.; Sartori, S.; Schoos, M.M.; Sillesen, H.; Muntendam, P.; Garcia, M.J.; Gregson, J.; Pocock, S.; Falk, E.; et al. Prevalence, impact, and predictive value of detecting subclinical coronary and carotid atherosclerosis in asymptomatic adults: The BioImage study. *J. Am. Coll. Cardiol.* **2015**, *65*, 1065–1074. [CrossRef]
48. Witt, B.J.; Ballman, K.V.; Brown, R.D., Jr.; Meverden, R.A.; Jacobsen, S.J.; Roger, V.L. The incidence of stroke after myocardial infarction: A meta-analysis. *Am. J. Med.* **2006**, *119*, 354.e1–354.e9. [CrossRef]
49. Hata, J.; Kiyohara, Y. Epidemiology of stroke and coronary artery disease in Asia. *Circ. J.* **2013**, *77*, 1923–1932. [CrossRef]
50. Kim, J.Y.; Kang, K.; Kang, J.; Koo, J.; Kim, D.H.; Kim, B.J.; Kim, W.J.; Kim, E.G.; Kim, J.G.; Kim, J.M.; et al. Executive Summary of Stroke Statistics in Korea 2018: A Report from the Epidemiology Research Council of the Korean Stroke Society. *J. Stroke* **2019**, *21*, 42–59. [CrossRef]
51. Hwang, I.C.; Lee, H.; Yoon, Y.E.; Choi, I.S.; Kim, H.L.; Chang, H.J.; Lee, J.Y.; Choi, J.A.; Kim, H.J.; Cho, G.Y.; et al. Risk stratification of non-obstructive coronary artery disease for guidance of preventive medical therapy. *Atherosclerosis* **2019**, *290*, 66–73. [CrossRef]
52. Handberg, E.M.; Merz, C.N.B.; Cooper-Dehoff, R.M.; Wei, J.; Conlon, M.; Lo, M.C.; Boden, W.; Frayne, S.M.; Villines, T.; Spertus, J.A.; et al. Rationale and design of the Women's Ischemia Trial to Reduce Events in Nonobstructive CAD (WARRIOR) trial. *Am. Heart J.* **2021**, *237*, 90–103. [CrossRef]

Disclaimer/Publisher's Note: The statements, opinions and data contained in all publications are solely those of the individual author(s) and contributor(s) and not of MDPI and/or the editor(s). MDPI and/or the editor(s) disclaim responsibility for any injury to people or property resulting from any ideas, methods, instructions or products referred to in the content.

Article

Predictors of Readmission after the First Acute Coronary Syndrome and the Risk of Recurrent Cardiovascular Events—Seven Years of Patient Follow-Up

Cristiana Bustea [1,†], Delia Mirela Tit [2,3,*], Alexa Florina Bungau [1,3,*], Simona Gabriela Bungau [2,3,†], Vlad Alin Pantea [4,†], Elena Emilia Babes [5] and Larisa Renata Pantea-Roșan [5]

1. Department of Preclinical Disciplines, Faculty of Medicine and Pharmacy, University of Oradea, 410073 Oradea, Romania
2. Department of Pharmacy, Faculty of Medicine and Pharmacy, University of Oradea, 410028 Oradea, Romania
3. Doctoral School of Biomedical Sciences, University of Oradea, 410087 Oradea, Romania
4. Department of Dental Medicine, Faculty of Medicine and Pharmacy, University of Oradea, 410073 Oradea, Romania
5. Department of Medical Disciplines, Faculty of Medicine and Pharmacy, University of Oradea, 410073 Oradea, Romania

* Correspondence: mirela_tit@yahoo.com (D.M.T.); pradaalexaflorina@gmail.com (A.F.B.)
† These authors contributed equally to this work.

Abstract: Recurrent hospitalization after acute coronary syndromes (ACS) is common. Identifying risk factors associated with subsequent cardiovascular events and hospitalization is essential for the management of these patients. Our research consisted in observing the outcomes of subjects after they suffered an acute coronary event and identifying the factors that can predict rehospitalization in the first 12 months and the recurrence of another acute coronary episode. Data from 362 patients admitted with ACS during 2013 were studied. Recurrent hospitalizations were retrospectively reviewed from medical charts and electronic hospital archives over a period of seven years. The mean age of the studied population was 64.57 ± 11.79 years, 64.36% of them being males. The diagnosis of ACS without ST elevation was registered in 53.87% of the patients at index hospitalization. More than half had recurrent hospitalization in the first year after the first ACS episode. Patients with lower ejection fraction (39.20 ± 6.85 vs. 42.24 ± 6.26, $p < 0.001$), acute pulmonary edema during the first hospitalization (6.47% vs. 1.24%, $p = 0.022$), coexistent valvular heart disease (69.15% vs. 55.90%, $p = 0.017$), and three-vessel disease (18.90% vs. 7.45%, $p = 0.002$) were more frequently readmitted in the following twelve months after their first acute coronary event, while those with complete revascularization were less frequently admitted (24.87% vs. 34.78%, $p = 0.005$). In multiple regression, complete revascularization during the index event (HR = 0.58, 95% CI 0.35–0.95, $p = 0.03$) and a higher LVEF (left ventricular ejection fraction) (HR = 0.95, 95% CI 0.92–0.988, $p = 0.009$) remained independent predictors of fewer early readmissions. Complete revascularization of the coronary lesions at the time of the first event and a preserved LVEF were found to be the predictors of reduced hospitalizations in the first year after an acute coronary event.

Keywords: recurrent cardiovascular events; predictors; hospital readmission; first acute coronary syndrome; complete revascularization; STEMI

1. Introduction

Cardiovascular diseases (CVD) represent the main factor in increasing incidence of death among the population, becoming the most common cause of death worldwide [1]. Ischemic coronary artery diseases (CADs) are among the cardiovascular diseases with increased risk of death, through the appearance of acute coronary syndromes (ACS). Acute myocardial ischemia, which results from inadequate blood flow across the coronary tree, determines the cluster of symptoms known as ACS [2]. Acute thoracic discomfort, which can be characterized as pressure, pain, burning, or tightness, is the primary sign that starts the diagnostic and therapeutic process in patients with presumed ACS. Dyspnea, discomfort in the epigastric area, and left arm pain are typical signs that are comparable to pain in the chest [3].

Three distinct categories of medical symptoms are typically covered by ACS. These are classified based on the ST-segment on the electrocardiogram (ECG) trace as non-ST-segment elevation, such as unstable angina (UA) and non-ST-segment elevation myocardial infarction (NSTEMI), or as ST-segment elevation, such as acute ST-segment elevation myocardial infarction (STEMI) [4].

ACS occurs several years after the development and progression of atheromatous plaque [5]. Atherosclerosis is inextricably linked to development/appearance of vulnerable atherosclerotic plaques and of ACS.

After formation, the atheromatous plaques may be stable for a long time. Their destabilization due to the appearance of a rupture of a vulnerable atheromatous plaque leads to ACS. The rupture of the atheromatous plaque induces platelet activation that results in the formation of the initial white thrombus, and then of the red thrombus, due to the hematologic elements in the fibrin network, which can partially or completely block the coronary artery lumen. Significant partial blockage of the lumen causes UA or NSTEMI, while complete blockage causes STEMI [6].

An unhealthy lifestyle, associated with non-modifiable CVD risk factors (like gender, age, genetic factors) or modifiable ones (like dyslipidemia, hypertension, diabetes, obesity, chronic kidney disease (CKD), or psycho-emotional stress), facilitates and stimulates atheromatous plaques [7]. Unhealthy diet/eating habits, a sedentary lifestyle, and/or smoking are associated with high plasma total cholesterol levels which trigger the atherogenic cascade and, in time, the development of CAD with the appearance of ACS [8]. Furthermore, the findings of a recent investigation revealed that a body mass index (BMI) of more than 25 kg/m^2 is a significant indicator for increased on-treatment platelet reactivity in patients with STEMI receiving dual antiplatelet medication with ticagrelor or prasugrel and is correlated with tardy pharmacodynamic response to oral third-generation P2Y12 inhibitor loading dose [9].

Despite recent improvements in ACS treatment, CAD remains a major public health problem. Patients having ACS can be considered as also having a much higher risk (both short- and long-term) of recurrent CV events and hospitalizations. The possibility of such a recurrent CV event occurrence, or even the death of the subject, is most likely immediately after occurrence of ACS or in the next 12 months [10–12], and continues to be elevated in the following few years [12,13]. Comparing the data of a representative US population with an ACS event as the follow-up criterion, the event rate/5 years (representing non-fatal stroke or MI, or cardiovascular death) was 33.4%. Immediately following the index ACS, the risk was ≈six-fold higher compared to more than a year after leaving the hospital [14].

The overall goal of the management of patients with ACS is to re-establish and stabilize coronary blood flow and to initiate appropriate treatment to reduce the likelihood of recurrent CV events [15]. To prevent readmission and recurrent ACS, evidence-based post-discharge recommendations including medication, patient education, cardiac rehabilitation, and regular follow-up are required. Evidence from representative ACS populations from a current clinical practice setting will help in identifying strategies for improving patient outcomes. Considering the above-mentioned points, it is mandatory to understand in detail not only the studied populations' characteristics, the chances of risk with the passage of time, the perception of the patterns, and the results of the current medical practice, but also the method for choosing the secondary prevention strategy (which is optimal for additional risk mitigation).

Therefore, we decided to focus on observing the short-/long-term evolution of subjects who had suffered an acute coronary event and identifying those factors that can predict rehospitalization in the first twelve months after ACS due to a recurrence of another acute coronary episode. In order to give importance to this research and to provide relevant results, the observations took place over seven years. This topic is rarely discussed in the literature, especially with this approach. The study design allows the identification of factors associated with readmission as well as the determination of independent predictors of reduced hospitalizations in the first year after an acute coronary event. The obtained findings can assist healthcare professionals in deciding what steps to take to lessen the possibility of readmission for patients who are affected.

2. Materials and Methods

2.1. Patient Selection

This retrospective study was carried out by following 362 patients who had been admitted to the Oradea County Emergency Clinical Hospital, Unit for Advanced Monitoring and Treatment of Critical Cardiac Patients for ACS, between 1 January 2013 and 31 December 2013. The outcome and recurrent hospitalizations were reviewed from medical charts and the electronic hospital archive during a 7-year period, until 30 June 2020.

The study included patients who presented with ACS in 2013 and who were readmitted at least once in the following 7 years. The exclusion criteria used for patient selection were as follows:

- Patients who had stable angina pectoris;
- Patients with ACS at the hospital admission moment who could not be dynamically monitored due to insufficient data;
- Patients with oncological conditions (they are at risk of cardiovascular complications due to cancer treatment that can influence the rate of hospital readmission [16]), or psychiatric conditions (which imply a reduced compliance with treatment that can influence recurrent hospitalization rate [17]) at the time of hospitalization for ACS;
- Pregnant or lactating patients.

Initially, 574 patients were considered for potential inclusion in the study. However, only 362 patients met both of the aforementioned inclusion criteria. Figure 1 contains the flow chart describing the patient selection process. All 362 patients were readmitted at least once during the 7 years of follow-up. They were analyzed by comparing early (1 year) vs. late (more than 1 year) rehospitalizations.

ACS was diagnosed referencing the current European Society of Cardiology (ESC) Clinical Practice Guidelines. Acute myocardial infarction (AMI) was diagnosed when the following criteria were met:

- Typical angina clinical picture included suffering from myocardial ischemia accompanied by a rise in biomarkers of myocardial necrosis above the 99th percentile of the upper reference;
- Considering the level of the electrocardiographic (ECK) trace: new major left bundle branch block, ST-segment elevation, or the presence of a new Q wave;
- Checking the ECG, the presence of parietal kinetic disorders was observed;
- Angiographically: total occlusion of the coronary artery affected in the infarction [18].

Differentiation of STEMI from NSTEMI is based on ECG trace criteria. Thus, STEMI is considered to be present when a new ST-segment elevation or J-point elevation ≥ 1 mm is observed on the ECG trace in at least two contiguous leads other than V2 and V3, with the following particularities regarding V2–V3 leads:

- ≥ 2 mm (in men >40-years-old);
- ≥ 2.5 mm (in men <40-years-old);
- ≥ 1.5 mm (in women).

NSTEMI is considered to have occurred when ST-segment elevation ≥ 0.5 mm in two contiguous leads or when negative T-wave > 1 mm in two contiguous leads is present on the ECG trace [18]. At the same time, recurrent myocardial infarction is considered to be an AMI that occurs more than 28 days after a first AMI [18]. Unstable angina is considered to be part of ACS with no ST-segment elevation, along with NSTEMI; the difference between the two is based on the presence of myocyte necrosis revealed by the elevated levels of myocardial necrosis enzymes in the case of NSTEMI [19].

All patients were discharged after the first hospitalization with medication recommended by ESC guidelines for secondary prevention after acute coronary syndrome consisting of statins, P2Y12 inhibitors, β-blockers, aspirin, and angiotensin-receptor blockers or angiotensin-converting enzyme inhibitors.

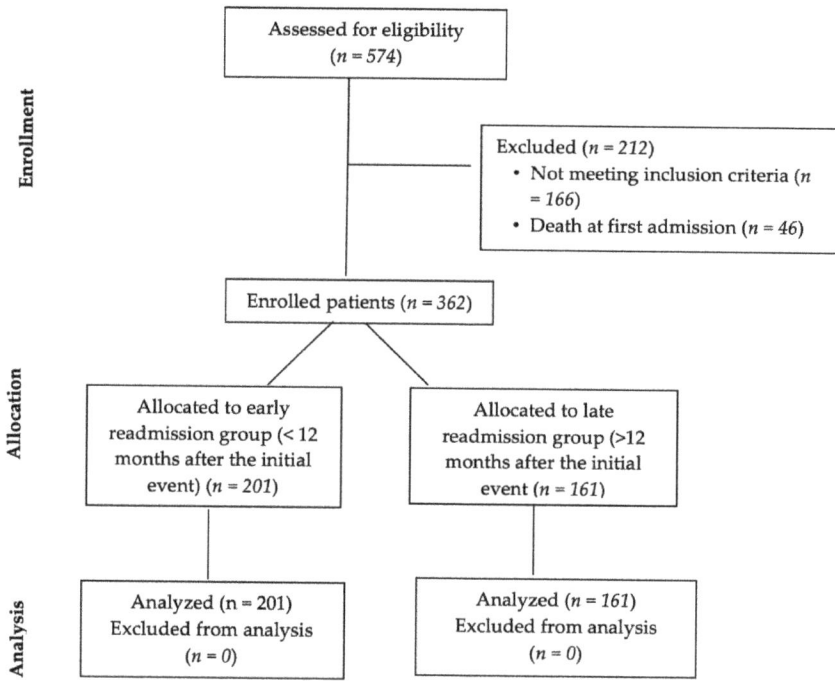

Figure 1. Type CONSORT diagram.

2.2. Statistical Analysis

Excel (2019 version) tabulated data were processed using the SPSS statistical package (version 25 statistical software) [20]. The obtained results are described as mean ± SD (for continuous variables), and as frequencies and % (for categorical variables). Additionally, the 2 groups were compared through the independent sample t-test (in the case of continuous variables) or the Kruskal–Wallis test (in the case of the categorical variables). The Pearson bivariate correlation test allowed the analysis of the relationship between the continuous variables, and the Spearman bivariate correlation test was performed for the categorical variables.

In the case of significantly different parameters for the 2 groups with rehospitalization in the first year and more than one year after the first event, a multiple-regression type analysis was used in order to calculate each parameter's value as an independent predictor for readmission in the first 12 months ($p < 0.05$ being considered statistically significant).

3. Results

A total of 362 patients was enrolled in the study; 233 were males; the mean age was 64.57 ± 11.79 years at first hospitalization for ACS. Regarding the type of ACS at first presentation, the diagnosis of ACS without ST elevation was more frequent, found in 195 patients (53.87%). For the group of patients with ACS without ST elevation, most had unstable angina (UA).

At the first hospitalization for ACS, patients presented with various cardiovascular risk factors and/or history of cardiovascular diseases. Most of them had dyslipidemia and hypertension, and many of them had diabetes and CKD (Table 1). A history of previous (old) myocardial infarction was registered in 21.5% of patients, and a large proportion of them had valvular heart disease and heart failure, or history of stroke (Table 1).

Coronarography was performed in 56% of patients and revealed mostly single-vessel disease. The artery most frequently affected was the left anterior descending artery, corresponding to the involvement of the anterior wall of the left ventricle and with ECG changes in the anterior territory. Most of the patients were treated with interventional revascularization, and only a limited number of patients with STEMI were subjected to thrombolysis. The patients with thrombolytic reperfusion therapy refused interventional investigation and treatment (10.5%). Five patients originating from geographic areas without hospitals containing percutaneous intervention (PCI) facilities were initially treated with thrombolytic therapy and then transferred to our hospital, where interventional revascularization was completed (they were eventually included in the PCI group).

Table 1. Baseline first-admission characteristics of patients enrolled in the study.

Demographic Baseline Characteristics		No. (%)
Patients (number)		362
Age (year)		64.57 ± 11.79
Sex (Male)		233 (64.36)
Urban environment		190 (52.6)
Type of Acute Coronary Syndrome		
ST-elevation myocardial infarction		167 (46.13)
Non-ST elevation myocardial infarction		64 (17.68)
Unstable angina		131 (36.2)
Cardiovascular Risk Factors and Comorbidities		
Smoking		122 (33,7)
Previous MI		78 (21.55)
Hypertension		254 (70.16)
	Grade I	30 (8.29)
	Grade II	196 (54.14)
	Grade III	28 (7.73)
Dyslipidemia		274 (75.7)
Chronic heart failure (according to New York Heart Association functional classification of heart failure, NYHA)		184 (50.82)
	I	12 (3.31)
	II	118 (32.59)
	III	44 (12.15)
	IV	12 (3.31)
Valvular heart disease		229 (63.26)
Chronic kidney disease		103 (28.45)
Diabetes type 2		141 (38.95)
	Oral therapy	69 (19.06)
	Insulin	72 (19.89)
History of stroke		27 (7.45)

Table 1. Cont.

ECG Territory Changes	
Anterior	98 (27.07)
Anterior and inferior	14 (3.87)
Anterior and lateral	10 (2.76)
Anterior septum	16 (4.41)
Inferior	64 (17.68)
Inferior and right leads	8 (2.21)
Inferior and lateral	16 (4.42)
Posterior and inferior	4 (1.10)
Echocardiography	
Left ventricular ejection fraction	40.45 ± 6.73
Coronary Angiography	
Not performed	159 (43.92)
Single-vessel disease	83 (22.92)
Left anterior descending artery	54 (14.9)
Circumflex artery	6 (1.6)
Right coronary artery	23 (8.8)
Two-vessel disease	70 (19.34)
Left main	6 (1.7)
Left anterior descending artery—circumflex coronary artery	30 (8.3)
Left anterior descending artery—right coronary artery	20 (5.5)
Circumflex coronary artery—right coronary artery	14 (3.9)
Three-vessel disease	50 (13.8)
Myocardial Revascularization Procedure	
Thrombolysis	38 (10.5)
Interventional or surgical revascularization	
Percutaneous coronary intervention	176 (48.62)
Coronary artery bypass graft	4 (1.10)
Not performed	182 (50.28)

During the first episode of hospitalization, the most frequent complications were rhythm disturbances, followed by cardiogenic shock and acute pulmonary edema (Table 2). A reduced number of patients presented at first admission with a hemorrhagic complication possibly related to antiplatelet, anticoagulant thrombolytic therapy: six patients had UGB, and 0.98% had a hemorrhagic stroke (Table 2).

During a follow-up period of seven years, all the patients were readmitted at least once. They registered a mean number of 4.46 ± 2.37 rehospitalizations during follow-up. More than half of the patients had recurrent hospitalization in the first year after the first ACS episode, and 44.5% of the patients were readmitted more than 12 months after the first acute coronary event (Figure 2).

Table 2. In-hospital complications of patients with acute coronary syndrome, at their first admission.

In-Hospital Complications	No (%)
Rhythm disturbances	95 (26.24)
Atrio-ventricular block, first degree	2 (0.55)
Atrio-ventricular block, first degree + left bundle branch block	2 (0.55)
Third-degree atrio-ventricular block	2 (0.55)
Left bundle branch block	4 (1.1)
Premature atrial beats	12 (3.31)
Premature ventricular beats	13 (3.59)
Paroxysmal atrial fibrillation	4 (1.1)
Persistent atrial fibrillation	38 (10.5)
Atrial fibrillation + third-degree atrio-ventricular block	2 (0.55)
Ventricular tachycardia non-sustained	4 (1.1)
Sustained ventricular tachycardia	6 (1.66)
Ventricular fibrillation	6 (1.7)
Acute pulmonary edema	15 (4.14)
Cardiogenic shock	20 (5.52)
Resuscitated cardiac arrest	15 (4.14)
Upper gastrointestinal bleeding	6 (1.65)
Acute stroke	6 (1.65)
Ischemic	2 (0.55)
Hemorrhagic	4 (1.1)

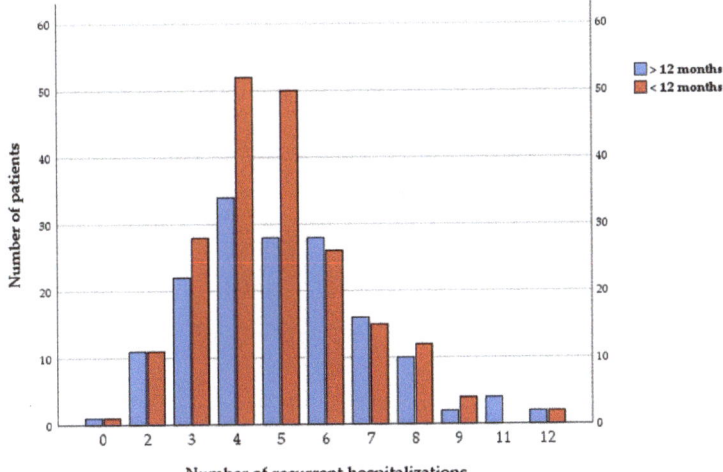

Figure 2. Number of recurrent hospitalizations.

No statistically significant differences existed between patients readmitted in the first 12 months compared to those readmitted after the first year, regarding associated cardiovascular risk factors. Patients with acute heart failure (specifically, acute pulmonary edema) during the first hospitalization were more frequently readmitted in the following 12 months after the first acute coronary event. Moreover, those with early readmission in the first 12 months had lower ejection fractions and more frequently associated valvular diseases (Table 3).

Angiographic characteristics at first admission that significantly correlated with recurrent hospitalization in the first 12 months were three-vessel involvement and incomplete revascularization during the first interventional procedure.

Table 3. Comparison between patients with early readmission (in the next 12 months following the initial event) and late readmission (>12 months after the initial event).

Demographic Parameters	Readmission < 12 Months —No. (%)	Readmission > 12 Months —No. (%)	p
	201 (55.52)	161 (44.48)	
Age (Y)	64.23 ± 10.871	64.18 ± 12.363	0.969
Sex (F)	76/201 (37.81)	53/161 (32.92)	0.432
Type of Acute Coronary Syndromes at First Admission			
ST-elevation myocardial infarction	93/201 (46.28)	74/161 (45.96)	0.954
non-ST elevation myocardial infarction	39/201 (19.40)	25/161 (15.53)	0.415
Unstable angina	70/201 (34.83)	61/161 (37.89)	0.485
Risk Factors and Comorbidities			
History of previous myocardial infarction	41/201 (20.39)	37/161 (22.98)	0.514
Hypertension	141/201 (70.14)	113/161 (70.19)	0.62
Dyslipidemia	154/201 (76.61)	120/161 (74.5)	0.497
Diabetes	81/201 (40.29)	60/161 (37.26)	0.682
Chronic kidney disease	65/201 (32.33)	38/161 (23.60)	0.055
Chronic heart failure	115/201 (57.21)	69/161 (42.86)	0.191
Acute pulmonary edema at first admission	13/201 (6.47)	2/161 (1.24)	0.022 *
Cardiogenic shock at first admission	15/201 (7.46)	5/161 (3.11)	0.056
Valvular heart disease	139/201 (69.15)	90/161 (55.90)	0.017 *
Left ventricular ejection fraction %	39.20 ± 6.85	42.24 ± 6.26	<0.001 *
Arrhythmias	53/201 (26.37)	42/161 (26.09)	0.889
History of stroke	15/201 (7.46)	12/161 (7.45)	0.541
Upper gastrointestinal bleeding	4/201 (1.99)	2/161 (1.24)	0.594
Resuscitated cardiac arrest	11/201 (5.47)	4/161 (2.48)	0.052
Thrombolysis at first admission	18/201 (8.96)	20/161 (12.42)	0.262
Coronarography Characteristics at First Admission			
Single-vessel disease	39/201 (19.40)	44/161 (27.33)	0.065
Two-vessel disease	40/201 (19.9)	30/161 (18.63)	0.806
Three-vessel disease	38/201 (18.90)	12/161 (7.45)	0.002 *
Revascularization Type of Procedure at First Admission			
Percutaneous coronary intervention	102/201 (50.74)	74/161 (45.96)	0.81
Coronary artery bypass graft	-	4/161 (2.48)	-
Complete revascularization at first admission	50/201 (24.87)	56/161 (34.78)	0.005 *

* p values < 0.05.

Multiple regression was used to analyze parameters significantly different between the two groups. Independent predictors for fewer early readmissions in the first 12 months after a first episode of ACS remained complete revascularization procedure at first hospitalization (HR = 0.58, 95% CI 0.35–0.95, p = 0.03) and a higher LVEF (HR = 0.95, 95% CI 0.92–0.988, p = 0.009) (Figure 3).

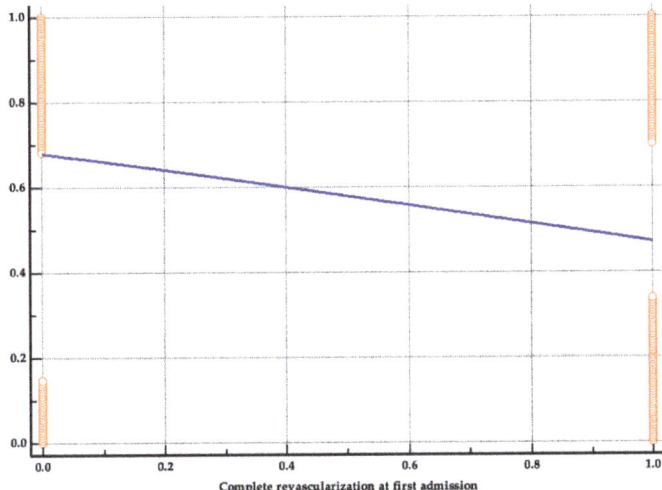

Figure 3. Regression analysis for complete revascularization procedure.

In 151 patients (41.71%), the second hospitalization readmission was due to ACS. The type of ACS was STEMI in 26 (17.21%) patients, NSTEMI in 22 patients (14.57%), and UA in 103 patients (68.21%). Of those patients with second admission due to STEMI, 12 patients (46.15%) presented in the first year after the first acute coronary event. Of the patients with NSTEMI, 12 (54.54%) were readmitted in the first year after the first acute coronary event. For most of the patients who presented with UA at the second admission (69 (66.99%)), symptoms occurred in the first 12 months after the first event.

Readmission for STEMI diagnosis was significantly correlated with both the existence of three-vessel CAD and the diagnosis of UA at first admission. Moreover, patients readmitted for STEMI had a lower ejection fraction at initial evaluation (Table 4). Readmission with NSTEMI diagnosis was more common in those having a previous old MI in their medical history, with two-vessel CAD, or with revascularization limited to the culprit lesion during first admission to the hospital.

Readmission for UA was more common in those subjects with associated heart failure, a lower ejection fraction, and associated CKD (Table 4). UGB at first hospitalization was significantly associated with readmission for STEMI or NSTEMI, probably due to inadequate dual antiplatelet therapy in the context of hemorrhagic complications during the first hospitalization. The obtained results indicate a weak-to-average correlation between the studied variables, which is nevertheless significant from a statistical point of view. Thus, it can be stated that the association between the variables is found at the same intensity, both in the sample and in the entire population.

Table 4. Significant correlations between parameters (at index hospitalization) and acute coronary syndrome type (at the second admission).

Significant Correlations for ST-Elevation Myocardial Infarction	p	r
Three-vessel disease	0.034	0.364
Left ventricular ejection fraction	0.013	0.359
Upper gastrointestinal bleeding at first hospitalization	0.012	0.361
Unstable angina at first hospitalization	0.002	0.361

Table 4. Cont.

Significant Correlation for Non-ST Elevation Myocardial Infarction		
Culprit-lesion-only revascularization	0.028	0.351
Two-vessel coronary artery disease	0.018	0.361
Previous myocardial infarction	0.004	0.361
Upper gastrointestinal bleeding at first hospitalization	0.005	0.361
Significant Correlation for Unstable Angina Pectoris		
Heart failure	0.005	0.361
Left ventricular ejection fraction	0.002	0.359
Chronic kidney disease	0.0018	0.361

4. Discussion

Because of its prevalence and the consequent elevated risk of repeated ischemic cardiovascular events, ACS remains a significant difficulty for specialists. Patients still experience a surprisingly increased risk of early repetitive ischemic episodes after ACS, regardless of recent improvements in both medical and interventional treatments.

There were fewer women than men with ACS in the present study, but no significant difference resulted between the two sexes with respect to recurrent hospitalization in the first 12 months after the index event. Although CHD is traditionally considered a male disease, clinical data (including reinfarction rates and MI mortality) reveal worse outcomes in women [21]. Similar results were presented in another observational multicenter retrospective study that included 1308 women and 2437 men. Both in the short and long term, no significant differences were found between the sexes, neither related to mortality, nor regarding the combined end point (reinfarction, cardiogenic shock, bleeding, stroke, or death) [22]. Additionally, a group of subjects from Canada, hospitalized with ACS and under follow-up for up to 2 years, highlighted the increased risk of adverse clinical outcomes in the case of women with ACS (who benefited from an early, invasive strategy, and from coronary revascularization) vs. men, although these differences were not seen in those treated with medical therapy alone [23].

Almost half of the ACS patients were initially admitted with STEMI, followed by UA, and only after that by NSTEMI. However, if ACS were categorized based only on the presence/absence of ST-segment elevation, the ratio of patients reverses, with more than half of them presenting with ACS without ST-segment elevation. Most studies on ACS define ACS as with/without ST-segment elevation and thus consider the frequency of non-ST-segment elevation ACS to be predominant, when, in fact, the differentiation of UA from NSTEMI in the case of ACS without ST-segment elevation is mostly omitted. This ignores the importance of the incidence of STEMI, though the presence of patients with STEMI is much higher compared to patients who develop NSTEMI or UA [24–26].

According to McManus DD [27], the incidence rates of STEMI are continuously declining compared to the previous data, while the incidence of NSTEMI has started to increase significantly lately. Neumann JT [28] believes that both the incidence rates of STEMI and UAP are declining, and only the incidence rates of NSTEMI are increasing.

However, the incidence rates of STEMI continue to be high among patients with CAD, but one should not ignore the incidence of ACS without ST-segment elevation which, as our research also shows, presents an increased ratio in terms of the incidence of patients with NSTEMI and UAP.

According to Wang TKM [29], NSTEMI patient mortality rates are low, despite the increased incidence of non-ST-elevation ACS vs. STEMI or UA patient mortality rates, which are increasing.

Percutaneous or surgical coronary intervention for myocardial revascularization was indicated for patients with STEMI and NSTEMI, respectively, and less indicated for patients with UAP. Thus, most patients underwent PCI for myocardial revascularization, and only a very few patients underwent CAGB. According to Spadaccio [30], the decision to perform PCI vs. CAGB must be made by the heart team, which assesses the individualized risks and benefits for the patient [31]. However, there was no significant difference in terms of in-hospital mortality and survival among patients who underwent PCI or CAGB [32].

Thrombolysis was performed in less than a quarter of the patients, because our medical center owns a catheterization laboratory where PCI can be carried out and, as current guidelines [33] recommend, thrombolysis was carried out only in patients transferred from other medical centers where coronary angiography could not be performed and in patients who refused interventional therapy. Short- and long-term outcomes proved to be more favorable in subjects who underwent PCI, compared to cases where thrombolytic therapy was performed [34].

The anterior topographic territory was the preferred territory of myocardial infarctions (regardless of ST-segment elevation), followed by the inferior territory. Having the LAD (left anterior descending artery) as the epicardial coronary artery responsible for acute myocardial infarction is consistent with existing data that also implicate the LAD, along with the anterior territory, as responsible for the majority of MI [35–37].

Most patients who underwent PCI presented with single-vessel CAD, followed by two-vessel CAD, where the left coronary artery and the LAD-circumflex artery, respectively, were mainly involved. Less than a quarter of the patients presented with three-vessel ischemic coronary disease. These subjects were recommended to undergo CAGB if they presented with UAP upon hospital admission and revascularization of the culprit lesion in case they presented with MI. They were recommended to undergo subsequent complete myocardial revascularization by surgical revascularization of the remaining lesions.

All patients included in the study presented with classic cardiovascular risk factors or were known to have a personal history of cardiovascular pathology.

Dyslipidemia was the most frequent cardiovascular risk factor involved in the incidence of ACS and, at the same time, in the development of atheromatous plaques, being present in three quarters of the patients. Arterial hypertension is another important cardiovascular risk factor involved in atherogenesis, being present in more than half of the patients. Published data [38] are even more emphatic than that, stating that dyslipidemia and arterial hypertension are predictors of ACS, especially of the occurrence of UAP, followed by ACS + ST-segment elevation (specifically of STEMI rather than of NSTEMI).

Both diabetes mellitus and CKD are not at all negligible in the development of ischemic coronary diseases, as their involvement in the steps leading to the onset of ACS is known [39,40]. Existence of CAD in subjects who continued to present with ACS is another predictor of the development of this pathology [41]. Thus, the study also included patients with previous MI and previous stroke. Ischemic cardiovascular disease occurred quite frequently among patients who subsequently suffered a case of ACS, and mortality among these patients remained high [5,41,42].

Most patients admitted for ACS presented with congestive heart failure and significant valve regurgitations. Heart failure is considered to be frequently encountered together with ischemic coronary disease; gradually, through the presence of advanced atherosclerosis, the endothelial dysfunction present in patients with an increased risk of ACS will aggravate the already existing myocyte injury [43]. ACS is a precipitant of acute heart failure. These patients require special care, because, in the absence of prompt treatment, the mortality rate in this category of patients is high [44].

In ACS patients, the accurate determination of LVEF is extremely important, as impaired LVEF represents a predictor of an unfavorable short-term outcome, showing increased mortality 1 year after the first ACS event [45].

Arrhythmias occur frequently in patients with ACS, especially in those who develop an MI. The emergency requires prompt treatment, as it is known that these patients are more prone to malignant arrhythmias which, in the absence of adequate treatment, can lead to death [46,47].

The rate of readmission within a year was higher compared to readmission after more than one year after an acute coronary event. An increased risk of a recurrent cardiovascular event was also observed in numerous other published studies, especially in the first year after a case of ACS [10–12]. The risk of a nonfatal MI, nonfatal ischemic stroke, or cardiovascular death at 5 years after a first ACS was 33.4%, being six-fold higher in the first year after ACS compared with more than 1 year after the index ACS event in a very large US study [14]. Published research [10] shares the findings with our research, stating that the risk of ACS recurrence after a first acute episode is high.

ACS recurrence is also common within a year after onset in the OACIS (Osaka Acute Coronary Insufficiency Study) registry. The results of the study emphasized that the incidence of recurrent MI/year decreased from the first year (2.65%) in all subsequent years, up to 5 years (0.91–1.42%) [48]. Namiuchi et al. revealed in their research that the recurrence rate of ACS in the second year after a first MI (2.1%) was lower than in the year immediately following the MI (4.2%), concluding that the high recurrence rate can persist in cases having multiple MIs [49].

The Optum database (recording 239,234 patients with evidence of an ACS hospitalization over 14 years, beginning in 2005) revealed these patients as having a hugely increased risk (6.4% after the first year), in the short-term, after ACS hospitalization. This observation provides an additional argument for the utility of the guideline-based treatments strategies to be initiated during hospitalization for ACS [14].

The results of a study conducted in 2016 concluded that approximately 25% of patients who survive a case of ACS will suffer a stroke, AMI, or cardiovascular death in the next 5 years, particularly in the first year (34.8% risk) [10].

In the first year following discharge, 18.3% of the patients experienced an AMI, stroke, or cardiovascular death, according to a Swedish study (>90,000 patients with AMI), of whom around 50% had undergone revascularization. Of patients who had no occurrences during the first year of follow-up, 20% experienced an event after three years [50]. In the same direction, 21,890 individuals with a background of ACS were included in the REACH registry between 2003 and 2004, being monitored over the next five years (until 2009). Outcomes at one and four years showed that the overall incidence of stroke, AMI, or cardiovascular mortality was roughly 6% and 16%, respectively [51]. Between 2005 and 2010, another study on >15,000 United Kingdom patients resulted in a cumulative incidence of stroke, AMI, and cardiovascular death of 7.3% (at one year), 12.3% (after the second year) and 17.7% at three years [52]. All the studies above imply that there is a high probability of serious cardiovascular problems recurring following a case of ACS.

There were significantly more patients who experienced a rehospitalization in less than 12 months after the first one if they experienced three-vessel disease and incomplete revascularization during the index event, compared to patients who developed the event after 1 year from the first event. This may have happened because the culprit lesion was treated in the first ACS event, and the remaining lesions were to be revascularized later. However, due to other events, the remaining lesions were deferred, and, subsequently, patients developed a second ACS event within a year after the first ACS event. Rathod KS [53] claims that performing complete coronary revascularization at a safe stage is far superior to revascularizing only the culprit lesion, as patients who undergo complete revascularization have a better long-term prognosis compared to patients in whom the other stenotic lesions were deferred or revascularized later.

Another extensive analysis that should be mentioned, carried out between 2004 and 2005, refers to the so-called Melbourne Interventional Group registry. There are 9615 patients who received PCI for the index MI. In the next year after their index PCI, 12.2% of the patient surviving to discharge had a history of ACS or unplanned revascularization requiring hospitalization. Following them for 10 years, it was found that the number of unplanned hospitalizations decreased significantly, the rate of hospitalization/12 months falling from 15.3 to 7.6% ($p < 0.001$). Additionally, for hospitalization, the authors detailed in the study several independent predictors both in cases with recurrent ACS and in cases with unplanned revascularization, as follows: female sex, multivessel CAD, LV dysfunction, heart failure, diabetes, sleep apnea, etc. Finally, the paper concluded that, in the case of multi-vessel CAD subjects, optimizing therapeutic management of LV dysfunction, non-culprit vessel PCI, or diabetes can prevent hospitalization [54], these disorders being identified as predictors for recurrent admission within 12 months in our study as well.

Patients with severe heart failure (acute pulmonary edema during first hospitalization), associated valvular diseases, and lower ejection fraction were more frequently hospitalized during the first month after ACS.

Thus, the short-term prognosis for patients with ACS is unfavorable, especially in the first 12 months after the ACS event. According to the specialized literature, more than half of the patients with a first ACS event require hospitalization within the first year, and most of them require lifetime readmission due to an acute cardiovascular event [55–58].

Two-vessel or three-vessel disease, reduced LVEF after myocardial revascularization, acute or chronic heart failure, or upper gastrointestinal bleeding present in patients hospitalized with ACS are predictors of hospital readmission due to a new acute cardiovascular event.

Figure 4 suggests a strategy for the management of the main predictors associated with second readmission in patients with ACS, according to the recommendations developed by the most current guidelines. The objective of these strategies is to optimize the evolution of the subjects, and the interventions are intended to influence the main predictors or complications that are associated with a negative prognosis.

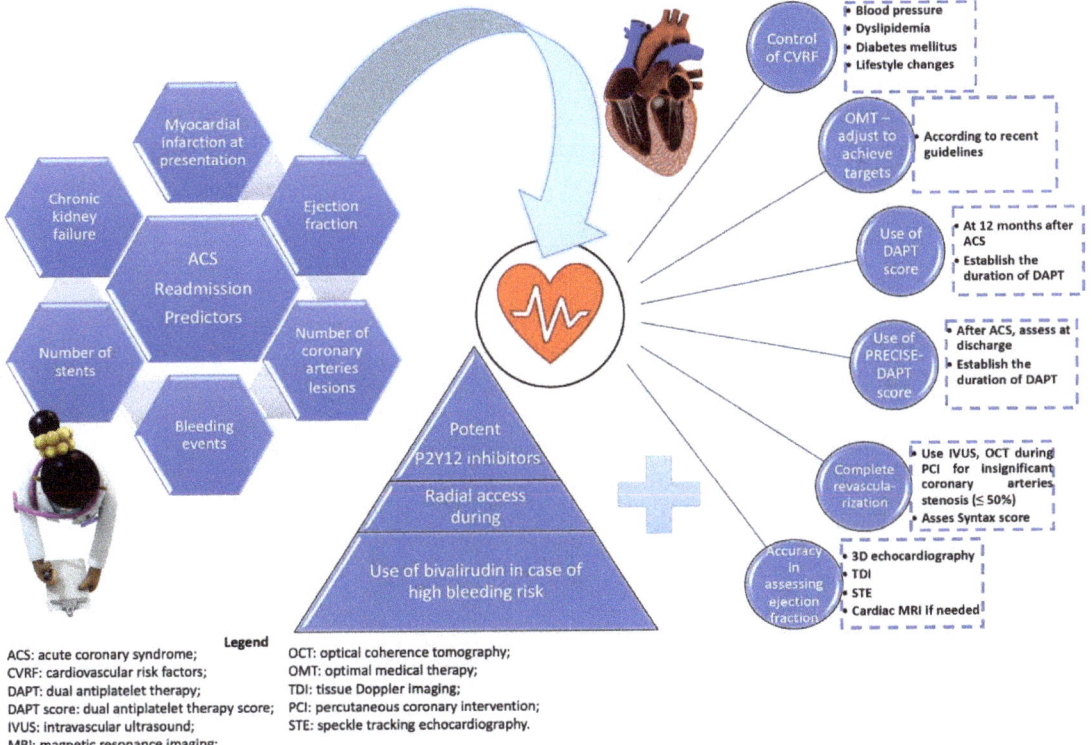

Figure 4. Main parameters and predictors of readmission in acute coronary syndrome subjects and a proposed algorithm for improving the outcome.

By highlighting factors associated with readmission, as well as independent predictors of reduced hospitalizations in the first year after an acute coronary event, the results obtained in this study provide relevant information for clinicians. These data also allow the optimization of both the clinical management of patients with ACS and their evolution, through interventions that can influence the main predictors or complications that are associated with negative prognosis.

Limitations and Strengths

Our study has some limitations that require consideration. The limited number of patients from a single center and the retrospective design together represent a significant shortcoming. The absence of specific data regarding the patients' adherence to their medication regimens as well as potential follow-up failure are additional drawbacks. Only the city's emergency public hospital underwent the readmission evaluation; neither other hospitals in the city nor hospitals in other regions were considered. These variables might have caused the number of readmissions to be underestimated. The benefit of this solely hospital-based strategy, on the other hand, is that it favored prospective enrollment of all eligible patients who had their first hospitalization for ACS and their close monitorization for a such a long period of seven years.

5. Conclusions

ACS represents the main cause of mortality and morbidity among patients with cardiovascular diseases. The incidence of STEMI increases in patients with ACS, but the incidence of non-ST-segment elevation acute coronary syndrome predominates both in patients developing ACS for the first time and in patients experiencing a second acute coronary event. Short- and long-term results in ACS patients remain unfavorable, most patients requiring rehospitalization within less than 12 months. Complete revascularization of the coronary lesions from the first event and a preserved LVEF were found to be the independent predictors of reduced hospitalizations in the following year after an acute coronary event.

Author Contributions: Conceptualization, C.B. and L.R.P.-R.; Data curation, D.M.T. and E.E.B.; Formal analysis, C.B. and S.G.B.; Investigation, C.B., A.F.B. and E.E.B.; Methodology, D.M.T.; Software, V.A.P.; Supervision, L.R.P.-R.; Validation, V.A.P.; Visualization, V.A.P.; Writing—original draft, D.M.T., A.F.B., E.E.B. and L.R.P.-R.; Writing—review and editing, S.G.B. All authors have read and agreed to the published version of the manuscript.

Funding: This research received no external funding.

Institutional Review Board Statement: The study was conducted in accordance with the Declaration of Helsinki and approved by the Ethics Committee of County Emergency Clinical Hospital of Oradea, Bihor, Romania (22884/08.10.2020).

Informed Consent Statement: Informed consent was obtained from all subjects involved in the study on the day of readmission.

Data Availability Statement: Data of the patients are available in the archive of the hospital in the study.

Conflicts of Interest: The authors declare no conflict of interest.

References

1. Balakumar, P.; Maung-U, K.; Jagadeesh, G. Prevalence and prevention of cardiovascular disease and diabetes mellitus. *Pharmacol. Res.* **2016**, *113*, 600–609. [CrossRef] [PubMed]
2. Cioni, G.; Abouzaki, N.A.; Jovin, I.S. Chapter 10—Acute Coronary Syndrome: Thrombotic Lesions in Patients with Unstable Angina. In *Cardiovascular Thrombus*; Topaz, O., Ed.; Academic Press: Cambridge, MA, USA, 2018; pp. 147–161. [CrossRef]
3. Corrigendum to: 2020 ESC Guidelines for the management of acute coronary syndromes in patients presenting without persistent ST-segment elevation: The Task Force for the management of acute coronary syndromes in patients presenting without persistent ST-segment elevation of the European Society of Cardiology (ESC). *Eur. Heart J.* **2021**, *42*, 2298. [CrossRef]
4. Birnbaum, Y.; Wilson, J.M.; Fiol, M.; de Luna, A.B.; Eskola, M.; Nikus, K. ECG diagnosis and classification of acute coronary syndromes. *Ann. Noninvasive Electrocardiol.* **2014**, *19*, 4–14. [CrossRef] [PubMed]
5. Fuster, V.; Badimon, L.; Badimon, J.J.; Chesebro, J.H.; Epstein, F.H. The Pathogenesis of Coronary Artery Disease and the Acute Coronary Syndromes. *N. Engl. J. Med.* **2010**, *326*, 310–318.

6. Libby, P.; Pasterkamp, G.; Crea, F.; Jang, I.-K. Reassessing the mechanisms of acute coronary syndromes: The "vulnerable plaque" and superficial erosion. *Circ. Res.* **2019**, *124*, 150–160. [CrossRef]
7. Rafieian-Kopaei, M.; Setorki, M.; Doudi, M.; Baradaran, A.; Nasri, H. Atherosclerosis: Process, indicators, risk factors and new hopes. *Int. J. Prev. Med.* **2014**, *5*, 927.
8. Ravnskov, U. Is atherosclerosis caused by high cholesterol? *Qjm* **2002**, *95*, 397–403. [CrossRef]
9. Scudiero, F.; Canonico, M.E.; Sanna, G.D.; Dossi, F.; Silverio, A.; Galasso, G.; Esposito, G.; Porto, I.; Parodi, G. Dual Antiplatelet Therapy with 3(rd) Generation P2Y(12) Inhibitors in STEMI Patients: Impact of Body Mass Index on Loading Dose-Response. *Cardiovasc. Drugs Ther.* **2022**. [CrossRef]
10. Abu-Assi, E.; López-López, A.; González-Salvado, V.; Redondo-Diéguez, A.; Peña-Gil, C.; Bouzas-Cruz, N.; Raposeiras-Roubín, S.; Abumuaileq, R.R.-Y.; García-Acuña, J.M.; González-Juanatey, J.R. The risk of cardiovascular events after an acute coronary event remains high, especially during the first year, despite revascularization. *Rev. Española De Cardiol.* **2016**, *69*, 11–18. [CrossRef]
11. Doost Hosseiny, A.; Moloi, S.; Chandrasekhar, J.; Farshid, A. Mortality pattern and cause of death in a long-term follow-up of patients with STEMI treated with primary PCI. *Open Heart* **2016**, *3*, e000405. [CrossRef]
12. Norgaard, M.L.; Andersen, S.S.; Schramm, T.K.; Folke, F.; Jørgensen, C.H.; Hansen, M.L.; Andersson, C.; Bretler, D.M.; Vaag, A.; Køber, L.; et al. Changes in short- and long-term cardiovascular risk of incident diabetes and incident myocardial infarction—A nationwide study. *Diabetologia* **2010**, *53*, 1612–1619. [CrossRef] [PubMed]
13. Rapsomaniki, E.; Thuresson, M.; Yang, E.; Blin, P.; Hunt, P.; Chung, S.-C.; Stogiannis, D.; Pujades-Rodriguez, M.; Timmis, A.; Denaxas, S.C.; et al. Using big data from health records from four countries to evaluate chronic disease outcomes: A study in 114 364 survivors of myocardial infarction. *Eur. Heart J. -Qual. Care Clin. Outcomes* **2016**, *2*, 172–183. [CrossRef] [PubMed]
14. Steen, D.L.; Khan, I.; Andrade, K.; Koumas, A.; Giugliano, R.P. Event Rates and Risk Factors for Recurrent Cardiovascular Events and Mortality in a Contemporary Post Acute Coronary Syndrome Population Representing 239 234 Patients During 2005 to 2018 in the United States. *J. Am. Heart Assoc.* **2022**, *11*, e022198. [CrossRef] [PubMed]
15. Goldman, J.D.; Harte, F.M. Transition of care to prevent recurrence after acute coronary syndrome: The critical role of the primary care provider and pharmacist. *Postgrad. Med.* **2020**, *132*, 426–432. [CrossRef]
16. Koene, R.J.; Prizment, A.E.; Blaes, A.; Konety, S.H. Shared Risk Factors in Cardiovascular Disease and Cancer. *Circulation* **2016**, *133*, 1104–1114. [CrossRef]
17. Penzenstadler, L.; Gentil, L.; Grenier, G.; Khazaal, Y.; Fleury, M.-J. Risk factors of hospitalization for any medical condition among patients with prior emergency department visits for mental health conditions. *BMC Psychiatry* **2020**, *20*, 431. [CrossRef]
18. Thygesen, K.; Alpert, J.S.; Jaffe, A.S.; Chaitman, B.R.; Bax, J.J.; Morrow, D.A.; White, H.D.; Mickley, H.; Crea, F.; Van de Werf, F. Fourth universal definition of myocardial infarction (2018). *Eur. Heart J.* **2019**, *40*, 237–269. [CrossRef]
19. Weber, M.; Hamm, C. Unstable angina pectoris (UIP) after a new classification: Which diagnosis, which treatment? *Deutsche Medizinische Wochenschrift (1946)* **2004**, *129*, 1082–1088.
20. Wagner, W.E., III. *Using IBM®SPSS®Statistics for Research Methods and Social Science Statistics*; Sage Publications: Thousand Oaks, CA, USA, 2019.
21. Shah, T.; Palaskas, N.; Ahmed, A. An Update on Gender Disparities in Coronary Heart Disease Care. *Curr. Atheroscler. Rep.* **2016**, *18*, 28. [CrossRef]
22. Soeiro, A.d.M.; Silva, P.G.M.d.B.e.; Roque, E.A.d.C.; Bossa, A.S.; Biselli, B.; Leal, T.d.C.A.T.; Soeiro, M.C.F.d.A.; Pitta, F.G.; Serrano, C.V., Jr.; Oliveira, M.T., Jr. Prognostic Differences between Men and Women with Acute Coronary Syndrome. Data from a Brazilian Registry. *Arq. Bras. De Cardiol.* **2018**, *111*, 648–653. [CrossRef]
23. Huber, E.; Le Pogam, M.-A.; Clair, C. Sex related inequalities in the management and prognosis of acute coronary syndrome in Switzerland: Cross sectional study. *BMJ Med.* **2022**, *1*, e000300. [CrossRef] [PubMed]
24. Ren, L.; Ye, H.; Wang, P.; Cui, Y.; Cao, S.; Lv, S. Comparison of long-term mortality of acute ST-segment elevation myocardial infarction and non-ST-segment elevation acute coronary syndrome patients after percutaneous coronary intervention. *Int. J. Clin. Exp. Med.* **2014**, *7*, 5588. [PubMed]
25. Chang, A.M.; Fischman, D.L.; Hollander, J.E. Evaluation of chest pain and acute coronary syndromes. *Cardiol. Clin.* **2018**, *36*, 1–12. [CrossRef] [PubMed]
26. Zhang, Q.; Zhao, D.; Xie, W.; Xie, X.; Guo, M.; Wang, M.; Wang, W.; Liu, W.; Liu, J. Recent trends in hospitalization for acute myocardial infarction in Beijing: Increasing overall burden and a transition from ST-segment elevation to non-ST-segment elevation myocardial infarction in a population-based study. *Medicine* **2016**, *95*, e2677. [CrossRef]
27. McManus, D.D.; Gore, J.; Yarzebski, J.; Spencer, F.; Lessard, D.; Goldberg, R.J. Recent trends in the incidence, treatment, and outcomes of patients with STEMI and NSTEMI. *Am. J. Med.* **2011**, *124*, 40–47. [CrossRef]
28. Neumann, J.T.; Gößling, A.; Sörensen, N.A.; Blankenberg, S.; Magnussen, C.; Westermann, D. Temporal trends in incidence and outcome of acute coronary syndrome. *Clin. Res. Cardiol.* **2020**, *109*, 1186–1192. [CrossRef]
29. Wang, T.K.M.; Grey, C.; Jiang, Y.; Jackson, R.T.; Kerr, A.J. Nationwide trends in acute coronary syndrome by subtype in New Zealand 2006–2016. *Heart* **2020**, *106*, 221–227. [CrossRef]
30. Spadaccio, C.; Benedetto, U. Coronary artery bypass grafting (CABG) vs. percutaneous coronary intervention (PCI) in the treatment of multivessel coronary disease: Quo vadis?—A review of the evidences on coronary artery disease. *Ann. Cardiothorac. Surg.* **2018**, *7*, 506. [CrossRef]

31. Granger, C.B.; Krychtiuk, K.A.; Gersh, B.J. Personalizing Choice of CABG vs PCI for Multivessel Disease: Predictive Model Falls Short. *J. Am. Coll. Cardiol.* **2022**, *79*, 1474–1476. [CrossRef]
32. Šerpytis, R.; Puodžiukaitė, L.; Petrauskas, S.; Misonis, N.; Kurminas, M.; Laucevičius, A.; Šerpytis, P. Outcomes of a percutaneous coronary intervention versus coronary artery bypass grafting in octogenarians. *Acta Med. Litu.* **2018**, *25*, 132. [CrossRef]
33. Neumann, F.-J.; Sousa-Uva, M.; Ahlsson, A.; Alfonso, F.; Banning, A.P.; Benedetto, U.; Byrne, R.A.; Collet, J.-P.; Falk, V.; Head, S.J.; et al. 2018 ESC/EACTS Guidelines on myocardial revascularization. *Eur. Heart J.* **2019**, *40*, 87–165. [CrossRef] [PubMed]
34. Aversano, T.; Aversano, L.; Passamani, E.; Knatterud, G.; Terrin, M.; Williams, D.; Forman, S. Atlantic Cardiovascular Patient Outcomes Research Team (CPORT). Thrombolytic therapy vs primary percutaneous coronary intervention for myocardial infarction in patients presenting to hospitals without on-site cardiac surgery: A randomized controlled trial. *Jama* **2002**, *287*, 1943–1951. [CrossRef] [PubMed]
35. Moisi, M.I.; Rus, M.; Bungau, S.; Zaha, D.C.; Uivarosan, D.; Fratila, O.; Tit, D.M.; Endres, L.; Nistor-Cseppento, D.C.; Popescu, M.I. Acute Coronary Syndromes in Chronic Kidney Disease: Clinical and Therapeutic Characteristics. *Medicina* **2020**, *56*, 118. [CrossRef] [PubMed]
36. Pantea-Roșan, L.R.; Pantea, V.A.; Bungau, S.; Tit, D.M.; Behl, T.; Vesa, C.M.; Bustea, C.; Moleriu, R.D.; Rus, M.; Popescu, M.I.; et al. No-Reflow after PPCI—A Predictor of Short-Term Outcomes in STEMI Patients. *J. Clin. Med.* **2020**, *9*, 2956. [CrossRef]
37. Kumar, A.; Cannon, C.P. Acute coronary syndromes: Diagnosis and management, part I. In Proceedings of the Mayo Clinic Proceedings; Elsevier: Amsterdam, The Netherlands, 2009; pp. 917–938.
38. Brunori, E.H.F.R.; Lopes, C.T.; Cavalcante, A.M.R.Z.; Santos, V.B.; Lopes, J.d.L.; Barros, A.L.B.L.d. Association of cardiovascular risk factors with the different presentations of acute coronary syndrome. *Rev. Lat. -Am. De Enferm.* **2014**, *22*, 538–546. [CrossRef]
39. Reriani, M.K.; Flammer, A.J.; Jama, A.; Lerman, L.O.; Lerman, A. Novel functional risk factors for the prediction of cardiovascular events in vulnerable patients following acute coronary syndrome. *Circ. J.* **2012**, *76*, 778–783. [CrossRef]
40. Babes, E.E.; Bustea, C.; Behl, T.; Abdel-Daim, M.M.; Nechifor, A.C.; Stoicescu, M.; Brisc, C.M.; Moisi, M.; Gitea, D.; Iovanovici, D.C.; et al. Acute coronary syndromes in diabetic patients, outcome, revascularization, and antithrombotic therapy. *Biomed. Pharmacother.* **2022**, *148*, 112772. [CrossRef]
41. Sanchis-Gomar, F.; Perez-Quilis, C.; Leischik, R.; Lucia, A. Epidemiology of coronary heart disease and acute coronary syndrome. *Ann. Transl. Med.* **2016**, *4*, 256. [CrossRef]
42. Rosengren, A.; Wallentin, L.; Simoons, M.; Gitt, A.; Behar, S.; Battler, A.; Hasdai, D. Cardiovascular risk factors and clinical presentation in acute coronary syndromes. *Heart* **2005**, *91*, 1141–1147. [CrossRef]
43. Hernandez-Leiva, E. Epidemiology of acute coronary syndrome and heart failure in Latin America. *Rev. Esp. De Cardiol.* **2011**, *64*, 34–43.
44. Harjola, V.P.; Parissis, J.; Bauersachs, J.; Brunner-La Rocca, H.P.; Bueno, H.; Čelutkienė, J.; Chioncel, O.; Coats, A.J.; Collins, S.P.; de Boer, R.A. Acute coronary syndromes and acute heart failure: A diagnostic dilemma and high-risk combination. A statement from the Acute Heart Failure Committee of the Heart Failure Association of the European Society of Cardiology. *Eur. J. Heart Fail.* **2020**, *22*, 1298–1314. [CrossRef] [PubMed]
45. Khaled, S.; Matahen, R. Cardiovascular risk factors profile in patients with acute coronary syndrome with particular reference to left ventricular ejection fraction. *Indian Heart J.* **2018**, *70*, 45–49. [CrossRef] [PubMed]
46. Trappe, H.-J. Tachyarrhythmias, bradyarrhythmias and acute coronary syndromes. *J. Emerg. Trauma Shock* **2010**, *3*, 137. [CrossRef] [PubMed]
47. Chiwhane, A. Study of Rhythm Disturbances in Acute Myocardial Infarction. *J. Assoc. Phys. India* **2018**, *66*, 54–58.
48. Nakatani, D.; Sakata, Y.; Suna, S.; Usami, M.; Matsumoto, S.; Shimizu, M.; Sumitsuji, S.; Kawano, S.; Ueda, Y.; Hamasaki, T.; et al. Incidence, predictors, and subsequent mortality risk of recurrent myocardial infarction in patients following discharge for acute myocardial infarction. *Circ. J.* **2013**, *77*, 439–446. [CrossRef] [PubMed]
49. Namiuchi, S.; Sunamura, S.; Tanita, A.; Ushigome, R.; Noda, K.; Takii, T. Higher Recurrence Rate of Acute Coronary Syndrome in Patients with Multiple-Time Myocardial Infarction. *Int. Heart J.* **2021**, *62*, 493–498. [CrossRef]
50. Jernberg, T.; Hasvold, P.; Henriksson, M.; Hjelm, H.; Thuresson, M.; Janzon, M. Cardiovascular risk in post-myocardial infarction patients: Nationwide real world data demonstrate the importance of a long-term perspective. *Eur. Heart J.* **2015**, *36*, 1163–1170. [CrossRef]
51. Bhatt, D.L.; Eagle, K.A.; Ohman, E.M.; Hirsch, A.T.; Goto, S.; Mahoney, E.M.; Wilson, P.W.F.; Alberts, M.J.; D'Agostino, R.; Liau, C.-S.; et al. Comparative Determinants of 4-Year Cardiovascular Event Rates in Stable Outpatients at Risk of or With Atherothrombosis. *JAMA* **2010**, *304*, 1350–1357. [CrossRef]
52. Rapsomaniki, E.; Stogiannis, D.; Emmas, C.; Chung, S.; Pasea, L.; Denaxas, S.; Shah, A.; Pujades-Rodriguez, M.; Timmis, A.; Hemingway, H. Health outcomes in patients with stable coronary artery disease following myocardial infarction; construction of a PEGASUS-TIMI-54 like population in UK linked electronic health records. In *Proceedings of the European Heart Journal*; Oxford University Press: Oxford, UK, 2014; p. 363.
53. Rathod, K.S.; Koganti, S.; Jain, A.K.; Astroulakis, Z.; Lim, P.; Rakhit, R.; Kalra, S.S.; Dalby, M.C.; O'Mahony, C.; Malik, I.S. Complete versus culprit-only lesion intervention in patients with acute coronary syndromes. *J. Am. Coll. Cardiol.* **2018**, *72*, 1989–1999. [CrossRef]

54. Yudi, M.B.; Clark, D.J.; Farouque, O.; Andrianopoulos, N.; Ajani, A.E.; Brennan, A.; Lefkovits, J.; Freeman, M.; Hiew, C.; Selkrig, L.A.; et al. Trends and predictors of recurrent acute coronary syndrome hospitalizations and unplanned revascularization after index acute myocardial infarction treated with percutaneous coronary intervention. *Am. Heart J.* **2019**, *212*, 134–143. [CrossRef]
55. Kolansky, D.M. Acute coronary syndromes: Morbidity, mortality, and pharmacoeconomic burden. *Am. J. Manag. Care* **2009**, *15*, S36. [PubMed]
56. Babes, E.E.; Zaha, D.C.; Tit, D.M.; Nechifor, A.C.; Bungau, S.; Andronie-Cioara, F.L.; Behl, T.; Stoicescu, M.; Munteanu, M.A.; Rus, M.; et al. Value of Hematological and Coagulation Parameters as Prognostic Factors in Acute Coronary Syndromes. *Diagnostics* **2021**, *11*, 850. [CrossRef] [PubMed]
57. Mansur, A.J. Hospital Readmissions after Acute Coronary Syndromes. *Arq. Brasileiros Cardiol.* **2019**, *113*, 50–51. [CrossRef] [PubMed]
58. Babes, E.E.; Tit, D.M.; Bungau, A.F.; Bustea, C.; Rus, M.; Bungau, S.G.; Babes, V.V. Myocardial Viability Testing in the Management of Ischemic Heart Failure. *Life* **2022**, *12*, 1760. [CrossRef]

Disclaimer/Publisher's Note: The statements, opinions and data contained in all publications are solely those of the individual author(s) and contributor(s) and not of MDPI and/or the editor(s). MDPI and/or the editor(s) disclaim responsibility for any injury to people or property resulting from any ideas, methods, instructions or products referred to in the content.

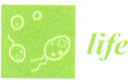 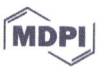

Review

TAVR Interventions and Coronary Access: How to Prevent Coronary Occlusion

Flavius-Alexandru Gherasie [1,*] and Alexandru Achim [2]

1. Department of Cardiology, University of Medicine and Pharmacy "Carol Davila", 050474 Bucharest, Romania
2. Department of Cardiology, Medizinische Universitätsklinik, Kantonsspital Baselland, Rheinstrasse 26, 4410 Liestal, Switzerland; alexandru.achim@ksbl.ch
* Correspondence: flavius.gherasie@drd.umfcd.ro

Abstract: Due to technological advancements during the past 20 years, transcatheter aortic valve replacements (TAVRs) have significantly improved the treatment of symptomatic and severe aortic stenosis, significantly improving patient outcomes. The continuous evolution of transcatheter valve models, refined imaging planning for enhanced accuracy, and the growing expertise of technicians have collectively contributed to increased safety and procedural success over time. These notable advancements have expanded the scope of TAVR to include patients with lower risk profiles as it has consistently demonstrated more favorable outcomes than surgical aortic valve replacement (SAVR). As the field progresses, coronary angiography is anticipated to become increasingly prevalent among patients who have previously undergone TAVR, particularly in younger cohorts. It is worth noting that aortic stenosis is often associated with coronary artery disease. While the task of re-accessing coronary artery access following TAVR is challenging, it is generally feasible. In the context of valve-in-valve procedures, several crucial factors must be carefully considered to optimize coronary re-access. To obtain successful coronary re-access, it is essential to align the prosthesis with the native coronary ostia. As part of preventive measures, strategies have been developed to safeguard against coronary obstruction during TAVR. One such approach involves placing wires and non-deployed coronary balloons or scaffolds inside an at-risk coronary artery, a procedure known as chimney stenting. Additionally, the bioprosthetic or native aortic scallops intentional laceration to prevent iatrogenic coronary artery obstruction (BASILICA) procedure offers an effective and safer alternative to prevent coronary artery obstructions. The key objective of our study was to evaluate the techniques and procedures employed to achieve commissural alignment in TAVR, as well as to assess the efficacy and measure the impact on coronary re-access in valve-in-valve procedures.

Keywords: coronary artery obstruction; transcatheter aortic valve replacement; valve-in-valve interventions

Citation: Gherasie, F.-A.; Achim, A. TAVR Interventions and Coronary Access: How to Prevent Coronary Occlusion. *Life* **2023**, *13*, 1605. https://doi.org/10.3390/life13071605

Academic Editor: Dimitris Tousoulis

Received: 19 June 2023
Revised: 6 July 2023
Accepted: 20 July 2023
Published: 21 July 2023

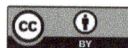

Copyright: © 2023 by the authors. Licensee MDPI, Basel, Switzerland. This article is an open access article distributed under the terms and conditions of the Creative Commons Attribution (CC BY) license (https://creativecommons.org/licenses/by/4.0/).

1. Introduction

Since 2002, transcatheter aortic valve replacement (TAVR) has become an increasingly popular and less invasive option for treating symptomatic severe aortic stenosis (AS) compared with conventional surgical aortic valve replacement (SAVR) [1]. Compared with SAVR, TAVR offers equal or superior patient outcomes regardless of risk. Moreover, it has been demonstrated to be cost-effective, providing excellent clinical outcomes and improved quality of life in patients with severe AS. As a result, TAVR has become the preferred intervention method for patients with symptomatic severe AS who are not suitable for standard SAVR [2–6]. It is essential to note that while surgical aortic valve replacement has been the cornerstone of care for severe symptomatic aortic stenosis for a long time, TAVR has now become the predominant treatment in the United States and Europe [7–9].

There is a high probability of simultaneously occurring coronary artery disease (CAD) in severe AS, accounting for approximately half of all patients undergoing TAVR. However, the rate has decreased as TAVR is increasingly performed on healthier patients [10,11].

When deciding whether to perform a percutaneous coronary intervention (PCI) before TAVR, it is important to consider integrated management of the case. This includes reducing the risk of ischemic events associated with valve replacement, especially when rapid pacing is needed, and ensuring that the coronary intervention can be easily performed without interference from the valve prosthesis.

Lateef et al. concluded that PCI for severe CAD before TAVR is not clinically advantageous [12,13]. Rather, it seems that patients with severe coronary artery disease who undergo TAVR may experience better outcomes if they undergo complete revascularization, which is determined by recalculating the SYNTAX scores after the procedure [14]. A recent European clinical consensus statement recommends that when considering the possibility of performing PCI after TAVR, it is crucial to select the appropriate transcatheter heart valve, self-expanding valve, or balloon-expandable valve and employ an implantation technique that prioritizes the preservation of unhindered coronary access. The same consensus states that although the available evidence is limited, it generally does not endorse the routine use of PCI before TAVR in asymptomatic lesions. Instead, the evidence indicates that a specific stepwise procedure performed prior to TAVR is a more promising approach when a percutaneous coronary procedure is deemed necessary. Presently, the ongoing COMPLETE TAVR trial (ClinicalTrials.gov: NCT04634240) is in the process of randomizing 4000 patients undergoing TAVR and presenting severe CAD. This encompasses individuals with more than one lesion in a coronary artery, exhibiting more than 70% angiographical diameter stenosis, with a diameter greater than 2.5 mm, while not including chronic total occlusions. The trial aims to compare the outcomes of staged complete revascularization following TAVR with a balloon-expandable valve with the outcomes of solely medical management. The ESC/European Association for Cardio-Thoracic Surgery (EACTS) Clinical Practice Guidelines on Myocardial Revascularization state that patients who have stenosis of over 70% in the proximal segments of their vessels and are scheduled for TAVR should consider coronary angioplasty. This guideline is in effect immediately and provides patients with a clear course of action for optimal treatment [15].

As the age and intensity of complications among TAVR patients decrease, they can enjoy longer and more active lives after undergoing valve intervention. As a consequence, patients may require supplementary diagnostic angiographies and angioplasties. In the meantime, patients could evolve newly developed or advanced coronary artery disease. Those who have undergone PCIs in the past may need to undergo inspection and new procedures due to stent restenosis.

Vilalta et al. reported from a study conducted over two years that acute coronary syndrome following TAVR occurs as frequently as in 10% of cases [16]. Coronary artery re-access may be compromised due to the anatomical alignment between the coronary ostia and prosthetic aortic valve. When planning a strategy for engaging the coronary arteries, it is important to consider the various design characteristics of the type of transcatheter aortic valves. Several studies have demonstrated the feasibility of coronary angiography and intervention following TAVR [17–20]. Even so, consistent reports of low success rates have been reported following the insertion of the Medtronic CoreValve (Medtronic Inc., Minneapolis, MN, USA), particularly in the right coronary artery [20–22]. An overview of valve deployment strategies is presented in this paper with particular emphasis on valve-in-valve procedures and catheter options to facilitate effective post-TAVR assessments and coronary angioplasties.

2. Overview of Strategies to Prevent Coronary Obstruction

Transcatheter aortic valve replacement is a way to replace a damaged aortic valve without undergoing surgery. It can be used to replace either native leaflets or bioprosthetic leaflets. During heart valve implantation, aortic leaflets can be displaced and impede coronary arteries in 0.7% of all cases, necessitating urgent percutaneous coronary interventions or coronary artery bypass grafts [23]. As such, it is important to avoid displacement of the aortic leaflets during implantation. Various techniques and tools can be used to ensure that the aortic valve is correctly placed and that the leaflets are not displaced. Additionally, TAVR valve designs that allow aortic leaflets to be positioned away from the coronary ostia, as well as those that allow the recapture of the leaflets, are being developed to reduce the risk of coronary artery obstruction. In summary, the careful planning and implementation of the TAVR procedure are essential to reduce the risk of aortic valve displacement into the coronary arteries. According to recently published studies, the valve-in-valve TAVR risk is higher (2.3%) [24].

The potential for obstruction of one or both of the major coronary arteries due to the coverage of the ostia due to very large native leaflets having been displaced from their positions by the body of the expandable heart valve is a very concerning issue. The leaflets' displacement results from the frame of the valve covering the ostia, blocking the native flaps from occupying their regular positions. This can result in the narrowing of the coronary artery, which can reduce and even completely obstruct blood flow to the heart. An obstruction of this nature has the potential to give rise to a variety of serious and potentially fatal cardiovascular complications, emphasizing the importance of recognizing the risks connected with this matter. It is important to be aware of the potential for the displacement of native leaflets due to the frame of the THV (transcatheter heart valve), particularly in bicuspid aortic valve interventions, and take the necessary steps to minimize this risk [25].

Valve-in-valve (VIV) procedures have become increasingly popular for treating patients with failing bioprosthetic valves. However, these procedures must be performed with caution, as the displacement of the bioprosthetic leaflets that cover the coronary ostia can lead to reduced coronary blood flow toward the sinus of Valsalva (SOV). This occurs if the displaced leaflets, both native and prosthetic, are pushed into contact with the sinotubular junction. Therefore, it is important to pay attention to the displacement of the leaflets and ensure that there is no contact between the leaflets and the sinotubular junction during VIV procedures. The skirt or commissural posts of transcatheter heart valves can obstruct coronary ostia. Less common causes include coronary dissection, hematomas, or embolizations caused by thrombotic or degenerative conditions. It has been reported that the 30-day mortality rate for acute CAO (coronary artery occlusion) during TAVR is high. During TAVR procedures for native aortic stenosis, the complication rate can vary from 8% to 41%. For valve-in-valve procedures, the complication rate can reach up to 53% [24,26].

Some factors can predict coronary occlusion during TAVR procedures, such as being female, having a short sinus of Valsalva, and having a distance from the valve to the coronary ostia that is less than 10 mm (Table 1) [27].

Table 1. Risk factors for coronary occlusion.

VIV	TAVR
Stentless valve design	Female gender
Stented prosthesis with leaflets outside	Coronary height of <10 mm
Distance of the bioprosthetic valve from the coronary artery of <4 mm	Sinus of Valsalva of <28 mm
	Leaflet elongation according to coronary height
	Masses of calcium
	Leaflet dimensions and placement

For the accurate measurement of aortic root dimensions, including the distance of the bioprosthetic valve from the coronary artery (VTC), CT angiography is essential. Dvir et al. suggested that having a final VTC size of 3 mm or less carries an increased risk of ostial occlusion [28]. The primary underlying factor in aortic valve-in-valve procedures is the coronary ostia's proximity to the expected placement of the shifted bioprosthetic leaflets following valve deployment. As a result, conditions that increase the likelihood of CAO may encompass a bioprosthetic valve positioned above the annulus, a sinotubular junction that is both narrow and positioned low, leaflets that are bulky in nature, and coronaries located in a narrow aortic root or those that have been re-implanted.

3. Commissural Alignment

Optimal transcatheter aortic valve function and coronary access are associated with commissural alignment. To achieve this, certain factors must be considered. Firstly, the orientation of the valve must be taken into account, as it directly affects the degree of commissural alignment. Secondly, the size and shape of the valve must be taken into consideration, as these can affect the alignment of the commissure. Thirdly, the depth at which the valve is to be inserted must be measured accurately, as too deep an insertion can cause an improper commissural alignment. Finally, the amount of force applied during the insertion must be monitored, as too much force can lead to improper commissural alignment. All these factors must be taken into account to ensure optimal coronary access through a proper commissural alignment [29].

To achieve optimal fluoroscopic angulation, pre-procedural MDCT (multidetector computed tomography) calculates the annular plane of the aortic valve based on the cusp hinge points. Multiple angulations are visualized across the S-curve of the valve until the designated hinge points for the LCC and RCC overlap, thus isolating the NCC on the opposite side. The cusp-overlap angulation is defined using the fluoroscopic angulation [30].

The right–left cusp overlap view is the preferred method for the commissural alignment of a transcatheter aortic valve. This view isolates the commissure, which is the 120-degree separation along the right and left cusps on the right of the fluoroscopic view. This view is important as it allows for a more accurate alignment of the THV, ensuring that it is properly secured in the aortic annulus. It is also ideal for the accurate sizing of the THV, as the commissural alignment can help to determine the optimal size of the valve. Proper alignment is essential for a successful THV procedure, and this view is an essential part of the process. The left–right cusp overlap view is an important imaging technique for assessing coronary access. For ideal commissural alignment, the left and right coronary arteries must emerge from the left–right commissure at an angle of 60 degrees. If the coronary arteries emerge at an angle smaller or larger than 60 degrees, this could indicate a misalignment. It is important to recognize misalignment, as it can indicate coronary artery disease or other vascular issues. The left and right coronary arteries must emerge from the left–right commissure at the correct angle to ensure that the best possible coronary access is achieved [31,32].

In cases where commissural alignment leads to coronary misalignment as a result of coronary ostium eccentricity, coronary alignment is recommended. In order to line up the nadir of the bioprosthetic leaflets with the coronary ostia in these cases, the operator must calculate an alternative THV rotation angle to preserve a 60-degree angle from the TAV commissural post and the coronary ostia [33,34].

Based on the method of deployment, TAVR devices can be categorized as either balloon-expandable or self-expandable (Table 2).

Table 2. Main TAVR devices and characteristics.

JenaValve JenaValve Technology GmbH	Lotus Boston Scientific Corporation	Portico St. Jude Medical, Inc.	Acurate Neo Symetis	Evolut R Medtronic	Sapiens 3 Edwards Lifesciences	Valve Name
Self-expandable porcine pericardial tissue	Self-expandable bovine pericardial tissue	Self-expandable bovine pericardial tissue	Self-expandable porcine pericardial tissue	Self-expandable porcine pericardial tissue	Balloon-expandable bovine pericardial tissue	Structure Type
-	≥6 mm for 23 mm device size ≥6.5 mm for 25 mm and 27 mm device size	≥6 mm	≥6 mm	≥5 mm for 23 mm for 26 mm and 29 mm device size ≥5.5 mm for 34 mm device size	≥5 mm for 23 mm and 26 mm device size ≥5.5 mm for 29 mm device size	Access Vessel Diameter
TA sheathless 32 F (23, 25, and 27 mm)	TF 18 F (23 mm) 20 F (25 and 27 mm)	TF, TAo, TSc 18 F (23 and 25 mm) 19 F (27 and 29 mm)	TF 18 F TA sheathless 28 F	TF, TAo, and TSc 14 F (23, 26, 29, and 34 mm)	TF 14 F (20, 23, and 26 mm), 16 F (26 mm) TA, TAo 18 F (20, 23, and 26 mm), 21 F (26 mm)	Access Type Device Size
Yes	Yes	Yes	No	Yes	No	Repositionable

TF, transfemoral; TA, transapical; TAo, transaortic; TSc, trans-subclavian.

Our next section focuses on the disparities in commissural alignment among the three major TAVR platforms.

3.1. CoreValve Evolut R and PRO Valves (Medtronic Minneapolis, MN, USA)

The CoreValve Evolut R and Pro devices are equipped with three commissural frame posts, each measuring 26 mm in height. One of these posts is positioned in line with the paddle on the C-Table. One way to predict the direction of the commissural alignment for the ostium is by observing the hat's orientation on the delivery catheter during deployment. This is due to the fact that the hat on the delivery catheter is always oriented in the same direction as the commissural frame posts, making it easy to identify the orientation of the coronary ostia.

A new study discovered that if the hat indicator of the CoreValve Evolut delivery system is aligned with the aortic curve and center front of the aorta on the coplanar three-cusp angiographic view, it can significantly reduce the incidence of severe coronary overlap. Out of all the positions, this one had the least amount of overlap, at only 23.2%. However, when the hat marker is oriented toward the inner curve and center back of the aorta, the overlap frequency increased to 75%. This finding is crucial as it helps to identify the most optimal system positioning for better overall patient outcomes. By directing the hat marker along the inside curve and center back of the aorta, the frequency of overlap increased to 75%. This discovery is critical in identifying the optimal system positioning for better patient outcomes [35].

For patients with severe AS who also have other conditions like chronic or acute coronary syndromes that require easy access to coronary arteries for additional coronary angiography, optimizing the alignment of the TAV commissures is important. This is especially crucial for younger patients who are at lower risk. For the CoreValve Evolut R/Pro implantation system, it is recommended to introduce it through the common femoral artery using flush ports at the 3 o'clock position. The hat marker is oriented to face the aortic root's outer curve when the delivery system passes through the aortic valve. This ensures proper commissural alignment and prevents overlap with the coronary ostia [36].

3.2. SAPIEN XT and SAPIEN 3 Valves (Edwards Lifesci-Ences, Irvine, California)

SAPIEN 3/Ultra is the only transcatheter heart valve authorized in Europe and the United States for a second TAVR procedure. Recently, an operative guidance consensus was published on procedural planning and techniques for this particular valve [37]. Compared with the CoreValve Evolut, the Sapien 3 has a 3 mm tab positioned on the commissural primary rows instead of a commissural post. Even though the Sapien 3 device has a lower frame height than the Evolut device, the commissural tabs may find themselves next to the coronary ostium, particularly if the coronary origin has a low origin. Crimping the Sapien 3 valve at different angles prevents the possibility of intentional commissural alignment. This is because the angle of the crimp has a direct effect on the alignment of the commissures. If the crimp is not consistent, the alignment of the commissures is affected, making it difficult to achieve an intentional alignment [38]. Compared with the Evolut device, which contains a supra-annular valve system, Sapiens 3 valves are balloon-expandable intra-annular valves, giving them an advantage in coronary occlusion prevention. Lopes et al. presented a report regarding the failure of a 34 mm Evolut Pro valve implantation, which led to coronary occlusion and cardiac arrest. The quick recognition of acute left main occlusion caused by the high valve implantation resulted in the immediate initiation of advanced life support. The valve was quickly pulled toward the ascending aorta utilizing the snare technique, which immediately restored the flow and facilitated effective cardiopulmonary resuscitation. Following this, a 29 mm balloon-expandable Sapiens 3 valve was implanted successfully [39]. In general, the position of the second valve should be chosen to improve the procedure's results and reduce the risk of coronary occlusion and sinus compression. It is important to implant the second valve at a low implanting depth to reduce the risk of coronary blockage, enabling various levels of overlap between the valve's leaflets. Before proceeding with the index transcatheter heart valve intervention, it is important to evaluate the alignment of the neo-commissure. This determines the technique's effectiveness, as significant misalignment during the first valve procedure could limit its benefits.

3.3. Acurate Neo Valve (Boston Scientific, Marlborough, MA, USA)

Accurate Neo is a self-expanding transcatheter valve with a supra-annular configuration and porcine pericardial leaflets available in Europe since 2014. The top-down positioning facilitates optimal positioning and limits flow obstruction upon deployment. A total of three stabilization pillars facilitate better coaxial alignment, and the superior crown enhances anchoring. As long as the upper crown keeps the native cusps away from the coronary ostia, there is a low risk of coronary obstruction.

The coronary re-access procedure is made less challenging by the top crown's short stent design and open-cell architecture. This design allows for easier and faster deployment, as well as improved stent visibility. Additionally, the open-cell design of the upper crown makes it easier to pass a guidewire distally, if needed. This makes the procedure easier and more efficient, resulting in shorter procedure times. Furthermore, the short stent profile and open-cell configuration of the top crown make it easier to access the distal vessel, which can be beneficial in certain cases. SAVI TF registry records report that there have been no cases of coronary obstruction that require intervention in 1000 patients [40].

Vanhaverbeke et al. reported a successful valve-in-valve replacement with a Sapiens valve in a degenerated ACURATE Neo prosthesis [41]. A typical THV is equipped with a complete frame, which allows the leaflet to form the neoskirt. The neoskirt of the ACURATE neo does not extend to the upper crown of the SAPIEN 3, which minimizes the risk of coronary obstruction and promotes optimal coronary access. ACURATE Neo also has the advantage of not overexpanding when it performs TAV-in-TAV. To confirm these encouraging observations, more SAPIEN-in-ACURATE cases in the real world are needed, despite the extensive modeling and testing that has been pre-procedurally conducted on the current TAV-in-TAV case and the clinical outcomes confirming both bench tests and computational models.

4. Angiograms and Interventions following TAVR

Understanding the location of the coronary arteries relative to the THV is the first step in the angiographic imaging of coronary arteries. When performing coronary catheterization, the catheter used is often chosen based on the shape and design of the transcatheter heart valve. Typically, the left main coronary artery and right coronary artery origins are seen in a left anterior oblique (LAO) projection.

For CoreValve Evolut coronary re-access, the standard JR4 or JL4 diagnostic catheters are generally the most suitable options. However, in some cases, a half-size smaller JL catheter may be preferable [42,43]. This is because it can provide a more comfortable fit while still offering the same degree of accuracy as larger catheters. Additionally, the smaller catheter may also be easier to maneuver in smaller lumens or vessels. In any case, it is important to consider the individual patient's anatomy and preferences when selecting a catheter. Ultimately, the choice of the right catheter helps ensure a successful re-access procedure. Although various catheters may be able to provide results, Ikari efficiently delivers for both coronary arteries. To perform sub-selective angiography, any cell above the coronary artery can be engaged. If selective imaging must be performed, inserting a wire into the vessel and guiding the catheter with the wire to introduce the catheter is extremely useful.

Edwards Sapien 3 valves are often placed above the coronary ostia, their frame is taller, and the upper cells are more prominent, resulting in less interference with coronary ostia access. It is uncommon to experience coronary obstruction when using the "high implant-90/10" implantation technique, which helps to minimize interference with the left ventricular outflow tract. In most cases, a specific catheter selection does not need to engage the coronary arteries with a Sapien 3 valve. To avoid altering the position of the

Sapien 3 valve or managing the task of disengaging the guiding wire post-intervention, a guide extender is recommended for percutaneous coronary interventions [44,45].

With the bench-testing of patient-specific 3D-printed models, it has been demonstrated that diagnostic angiography and PCI are highly feasible following ViV-TAVR using the ACURATE neo valve [46]. It was reported that 62/64 (97%) cannulations were suitable for the assessment of angiography. On average, only one attempt was needed for cannulation, and the procedure took approximately 1 min and 48 s to complete. Selective cannulation was achieved in 82% of cases (51 out of 62). As a rule, in most of the situations, no more than one cannulation attempt was needed (49/62, 79%). A total of 9 out of 62 (15%) cannulations involved complex cannulation techniques with 0.014" coronary wire-assisted cannulation being the most frequently used approach.

In terms of cannulation feasibility, selectivity, attempts, time, or technique, no significant disparities were noted between the LCA and RCA. It was viable to conduct the entire PCI procedure in 61/64 (95% of cases).

5. Basilica Procedure

During the valve deployment procedure, leaflets may be lacerated, or the coronary ostia may be protected with a guide catheter to prevent obstruction. Before a transcatheter heart valve implantation, a BASILICA (bioprosthetic or native aortic scallop intentional laceration to prevent iatrogenic coronary artery obstruction) procedure uses a transcatheter electrosurgical process. This involves crossing the aortic leaflet and lacerating it in line with the exposed coronary artery ostium to ensure blood flow to the coronary arteries is maintained after the valve implantation, thus avoiding coronary occlusion (Figure 1) [47,48].

During such a procedure, a wire loop is created by snagging the guidewire within the left ventricle. A non-insulated, non-coated portion of the wire is positioned at the leaflet to split the aortic leaflet, and electricity is applied. To reduce coronary obstruction following the valve implantation, the bioprosthetic leaflet or native leaflet is separated. It may be more challenging to lacerate leaflets with excessive calcification or thickening.

A prospective, multicenter registry named BASILICA tracks patients at risk for iatrogenic coronary occlusion following TAVR using the BASILICA technique. In North America and Europe, the registry enrolled 214 patients. 72.8 percent of patients had bioprosthetic aortic valves. There was a success rate of 94.9% and 94.4% for leaflet traversal and laceration, and the prevalence of coronary obstructions (partial or complete) was 4.7% [49–51].

In Europe, EURO-BASILICA provides the first multicenter study investigating the BASILICA technique. A one-year clinical study demonstrated that this technique was effective and viable in protecting against CAO caused by TAVR. There were 76 patients enrolled across ten centers in Europe, 5.3% of whom had native aortic valves, 92.1% had surgical bioprosthetic valves, and 2.6% had transcatheter valves. The proportion of patients who required double BASILICA (for both coronary cusps) was 11.8%. The BASILICA approach resulted in successful outcomes in 97.7% of cases, with only a small percentage (2.4%) experiencing complete coronary occlusion. Additionally, in 90.6% of situations, there were no instances of leaflet-associated coronary occlusion [52]. A total leaflet-induced occlusion was documented in two patients. In one case, the left coronary artery was occluded, and extracorporeal membrane oxygenation was needed for one hour. Using the chimney technique, the occlusion was treated with ostial stenting. In the second case, the left coronary artery ostium was completely obliterated by the partial avulsion of a bioprosthetic valve leaflet. Ostial stenting was used to treat the obstruction, and Impella was used to provide mechanical support.

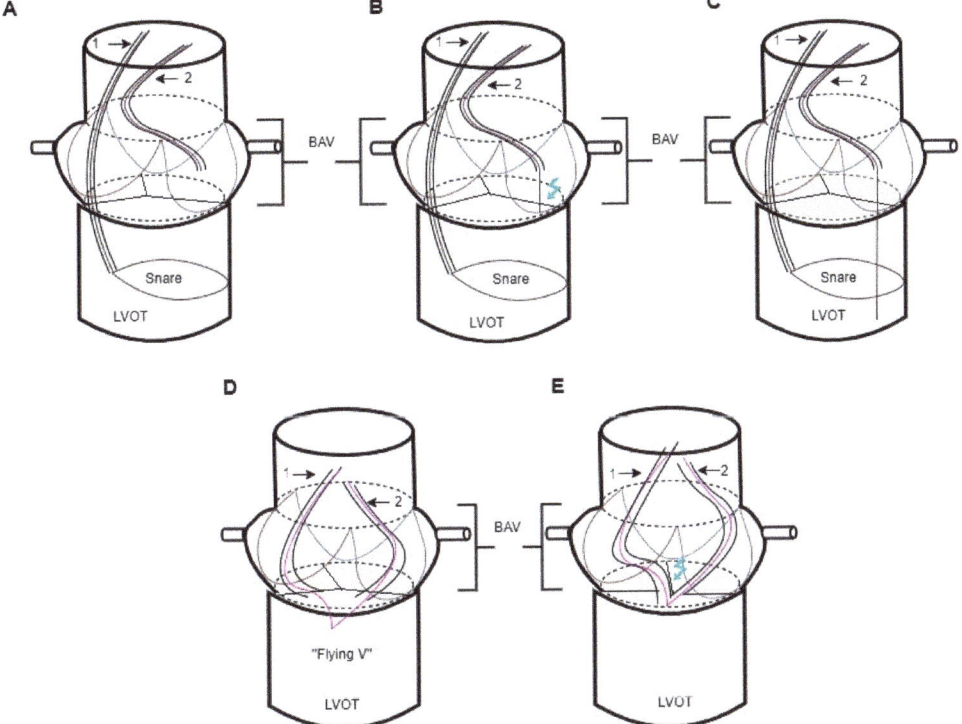

Figure 1. BASILICA procedure on the left aortic leaflet in a biological aortic valve. 1—MP1; 2—AL2. Steps: Amplatz Left 2 (AL2) guiding catheter is placed in the ascending aorta. Goose Neck snares are delivered into the LVOT through a Multipurpose 1 (MP1) guiding catheter (**A**). After the placement of an 0.014″ Astato wire into the AL2 until it reaches the lowest point of the left aortic leaflet, it is electrified before crossing over into the LVOT. (**B**). The 0.014″ Astato wire is snared (**C**). In the next step, the snare is externalized, and the "flying V" is placed (**D**). Injection of 5% dextrose water into both catheters results in laceration of the leaflet with the Astato wire, causing it to splay outward (**E**). LVOT, left ventricular outflow tract; BAV, biological aortic valve.

6. Chimney Stenting Procedure

Chimney stenting is an acceptable (and less laborious than the BASILICA) bailout technique among patients with established coronary artery occlusion and those without upfront coronary protection. Before expanding the valve, the "chimney" technique involves using a guide catheter and guide extender to engage the coronary artery (Figure 2).

The chimney stenting technique and flow chart is conducted as follows: Step 1, place an adequately dimensioned coronary stent in the mid-left anterior descending coronary artery before the implantation of the transcatheter heart valve. The scaffolding must be long enough to extend into the ascending aorta until it reaches the sinotubular junction. Step 2, when implanting the valve, withdraw the guide catheter and place it in the ascending aorta. Step 3, in case of compromised coronary blood flow, meticulously pull the non-deployed stent back over the coronary ostium and over the dislocated aortic leaflets and then implant it. Step 4, if the valve needs post-dilatation, complete simultaneous kissing balloon inflation with the chimney stent. Step 5, complete a final angiographic check.

Protecting the coronary artery during TAVR typically involves using additional arterial access to engage the guide catheter in the at-risk coronary artery. It is recommended to use Judkins left/right or multipurpose guiding catheters during THV deployment since these catheters allow quicker backup into the ascending aorta and can be moved closer to the ostium after THV deployment. Using other catheters (Ikari, EBU, or AL1) may also be successful. However, they may be more difficult to reposition after THV implantation. As a precaution against hemodynamic instability following balloon aortic valvuloplasty (BAV), a coronary guide catheter needs to be attached and a guidewire placed distally into the vessel. Having positioned a balloon or stent over the wire distally in the artery, the guide catheter is withdrawn slowly into the ascending aorta. The anatomical factors concerning the aortic root and the apprehension of the risk of CAO may influence the judgment to place a balloon or scaffold on the guidewire. Although using only a guide wire can save costs and time, it can be challenging to deliver a stent next to an implanted valve and dislocated native leaflets due to calcium build-up or the protection guidewire becoming stuck [53,54]. The failure rate of stent deployment was 10 to 20 percent in two observational trials in which stenting was attempted for the treatment of CAO during TAVR [26,55].

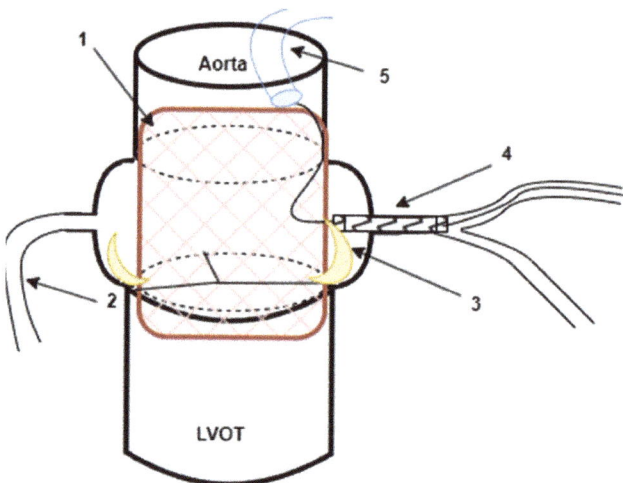

Figure 2. During TAVR implantation, a chimney stenting procedure is performed due to occlusion of the left coronary artery: 1—TAVR valve implanted; 2—the right coronary artery, 3—dislocated leaflet causing CAO; 4—left main stenting as a bailout strategy; and 5—Luncher guide catheter.

The International Chimney Registry was founded in October 2017, included 60 patients, and gathered retrospective data from 16 centers in North America, Europe, and the Middle East on individuals experiencing chimney stenting as part of transcatheter aortic valve interventions from May 2010 to July 2018. The database did not include data from cases with initial coronary protection involving no chimney scaffold implantation or patients with coronary artery obstruction resolved using other strategies. Among the arteries stented, the left main was more commonly treated by itself (49 cases; 81.6% of the total) or in conjunction with the right coronary artery (6 patients; 10% of the cases). In most cases (96.6%), drug-eluting stents were used, with an average stent size and diameter of 19 ± 7.8 and 4.1 ± 0.5 mm, according to the data. Many incomplete stent expansions were observed in 55% of cases, requiring further dilation or implantation of a second scaffold within the initially implanted stent (11 patients). A total of 2 patients (3.3%) underwent post-dilatation of the transcatheter heart valve with a kissing balloon technique. In 19 cases with mean gradients of over 20 mm Hg, 90% had experienced a valve-in-valve intervention. The number of patients with more than mild paravalvular leaks was 3 (5.0%). Out of the total number of patients, 3 (5.0%) died while in hospital. One patient was unresponsive after being removed from a cardiopulmonary bypass on the first day, another patient succumbed on the fifth day due to complications related to cardiogenic shock, and the third patient died on the eleventh day from septic shock following the intervention [56,57]. The COPROTAVR registry collected data on 236 patients at risk of coronary occlusion who had undergone transcatheter aortic valve implantation with a coronary safety guidewire in place [58]. Out of the total number of participants in the trial, 143 patients underwent coronary stenting, which makes up 60.6% of the total. Of these patients, 79% received chimney stenting, while 21% received ostial stenting. After a 3-year follow-up, patients who underwent stenting had positive outcomes with lower rates of cardiac mortality (7.8%), myocardial infarction (9.8%), and stroke (5.4%). Although stent thrombosis was infrequent (0.9%), it posed a life-threatening risk in every instance [58].

These trials provide initial indications of reasonably acceptable mid-term safety when it comes to chimney stenting. However, it is important to approach these retrospective findings with caution due to the limited number of patients involved. Consequently, we advise against employing chimney stenting as the primary strategy for younger individuals or those with more severe CAD. Instead, angioplasty should only be considered a rescue alternative in situations where a potential or existing coronary artery obstruction necessitates immediate intervention.

7. Conclusions

As part of selecting an appropriate THV, it is important to carefully consider the valve's shape and how it relates to the coronary arteries. It is also crucial to thoroughly examine the computer tomography study before the procedure to fully understand the anatomy of the coronary ostia, sinus of Valsalva, and sinotubular junction. Numerous factors need to be taken into account to facilitate coronary re-access in valve-in-valve procedures. Identifying the risk factors for coronary artery occlusion during TAVR is crucial, as this is a rare yet grave, life-threatening issue. If the valve neoskirt extends over at least one of the coronaries and the valve–aorta distance is less than 3–4 mm, it is recommended to use a coronary guide wire and a pre-mounted stent. This is particularly important if the additional transcatheter valve heart is planned to be placed high or if there is a risk of the index THV stent expanding excessively. Chimney stenting can be performed in order to restore coronary flow in the case of impending or established CAO. For patients who are at high risk of coronary occlusion, the BASILICA approach may be considered as an option. However, it is important to evaluate the positioning of the first implanted valve with the native aortic valve before the procedure. If there is severe misalignment, the outcome of the technique may be compromised. The long-term effectiveness (>12 months) of both CAO prevention techniques remains unknown.

Author Contributions: Conceptualization, F.-A.G. and A.A.; methodology, F.-A.G. and A.A.; writing—original draft preparation, F.-A.G. and A.A.; writing—review and editing, F.-A.G. and A.A.; visualization, F.-A.G. and A.A.; supervision, A.A.; project administration, F.-A.G. All authors have read and agreed to the published version of the manuscript.

Funding: This research received no external funding.

Institutional Review Board Statement: Not applicable.

Informed Consent Statement: Not applicable.

Data Availability Statement: Not applicable.

Conflicts of Interest: The authors declare no conflict of interest.

References

1. Figulla, H.R.; Franz, M.; Lauten, A. The History of Transcatheter Aortic Valve Implantation (TAVI)-A Personal View Over 25 Years of Development. *Cardiovasc. Revasc. Med.* **2020**, *21*, 398–403. [CrossRef] [PubMed]
2. Leon, M.B.; Smith, C.R.; Mack, M.; Miller, D.C.; Moses, J.W.; Svensson, L.G.; Tuzcu, E.M.; Webb, J.G.; Fontana, G.P.; Makkar, R.R.; et al. Transcatheter Aortic-Valve Implantation for Aortic Stenosis in Patients Who Cannot Undergo Surgery. *N. Engl. J. Med.* **2010**, *363*, 1597–1607. [CrossRef]
3. Smith, C.R.; Leon, M.B.; Mack, M.J.; Miller, D.C.; Moses, J.W.; Svensson, L.G.; Tuzcu, E.M.; Webb, J.G.; Fontana, G.P.; Makkar, R.R.; et al. Transcatheter versus Surgical Aortic-Valve Replacement in High-Risk Patients. *N. Engl. J. Med.* **2011**, *364*, 2187–2198. [CrossRef]

4. Reardon, M.J.; Van Mieghem, N.M.; Popma, J.J.; Kleiman, N.S.; Søndergaard, L.; Mumtaz, M.; Adams, D.H.; Deeb, G.M.; Maini, B.; Gada, H.; et al. Surgical or Transcatheter Aortic-Valve Replacement in Intermediate-Risk Patients. *N. Engl. J. Med.* **2017**, *376*, 1321–1331. [CrossRef]
5. Thourani, V.H.; Kodali, S.; Makkar, R.R.; Herrmann, H.C.; Williams, M.; Babaliaros, V.; Smalling, R.; Lim, S.; Malaisrie, S.C.; Kapadia, S.; et al. Transcatheter Aortic Valve Replacement versus Surgical Valve Replacement in Intermediate-Risk Patients: A Propensity Score Analysis. *Lancet* **2016**, *387*, 2218–2225. [CrossRef]
6. Popma, J.J.; Deeb, G.M.; Yakubov, S.J.; Mumtaz, M.; Gada, H.; O'Hair, D.; Bajwa, T.; Heiser, J.C.; Merhi, W.; Kleiman, N.S.; et al. Transcatheter Aortic-Valve Replacement with a Self-Expanding Valve in Low-Risk Patients. *N. Engl. J. Med.* **2019**, *380*, 1706–1715. [CrossRef] [PubMed]
7. Eggebrecht, H.; Mehta, R.H. Transcatheter Aortic Valve Implantation (TAVI) in Germany 2008-2014: On Its Way to Standard Therapy for Aortic Valve Stenosis in the Elderly? *EuroIntervention* **2016**, *11*, 1029–1033. [CrossRef] [PubMed]
8. Grover, F.L.; Vemulapalli, S.; Carroll, J.D.; Edwards, F.H.; Mack, M.J.; Thourani, V.H.; Brindis, R.G.; Shahian, D.M.; Ruiz, C.E.; Jacobs, J.P.; et al. 2016 Annual Report of The Society of Thoracic Surgeons/American College of Cardiology Transcatheter Valve Therapy Registry. *J. Am. Coll. Cardiol.* **2017**, *69*, 1215–1230. [CrossRef]
9. De Backer, O.; Luk, N.H.V.; Olsen, N.T.; Olsen, P.S.; Søndergaard, L. Choice of Treatment for Aortic Valve Stenosis in the Era of Transcatheter Aortic Valve Replacement in Eastern Denmark (2005 to 2015). *JACC. Cardiovasc. Interv.* **2016**, *9*, 1152–1158. [CrossRef] [PubMed]
10. Faroux, L.; Guimaraes, L.; Wintzer-Wehekind, J.; Junquera, L.; Ferreira-Neto, A.N.; del Val, D.; Muntané-Carol, G.; Mohammadi, S.; Paradis, J.M.; Rodés-Cabau, J. Coronary Artery Disease and Transcatheter Aortic Valve Replacement: JACC State-of-the-Art Review. *J. Am. Coll. Cardiol.* **2019**, *74*, 362–372. [CrossRef]
11. Paradis, J.M.; Labbé, B.; Rodés-Cabau, J. Coronary Artery Disease and Transcatheter Aortic Valve Replacement: Current Treatment Paradigms. *Coron. Artery Dis.* **2015**, *26*, 272–278. [CrossRef] [PubMed]
12. Lateef, N.; Khan, M.S.; Deo, S.V.; Yamani, N.; Riaz, H.; Virk, H.U.H.; Khan, S.U.; Hedrick, D.P.; Kanaan, A.; Reed, G.W.; et al. Meta-Analysis Comparing Outcomes in Patients Undergoing Transcatheter Aortic Valve Implantation With Versus Without Percutaneous Coronary Intervention. *Am. J. Cardiol.* **2019**, *124*, 1757–1764. [CrossRef] [PubMed]
13. Tarantini, G.; Tang, G.; Fovino, L.N.; Blackman, D.; Mieghem, N.V.; Kim, W.-K.; Karam, N.; Carrilho-Ferreira, P.; Fournier, S.; Pręgowski, J.; et al. Management of Coronary Artery Disease in Patients Undergoing Transcatheter Aortic Valve Implantation. A Clinical Consensus Statement from the European Association of Percutaneous Cardiovascular Interventions in Collaboration with the ESC Working Group on Cardiovascular Surgery. Available online: https://eurointervention.pcronline.com/article/management-of-coronary-artery-disease-in-patients-undergoing-transcatheter-aortic-valve-implantation-a-clinical-consensus-statement-from-the-european-association-of-percutaneous-cardiovascular-interventions-in-collaboration-with-the-esc-working-group-on-cardiovascular-surgery (accessed on 13 June 2023).
14. Witberg, G.; Regev, E.; Chen, S.; Assali, A.; Barbash, I.M.; Planer, D.; Vaknin-Assa, H.; Guetta, V.; Vukasinovic, V.; Orvin, K.; et al. The Prognostic Effects of Coronary Disease Severity and Completeness of Revascularization on Mortality in Patients Undergoing Transcatheter Aortic Valve Replacement. *JACC. Cardiovasc. Interv.* **2017**, *10*, 1428–1435. [CrossRef] [PubMed]
15. Neumann, F.-J.; Sousa-Uva, M.; Ahlsson, A.; Alfonso, F.; Banning, A.P.; Benedetto, U.; Byrne, R.A.; Collet, J.-P.; Falk, V.; Head, S.J.; et al. 2018 ESC/EACTS Guidelines on Myocardial Revascularization. *Eur. Heart J.* **2019**, *40*, 87–165. [CrossRef]
16. Vilalta, V.; Asmarats, L.; Ferreira-Neto, A.N.; Maes, F.; de Freitas Campos Guimarães, L.; Couture, T.; Paradis, J.M.; Mohammadi, S.; Dumont, E.; Kalavrouziotis, D.; et al. Incidence, Clinical Characteristics, and Impact of Acute Coronary Syndrome Following Transcatheter Aortic Valve Replacement. *JACC. Cardiovasc. Interv.* **2018**, *11*, 2523–2533. [CrossRef]
17. Allali, A.; El-Mawardy, M.; Schwarz, B.; Sato, T.; Geist, V.; Toelg, R.; Richardt, G.; Abdel-Wahab, M. Incidence, Feasibility and Outcome of Percutaneous Coronary Intervention after Transcatheter Aortic Valve Implantation with a Self-Expanding Prosthesis. Results from a Single Center Experience. *Cardiovasc. Revascularization Med. Incl. Mol. Interv.* **2016**, *17*, 391–398. [CrossRef]
18. Chetcuti, S.; Kleiman, N.; Matthews, R.; Popma, J.J.; Moore, J. TCT-743 Percutaneous Coronary Intervention after Self-Expanding Transcatheter Aortic Valve Replacement. *J. Am. Coll. Cardiol.* **2016**, *68*, B300–B301. [CrossRef]
19. Zivelonghi, C.; Pesarini, G.; Scarsini, R.; Lunardi, M.; Piccoli, A.; Ferrero, V.; Gottin, L.; Vassanelli, C.; Ribichini, F. Coronary Catheterization and Percutaneous Interventions After Transcatheter Aortic Valve Implantation. *Am. J. Cardiol.* **2017**, *120*, 625–631. [CrossRef]
20. Htun, W.W.; Grines, C.; Schreiber, T. Feasibility of Coronary Angiography and Percutaneous Coronary Intervention after Transcatheter Aortic Valve Replacement Using a Medtronic™ Self-Expandable Bioprosthetic Valve. *Catheter. Cardiovasc. Interv.* **2018**, *91*, 1339–1344. [CrossRef]
21. Boukantar, M.; Gallet, R.; Mouillet, G.; Belarbi, A.; Rubimbura, V.; Ternacle, J.; Dubois-Rande, J.L.; Teiger, E. Coronary Procedures After TAVI With the Self-Expanding Aortic Bioprosthesis Medtronic CoreValve™, Not an Easy Matter. *J. Interv. Cardiol.* **2017**, *30*, 56–62. [CrossRef]
22. Tanaka, A.; Jabbour, R.J.; Testa, L.; Agnifili, M.; Ettori, F.; Fiorina, C.; Adamo, M.; Bruschi, G.; Giannini, C.; Petronio, A.S.; et al. Incidence, Technical Safety, and Feasibility of Coronary Angiography and Intervention Following Self-Expanding Transcatheter Aortic Valve Replacement. *Cardiovasc. Revascularization Med.* **2019**, *20*, 371–375. [CrossRef] [PubMed]

23. Ribeiro, H.B.; Webb, J.G.; Makkar, R.R.; Cohen, M.G.; Kapadia, S.R.; Kodali, S.; Tamburino, C.; Barbanti, M.; Chakravarty, T.; Jilaihawi, H.; et al. Predictive Factors, Management, and Clinical Outcomes of Coronary Obstruction Following Transcatheter Aortic Valve Implantation: Insights from a Large Multicenter Registry. *J. Am. Coll. Cardiol.* **2013**, *62*, 1552–1562. [CrossRef] [PubMed]
24. Ribeiro, H.B.; Rodés-Cabau, J.; Blanke, P.; Leipsic, J.; Kwan Park, J.; Bapat, V.; Makkar, R.; Simonato, M.; Barbanti, M.; Schofer, J.; et al. Incidence, Predictors, and Clinical Outcomes of Coronary Obstruction Following Transcatheter Aortic Valve Replacement for Degenerative Bioprosthetic Surgical Valves: Insights from the VIVID Registry. *Eur. Heart J.* **2018**, *39*, 687–695. [CrossRef]
25. Gherasie, F.A.; Udroiu, C.A.; Davila, C. Bicuspid Aortic Valves and Transcatheter Valve Replacement: Feasibility and Safety. *Maedica* **2023**, *18*, 117. [PubMed]
26. Ribeiro, H.B.; Nombela-Franco, L.; Urena, M.; Mok, M.; Pasian, S.; Doyle, D.; Delarochellière, R.; Côté, M.; Laflamme, L.; Delarochellière, H.; et al. Coronary Obstruction Following Transcatheter Aortic Valve Implantation: A Systematic Review. *JACC Cardiovasc. Interv.* **2013**, *6*, 452–461. [CrossRef] [PubMed]
27. Nour, D.; Allahwala, U.; Hansen, P.; Brady, P.; Choong, C.; Bhindi, R. Cardiogenic Shock Due to Late Chimney Stent Failure Following Valve-in-Valve Transcatheter Aortic Valve Replacement. *JACC Case Rep.* **2019**, *1*, 313–318. [CrossRef]
28. Dvir, D.; Leipsic, J.; Blanke, P.; Ribeiro, H.B.; Kornowski, R.; Pichard, A.; Rodés-Cabau, J.; Wood, D.A.; Stub, D.; Ben-Dor, I.; et al. Coronary Obstruction in Transcatheter Aortic Valve-in-Valve Implantation Preprocedural Evaluation, Device Selection, Protection, and Treatment. *Circ. Cardiovasc. Interv.* **2015**, *8*, e002079. [CrossRef]
29. Khalid, A.M.; O'Sullivan, C.J. Commissural Alignment in Transcatheter Aortic Valve Replacement: A Literature Review. *Front. Cardiovasc. Med.* **2022**, *9*, 938653. [CrossRef]
30. Tchétché, D.; Siddiqui, S. Optimizing Fluoroscopic Projections for TAVR: Any Difference Between the Double S-Curve and the Cusp-Overlap Technique? *JACC Cardiovasc. Interv.* **2021**, *14*, 195–197. [CrossRef]
31. Ben-Shoshan, J.; Alosaimi, H.; Lauzier, P.T.; Pighi, M.; Talmor-Barkan, Y.; Overtchouk, P.; Martucci, G.; Spaziano, M.; Finkelstein, A.; Gada, H.; et al. Double S-Curve Versus Cusp-Overlap Technique: Defining the Optimal Fluoroscopic Projection for TAVR With a Self-Expanding Device. *JACC Cardiovasc. Interv.* **2021**, *14*, 185–194. [CrossRef]
32. Piazza, N.; Martucci, G.; Spaziano, M. Commissural or Coronary Alignment for TAVR? Align What and by How Much? *JACC Cardiovasc. Interv.* **2022**, *15*, 147–149. [CrossRef]
33. Redondo, A.; Baladrón Zorita, C.; Tchétché, D.; Santos-Martinez, S.; Delgado-Arana, J.R.; Barrero, A.; Gutiérrez, H.; Serrador Frutos, A.; Ybarra Falcón, C.; Gómez, M.G.; et al. Commissural Versus Coronary Optimized Alignment During Transcatheter Aortic Valve Replacement. *JACC Cardiovasc. Interv.* **2022**, *15*, 135–146. [CrossRef] [PubMed]
34. Wang, X.; De Backer, O.; Bieliauskas, G.; Wong, I.; Bajoras, V.; Xiong, T.Y.; Zhang, Y.; Kofoed, K.F.; Chen, M.; Sondergaard, L. Cusp Symmetry and Coronary Ostial Eccentricity and Its Impact on Coronary Access Following TAVR. *JACC: Cardiovasc. Interv.* **2022**, *15*, 123–134. [CrossRef] [PubMed]
35. Tang, G.H.L.; Zaid, S.; Gupta, E.; Ahmad, H.; Patel, N.; Khan, M.; Khan, A.; Kovacic, J.C.; Lansman, S.L.; Dangas, G.D.; et al. Impact of Initial Evolut Transcatheter Aortic Valve Replacement Deployment Orientation on Final Valve Orientation and Coronary Reaccess. *Circulation. Cardiovasc. Interv.* **2019**, *12*, e008044. [CrossRef] [PubMed]
36. Arshi, A.; Yakubov, S.J.; Stiver, K.L.; Sanchez, C.E. Overcoming the Transcatheter Aortic Valve Replacement Achilles Heel: Coronary Re-Access. *Ann. Cardiothorac. Surg.* **2020**, *9*, 468–477. [CrossRef] [PubMed]
37. Tarantini, G.; Delgado, V.; de Backer, O.; Sathananthan, J.; Treede, H.; Saia, F.; Blackman, D.; Parma, R. Redo-Transcatheter Aortic Valve Implantation Using the SAPIEN 3/Ultra Transcatheter Heart Valves—Expert Consensus on Procedural Planning and Techniques. *Am. J. Cardiol.* **2023**, *192*, 228–244. [CrossRef] [PubMed]
38. Yudi, M.B.; Sharma, S.K.; Tang, G.H.L.; Kini, A. Coronary Angiography and Percutaneous Coronary Intervention After Transcatheter Aortic Valve Replacement. *J. Am. Coll. Cardiol.* **2018**, *71*, 1360–1378. [CrossRef]
39. Lopes, P.M.; Brito, J.D.; Campante Teles, R.; Sousa Almeida, M. Acute Left Main Coronary Occlusion after Transcatheter Aortic Valve Implantation: Life-Saving Intervention Using the Snare Technique—A Case Report. *Eur. Heart J. Case Rep.* **2023**, *7*, ytac469. [CrossRef]
40. Möllmann, H.; Hengstenberg, C.; Hilker, M.; Kerber, S.; Schäfer, U.; Rudolph, T.; Linke, A.H.-P.; Franz, N.; Kuntze, T.; Nef, H.; et al. Real-World Experience Using the ACURATE Neo Prosthesis: 30-Day Outcomes of 1000 Patients Enrolled in the SAVI TF Registry. Available online: https://eurointervention.pcronline.com/article/real-world-experience-using-the-acurate-neo-prosthesis-30-day-outcomes-of-1000-patients-enrolled-in-the-savi-tf-registry (accessed on 2 May 2023).
41. Vanhaverbeke, M.; Kim, W.-K.; Mylotte, D.; Bieliauskas, G.; Janarthanan, S.; Sondergaard, L.; Backer, O.D. Procedural Considerations for Transcatheter Aortic Valve-in-Valve Implantation in a Degenerated ACURATE Neo Prosthesis. Available online: https://eurointervention.pcronline.com/article/procedural-considerations-for-transcatheter-aortic-valve-in-valve-implantation-in-a-degenerated-acurate-neo-prosthesis (accessed on 2 May 2023).
42. Kawamura, A.; Maeda, K.; Shimamura, K.; Yamashita, K.; Mukai, T.; Nakamura, M.; Mizote, I.; Sakata, Y.; Miyagawa, S. Coronary Access after Repeat Transcatheter Aortic Valve Replacement in Patients of Small Body Size: A Simulation Study. *J. Thorac. Cardiovasc. Surg.* **2022**, in press. [CrossRef]
43. Barbanti, M.; Costa, G.; Picci, A.; Criscione, E.; Reddavid, C.; Valvo, R.; Todaro, D.; Deste, W.; Condorelli, A.; Scalia, M.; et al. Coronary Cannulation After Transcatheter Aortic Valve Replacement: The RE-ACCESS Study. *JACC Cardiovasc. Interv.* **2020**, *13*, 2542–2555. [CrossRef]

44. Tarantini, G.; Nai Fovino, L.; Le Prince, P.; Darremont, O.; Urena, M.; Bartorelli, A.L.; Vincent, F.; Hovorka, T.; Alcalá Navarro, Y.; Dumonteil, N.; et al. Coronary Access and Percutaneous Coronary Intervention up to 3 Years after Transcatheter Aortic Valve Implantation with a Balloon-Expandable Valve. *Circ. Cardiovasc. Interv.* **2020**, *13*, e008972. [CrossRef]
45. Ochiai, T.; Chakravarty, T.; Yoon, S.H.; Kaewkes, D.; Flint, N.; Patel, V.; Mahani, S.; Tiwana, R.; Sekhon, N.; Nakamura, M.; et al. Coronary Access After TAVR. *JACC Cardiovasc. Interv.* **2020**, *13*, 693–705. [CrossRef]
46. Khokhar, A.A.; Ponticelli, F.; Zlahoda-Huzior, A.; Chandra, K.; Ruggiero, R.; Toselli, M.; Gallo, F.; Cereda, A.; Sticchi, A.; Laricchia, A.; et al. Coronary Access Following ACURATE Neo Implantation for Transcatheter Aortic Valve-in-Valve Implantation: Ex Vivo Analysis in Patient-Specific Anatomies. *Front. Cardiovasc. Med.* **2022**, *9*, 902564. [CrossRef]
47. Khan, J.M.; Dvir, D.; Greenbaum, A.B.; Babaliaros, V.C.; Rogers, T.; Aldea, G.; Reisman, M.; Mackensen, G.B.; Eng, M.H.K.; Paone, G.; et al. Transcatheter Laceration of Aortic Leaflets to Prevent Coronary Obstruction During Transcatheter Aortic Valve Replacement: Concept to First-in-Human. *JACC Cardiovasc. Interv.* **2018**, *11*, 677–689. [CrossRef] [PubMed]
48. Lederman, R.J.; Babaliaros, V.C.; Rogers, T.; Khan, J.M.; Kamioka, N.; Dvir, D.; Greenbaum, A.B. Preventing Coronary Obstruction During Transcatheter Aortic Valve Replacement: From Computed Tomography to BASILICA. *JACC Cardiovasc. Interv.* **2019**, *12*, 1197–1216. [CrossRef]
49. Khan, J.M.; Greenbaum, A.B.; Babaliaros, V.C.; Rogers, T.; Eng, M.H.; Paone, G.; Leshnower, B.G.; Reisman, M.; Satler, L.; Waksman, R.; et al. The BASILICA Trial: Prospective Multicenter Investigation of Intentional Leaflet Laceration to Prevent TAVR Coronary Obstruction. *JACC Cardiovasc. Interv.* **2019**, *12*, 1240–1252. [CrossRef] [PubMed]
50. Khan, J.M.; Greenbaum, A.B.; Babaliaros, V.C.; Dvir, D.; Reisman, M.; McCabe, J.M.; Satler, L.; Waksman, R.; Eng, M.H.; Paone, G.; et al. BASILICA Trial: One-Year Outcomes of Transcatheter Electrosurgical Leaflet Laceration to Prevent TAVR Coronary Obstruction. *Circ. Cardiovasc. Interv.* **2021**, *14*, E010238. [CrossRef] [PubMed]
51. Khan, J.M.; Babaliaros, V.C.; Greenbaum, A.B.; Spies, C.; Daniels, D.; Depta, J.P.; Oldemeyer, J.B.; Whisenant, B.; McCabe, J.M.; Muhammad, K.I.; et al. Preventing Coronary Obstruction During Transcatheter Aortic Valve Replacement: Results From the Multicenter International BASILICA Registry. *JACC Cardiovasc. Interv.* **2021**, *14*, 941–948. [CrossRef] [PubMed]
52. Abdel-Wahab, M.; Richter, I.; Taramasso, M.; Unbehaun, A.; Rudolph, T.; Ribichini, F.; Binder, R.; Schofer, J.; Mangner, N.-H.; Dambrink, J.-H.; et al. Procedural and One-Year Outcomes of the BASILICA Technique in Europe: The Multicentre EURO-BASILICA Registry. Available online: https://eurointervention.pcronline.com/article/procedural-and-one-year-outcomes-of-the-basilica-technique-in-europe-the-multicentre-euro-basilica-registry (accessed on 2 May 2023).
53. Rosseel, L.; Rosseel, M.; Hynes, B.; Bel, X.A.; Crilly, E.; Mylotte, D. Chimney Stenting during Transcatheter Aortic Valve Implantation. *Interv. Cardiol. Rev. Res. Resour.* **2020**, *15*, e09. [CrossRef] [PubMed]
54. Fetahovic, T.; Hayman, S.; Cox, S.; Cole, C.; Rafter, T.; Camuglia, A. The Prophylactic Chimney Snorkel Technique for the Prevention of Acute Coronary Occlusion in High Risk for Coronary Obstruction Transcatheter Aortic Valve Replacement/Implantation Cases. *Heart Lung Circ.* **2019**, *28*, e126–e130. [CrossRef]
55. Kappetein, A.P.; Head, S.J.; Généreux, P.; Piazza, N.; Van Mieghem, N.M.; Blackstone, E.H.; Brott, T.G.; Cohen, D.J.; Cutlip, D.E.; Van Es, G.A.; et al. Updated Standardized Endpoint Definitions for Transcatheter Aortic Valve Implantation: The Valve Academic Research Consortium-2 Consensus Document (VARC-2). *Eur. J. Cardio-Thorac. Surgery Off. J. Eur. Assoc. Cardio-Thorac. Surg.* **2012**, *42*, S45–S60. [CrossRef] [PubMed]
56. Mercanti, F.; Rosseel, L.; Neylon, A.; Bagur, R.; Sinning, J.M.; Nickenig, G.; Grube, E.; Hildick-Smith, D.; Tavano, D.; Wolf, A.; et al. Chimney Stenting for Coronary Occlusion During TAVR: Insights From the Chimney Registry. *JACC Cardiovasc. Interv.* **2020**, *13*, 751–761. [CrossRef] [PubMed]
57. Fernández Gonzalez, L.; Blanco Mata, R.; Fernandez Gonzalez, L.; Garcia, K.; Roman, S.; Villa, J.A. Emergent Chimney Stent to Treat Left Main Occlusion Following Valve-in-Valve Transfemoral Aortic Implantation Chimney Stent Following Valve-in-Valve TAVI. *J. Thorac. Cardiovasc. Surg.* **2018**, *in press*. [CrossRef]
58. Palmerini, T.; Chakravarty, T.; Saia, F.; Bruno, A.G.; Bacchi-Reggiani, M.-L.; Marrozzini, C.; Patel, C.; Patel, V.; Testa, L.; Bedogni, F.; et al. Coronary Protection to Prevent Coronary Obstruction During TAVR: A Multicenter International Registry. *JACC Cardiovasc. Interv.* **2020**, *13*, 739–747. [CrossRef]

Disclaimer/Publisher's Note: The statements, opinions and data contained in all publications are solely those of the individual author(s) and contributor(s) and not of MDPI and/or the editor(s). MDPI and/or the editor(s) disclaim responsibility for any injury to people or property resulting from any ideas, methods, instructions or products referred to in the content.

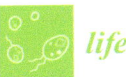

Review

Fighting Cardiac Thromboembolism during Transcatheter Procedures: An Update on the Use of Cerebral Protection Devices in Cath Labs and EP Labs

Alberto Preda [1,*], Claudio Montalto [2], Michele Galasso [2], Andrea Munafò [2], Ilaria Garofani [1], Matteo Baroni [1], Lorenzo Gigli [1], Sara Vargiu [1], Marisa Varrenti [1], Giulia Colombo [1], Marco Carbonaro [1], Domenico Giovanni Della Rocca [3,4], Jacopo Oreglia [2], Patrizio Mazzone [1] and Fabrizio Guarracini [5]

1. Electrophysiology Unit, De Gasperis Cardio Center, Niguarda Hospital, 20162 Milan, Italy
2. Interventional Cardiology Unit, De Gasperis Cardio Center, Niguarda Hospital, 20162 Milan, Italy; claudio.montalto@ospedaleniguarda.it (C.M.); andreamuna1993@gmail.com (A.M.)
3. Heart Rhythm Management Centre, Postgraduate Program in Cardiac Electrophysiology and Pacing, Universitair Ziekenhuis Brussel, Vrije Universiteit Brussel, European Reference Networks Guard-Heart, 1090 Brussels, Belgium
4. Texas Cardiac Arrhythmia Institute, St. David's Medical Center, Austin, TX 78705, USA
5. Department of Cardiology, Santa Chiara Hospital, 38122 Trento, Italy
* Correspondence: preda.alberto@hsr.it

Abstract: Intraprocedural stroke is a well-documented and feared potential risk of cardiovascular transcatheter procedures (TPs). Moreover, subclinical neurological events or covert central nervous system infarctions are concerns related to the development of dementia, future stroke, cognitive decline, and increased risk of mortality. Cerebral protection devices (CPDs) were developed to mitigate the risk of cardioembolic embolism during TPs. They are mechanical barriers designed to cover the ostium of the supra-aortic branches in the aortic arch, but newer devices are able to protect the descending aorta. CPDs have been mainly designed and tested to provide cerebral protection during transcatheter aortic valve replacement (TAVR), but their use in both Catheterization and Electrophysiology laboratories is rapidly increasing. CPDs have allowed us to perform procedures that were previously contraindicated due to high thromboembolic risk, such as in cases of intracardiac thrombosis identified at preprocedural assessment. However, several concerns related to their employment have to be defined. The selection of patients at high risk of thromboembolism is still a subjective choice of each center. The aim of this review is to update the evidence on the use of CPDs in either Cath labs or EP labs, providing an overview of their structural characteristics. Future perspectives focusing on their possible future employment are also discussed.

Keywords: cerebral protection; cerebral protection devices; left atrial appendage closure; ventricular tachycardia ablation; transcatheter procedures; stroke

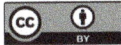

1. Introduction

The advent of cardiac transcatheter procedures (TPs) paved the way for minimally invasive approaches performed without the need for thoracotomy. Given the lower intraprocedural risk compared to cardiac surgery, these approaches allowed us to treat a lot of patients previously judged ineligible. To date, TPs have revolutionized the treatment of the most common heart diseases, such as ischemic heart diseases, valvopathies, heart failure (HF), and arrhythmias, leading to improved life expectancy, QoL, and functional status [1–4]. A number of transcatheter interventions are performed in both Catheterization labs (Cath labs) and Electrophysiology labs (EP labs) today. Percutaneous coronary interventions (PCI), transcatheter aortic valve replacement (TAVR), left atrial appendage closure (LAAC), atrial fibrillation (AF), and other arrhythmia ablations are among the most common TPs, covering approximately 90% of all interventional cardiology procedures.

However, these approaches, in particular those by intracardiac or arterial route, are not free from the risk of severe complications. Among all, stroke is a well-documented and feared potential risk of TPs [5–8], posing a tremendous strain on patients, their families, and the healthcare system [9]. Subclinical neurological events or covert central nervous system infarctions are also a significant risk and are related to the development of dementia, future stroke, cognitive decline, and increased risk of mortality [10–12]. Procedure-related stroke or new ischemic cerebral infarctions may result from a variety of patient- and disease-related causes, such as the severity of atherosclerosis, age, gender, dyslipidemia, history of AF, HF and/or technical aspects of the procedure itself, including mechanical manipulation of instruments or interventional devices. Because of their thrombogenic nature, acute thrombus may originate at any part of endovascular catheters. Thrombus formation on transseptal sheaths despite adequate anticoagulation was reported in 9% of cases [13], as well as the thrombogenicity of guidewires [14,15]. Therefore, the thrombogenicity of endovascular catheters cannot be avoided completely in every left-sided procedure despite an ACT level > 300 s, and the risk increases in long-lasting procedures, such as ventricular (VT) tachycardia ablation. Arterial wall tissue was frequently found in the filters, accompanied by smaller amounts of calcified and necrotic core tissue. The origin of this type of debris might be the manipulation of the ablation catheter within the aortic root, ascending aorta, and aortic arch. Debris may also originate from myocardial and valve tissue by advancing and manipulating the catheters into the left ventricle via the mitral valve [16]. Apart from biological tissue, foreign material was found in the filters of patients undergoing different TPs, probably arising from hydrophilic polymer coatings used on guidewires, catheters, previously implanted ICD leads, and transseptal sheaths, which have been shown to produce clinically relevant particles [14,17,18]. New medical devices are being developed to help mitigate this risk of cardioembolic embolism during TPs. Cerebral protection devices (CPDs) are mechanical barriers designed to cover the ostium of the supra-aortic branches in the aortic arch. They are characterized by a low-profile allowing the implantation by the radial or femoral artery, filter capabilities, and stability during the procedure. Their implantation is temporary and covers the duration of the procedure, after which, they are removed. CPDs have been designed and tested in particular to reduce the cardioembolic risk during TAVR, but their use in Cath labs and EP labs is rapidly increasing. According to recent studies and meta-analyses, CPD use is safe in terms of bleeding and vascular complications, but its real effectiveness in decreasing stroke rate and other major cardiovascular embolic events is still a matter of debate [19–21]. Significant reduction in MACE and mortality was sometimes reported, without differences in acute kidney injury. On the contrary, significantly lower subclinical brain lesions have been detected by diffusion-weighted magnetic resonance imaging (DW-MRI) in all studies [22,23]. Data on their use in clinical practice beyond TAVR is still limited. However, there is growing evidence of CPD safety in LAAC and VT ablation with concomitant left atrial appendage (LAA) or left ventricular thrombosis [18,24]. In this review, we aimed to present the technical characteristics of current available CPDs and update clinical evidence supporting their use in Cath labs or EP labs.

2. Cerebral Protection Devices

To reduce the risk of stroke, CPDs have been developed to prevent debris and clots from embolizing the brain [25]. Clots can already be present at the time of the procedure or can develop during it. CPDs are usually inserted throw a radial or femoral artery access. The positioning of the device can be challenging, particularly if atherosclerotic plaques are located in the vicinity of the ostium of supra-aortic vessels or aortic arch, hampering the implantation and positioning of the device which may even promote plaque disruption and, consequently, cerebral embolization. Therefore, in patients with several risk factors for atherosclerosis, such as smoking, diabetes, obesity, and kidney disease, a preprocedural chest computed tomography angiography (CTA) may be indicated [26]. CTA can also reveal some arteriopathies, such as vascular tortuosity or aneurysms, which can preclude the use of the device or its corrected deployment. The actual efficacy of the CPDs depends on the capacity to protect the three main branches of the aortic arch and the ability of the specialists to deploy it without disrupting aortic arch plaque. They can be classified as filters or deflectors: filter devices can retain embolic material, while deflector devices reject the debris towards the descending aorta [27]. Despite deflector systems not being capable of entraping embolic material but only diverting it towards the descending aorta, no cases of embolism in inferior districts have been reported so far. There are eight types of CPDs [28]. In general, all devices are constituted by various shapes of heparin-coated polyurethane membranes of around 100 μm size pores.

2.1. Deflector Systems

- Embrella (Edwards Lifesciences, Irvine, CA, USA) received a European CE mark approval in 2010. It was developed to deflect embolic material during TAVR [29]. This device is inserted by right radial or brachial approach with a 6 Fr sheath. The distal end is an umbrella-like device with two heparin-coated polyurethane membranes (pore size: 100 μm). The CPD is placed through the greater curvature of the aorta, safeguarding the brachiocephalic and left common carotid artery. Since the left subclavian artery is not covered by the device, Embrella provides only partial protection to supra-aortic vessels. According to the pilot study PROTAVI-C, the device was successfully positioned in 100% of the TAVR procedures (N = 41) [30]. Although its use was associated with a reduction in lesion volume evaluated by DW-MRI, it did not prevent the occurrence of new cerebral microemboli.
- TriGuard (Keystone Heart, Caesarea, Israel) received a European CE mark in 2014 [31]. It is advanced through a 9 Fr arterial sheath placed into the left femoral artery and deployed to cover the ostia of the three supra-aortic trunks. Its new generation, the TriGuard 3, incorporates a self-expanding deflection filter composed of a structural radiopaque nitinol frame and an ultra-thin polymer mesh (nominal pore size 115×145 μm). The device is heparin-coated to reduce thrombogenicity and increase lubricity. The full system includes a delivery subsystem for crimping and loading the device into an 8F sheath [32]. The device was primarily developed to provide cerebral protection during TAVR [33,34]. In recent years, its use in LAAC and VT ablation procedures has rapidly increased and provided encouraging results that could pave the way for new employment in electrophysiological procedures [35,36].
- ProtEmbo CPS (Protembis, Aachen, Germany, EU) received a European CE mark in 2014. This device covers all three supra-aortic vessels, and its low-profile design provides delivery by left radial access. The heparin-coated mesh has the smallest pore size (60 μm) among all available CPDs. For this reason, it might even safeguard the cerebrum from smaller-sized debris [32,37]. The PROTEMBO C trial evaluated the safety and performance of the ProtEmbo CPS in TAVR patients [38]. The CPD met the primary safety and performance endpoints compared to prespecified historical performance goals. Enrolled patients had smaller brain lesion volumes on DW-MRI compared to prior series and no large single lesions (>150 mm^3). The ongoing PROTEMBO SF (ClinicalTrials.gov Identifier: NCT03325283) is a prospective, observational, multicenter, intention-to-treat study of the safety and feasibility of the ProtEmbo CPS in subjects with severe symptomatic native aortic valve stenosis indicated for TAVR.

2.2. Filter Systems

2.2.1. Supra-Aortic Filters

- Sentinel (Boston Scientific, Marlborough, MA, USA) received a European CE mark in 2014 and is the most widely used CPD so far. It is formed by a dual system filter basket containing two polyurethane mesh filters with 140 μm pores. It is advanced through a 6 Fr delivery catheter from the right radial over a 0.014 inch guidewire. It consists of a proximal filter (diameter of 9–15 mm) delivered in the brachiocephalic artery and a distal filter (diameter of 6.5–10 mm) delivered in the left common carotid artery. Through an articulating sheath, the device can be sealed into the aortic arch according to its anatomy [27]. Since the Sentinel device is deployed into supra-aortic vessels, the diameter of the supra-aortic vessels must be previously measured by CTA, because proximal and distal filters are developed to be accommodated within a brachiocephalic artery of 9 to 15 mm, and a common carotid of more than 3 mm [39]. The left vertebral artery remains unprotected. Sentinel devices have only one available size, so complete sealing might not be obtained in all aortic anatomies. Several uses of this device for LAAC and VT ablation have been reported [18,36].

- The Wirion (Abbott, Chicago, IL, USA) is a single filter usually employed for carotid stenting and lower extremity endovascular interventions [40]. It consists of a distal filter (filter basket and locking mechanism) and a rapid exchange delivery catheter. The exchange catheter has a 1.1 mm crossing profile and can be mounted on any 0.014 inch guidewire and via 6F or greater guiding catheters. The filter basket is made of a self-expanding nitinol scaffold and a nylon filter membrane with 100 μm pores. The filter can efficiently be deployed in vessels with a diameter ranging from 3.5 to 6.0 mm and at any location along the guidewire, using a proprietary remote locking system (handle at the proximal end of the delivery catheter). Since this device protects only one vessel at a time, it cannot be used alone for TPs at high risk of cardioembolism. A study reported the utility of Wirion in combination with Sentinel to complete the protection of the left vertebral artery in patients undergoing TAVR [31].
- Emblok Embolic Protection System (EPS, Innovative Cardiovascular Solutions, Grand Rapids, MI, USA) is currently only for investigational use. It is formed by an 11 F sheath device containing a 4 Fr pigtail catheter advanced through femoral access. The filter system is a 125 μm pore-size nitinol that allows the embolic filter and a radiopaque pigtail catheter to be advanced simultaneously through femoral access. It fits in various anatomies of the aorta with a diameter of up to 35 mm. The prospective, nonrandomized, multicenter, first-in-man pilot study was designed to evaluate the efficacy and safety of cerebral embolic protection utilizing the EPS-enrolled 20 patients undergoing TAVR [41]. The device was successfully placed and retrieved in all cases, and no neurological events were observed. Cerebral total new lesion volume was similar to other trials on cerebral protection during TAVR. An ongoing prospective, multicenter, single-blind, randomized controlled trial enrolling >500 patients aims to evaluate the safety, effectiveness, and performance of the EMBLOK EPS during TAVR by randomized comparison with a commercially available embolic protection device (ClinicalTrials.gov Identifier: NCT05295628).

2.2.2. Full Body Filters

- Emboliner (Emboline, Santa Cruz, CA, USA) device system is currently only for investigational use. It is advanced from a 9 Fr transfemoral sheath used for the 6 Fr pigtail catheter for TAVR. It is engineered to protect all three cerebral vessels and the whole body. Early results from the SafePass 2 trial were presented in Transcatheter Cardiovascular Therapeutics 2019, reflecting no adverse events at 30 days with 100% procedural success.
- Captis (Filterlex Medical, Caesarea, Israel) is currently under development and carries a deflector mechanism with ipsilateral transfemoral access. Positioned in the aortic arch and descending aorta, it promises to provide full cerebral and body protection. The results of the prospective, single-arm, first-in-human study presented at EuroPCR 2022 involving 20 patients who underwent TAVR showed 100% technical device performance success, including deploy and retrieve and any interferences with the TAVR procedure. There were neither device-related complications nor cerebrovascular events (ClinicalTrials.gov Identifier: NCT04659538).

Figure 1 shows current CPDs used in cardiovascular TPs, while Table 1 summarizes the pros and cons of each device.

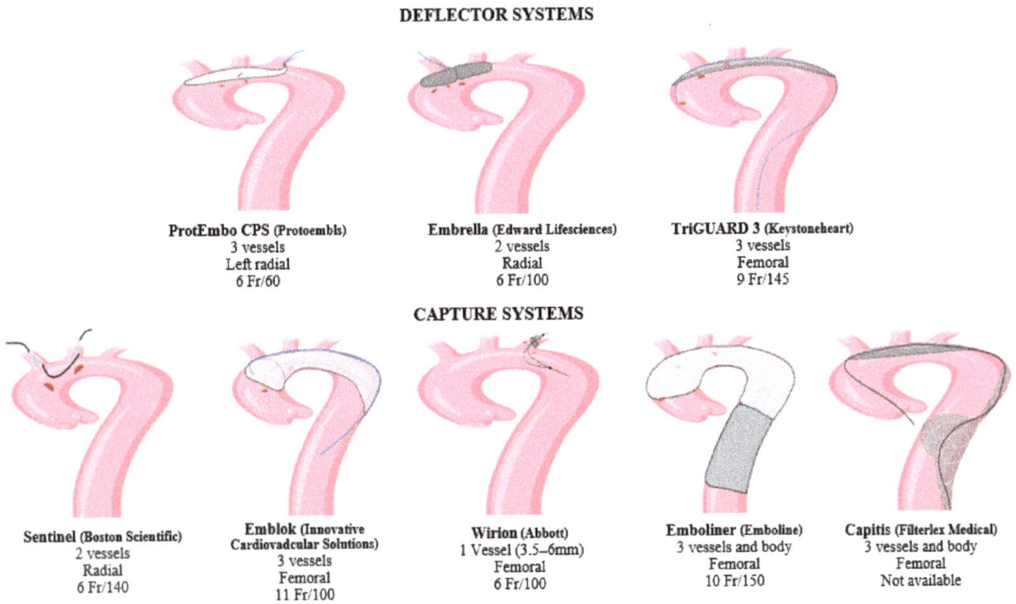

Figure 1. Current cerebral protection devices used in cardiovascular transcatheter procedures and main technical features (name, coverage, access site, sheath/pore size [mm]).

Table 1. Pros and cons of current cerebral protection devices.

Device	Pros	Cons
ProtEmbo CPS [38]	Small size sheath (6 Fr); Left radial/brachial access; Mesh with the smallest pore size available; 100% successful device positioning.	Partial coverage of the supra-aortic trunk; New cerebral lesions were detected, but smaller; Available evidence only for TAVR.
Embrella [30]	Small size sheath (6 Fr); Right radial/brachial access; 100% successful device positioning.	Partial coverage of the supra-aortic trunk; New cerebral lesions were detected, but smaller; Available evidence only for TAVR.
TriGuard 3 [36,42]	Intermedium size sheath (9 Fr); Implantable through both the left and right femoral arteries; Full coverage of the supra-aortic trunk; Can be left in the aortic arch for days; 100% successful device positioning; Large amount of evidence; Available evidence for TAVR, LAAC, and VT ablation.	Femoral access; Procedural concerns if transcatheter procedure performed through the retro-aortic path; New cerebral lesions were detected, but smaller.
Sentinel [36,43]	Small size sheath (6 Fr); Right radial/brachial access; 94.4% successful device positioning; Largest amount of evidence; Available evidence for TAVR, LAAC, and VT ablation.	Partial coverage of the supra-aortic trunk; New cerebral lesions were detected but smaller.
Emblok [41]	Implantable through both the left and right femoral arteries; 100% successful device positioning.	Intermedium size sheath (11 Fr); Femoral access; Procedural concerns if transcatheter procedure performed through the retro-aortic path; New cerebral lesions were detected, but smaller; Available evidence only for TAVR.

Table 1. Cont.

Device	Pros	Cons
Wirion [31]	Small size sheath (6 Fr); Right radial/brachial access; Very low amount of evidence.	Nonsufficient coverage of the supra-aortic trunk; Available evidence only for TAVR;
Emboliner	Coverage of the supra-aortic trunk and descending aorta; Implantable through both the left and right femoral arteries.	Data on the first-in-man study is not yet available.
Capitis	Coverage of the supra-aortic trunk and descending aorta; Implantable through both the left and right femoral arteries.	Data on the first-in-man study is not yet available.

3. Cerebral Protection in Cath Labs

As reported above, CPDs have been designed and tested to reduce the cardioembolic risk during TAVR. In fact, during TAVR, it is hypothesized that the manipulation of large devices into the aortic arch and through the calcified native valve might mobilize and fragment atherosclerotic plaques that are prone to embolization in the cerebral circulation [44]. Structural and procedural concerns are considered the major periprocedural risk conditions [45]: aortic valve area or aortic annulus size, the degree of aortic leaflet calcification, pure aortic stenosis, high gradients, the degree of aortic atherosclerotic burden (such as porcelain aorta), as well as procedure time, repositioning of the bioprosthesis, postdilation, the degree of anticoagulation, and the experience of the interventionalist. Ischemic stroke occurring >1 year from TAVR is named late stroke, and although its etiology is less understood, it seems to be mainly associated with patient characteristics: new-onset AF, HF, diabetes mellitus, systemic inflammatory diseases, thrombophilia, and chronic kidney disease. The disruption of the calcified native valve with denudation of endothelium and lack of endothelization of the stent-valve were also proposed among possible causes [46]. Direct evidence of embolized material in 99% of cases in dedicated trials [47] explains the high rates of peri-procedural strokes in the pivotal TAVR trials (5.5% at 30 days in intermediate-risk patients) [48]. Also, considering the expansion of TAVR to treat severe aortic stenosis in lower-risk patients [49,50], the rationale to minimize embolization and stroke is strong, and several trials tested the efficacy of different CPDs in this context, with two devices being particularly well-studied and more widely used. The Sentinel device is the most widely used CPD for cerebral protection during TAVR. As mentioned above, the whole cerebral circulation is not protected by this device, as the left vertebral artery, stemming from the left subclavian artery, is uncovered, leaving the posterior cerebral circulation prone to embolization. The Sentinel CPD has been studied extensively in earlier imaging studies and smaller trials, showing a reduction in ischemic lesions at cerebral DW-MRI (50% reduction of the number of new lesions and total lesion volume) but without a statistically significant reduction of clinical neurological events at follow-up [29]. In the larger, recent PROTECTED TAVR study [51], 3000 patients were randomly assigned to CPD or control. In this study, the incidence of peri-procedural stroke (within 72 h of TAVR) was 2.3% in the CPD group vs. 2.9% in the control group (difference: -0.6%; $p = 0.30$), thus failing to demonstrate a statistically significant advantage of CPDs. However, the incidence of disabling strokes was significantly lower in the CPD group (0.5% vs. 1.3%, difference: -0.8%; $p < 0.05$). The TriGuard 3 device offers a different mechanism of cerebral protection by deflection of debris to the lower systemic system. However, no clinical advantage has been demonstrated in the only randomized controlled trial that was prematurely halted after the commercial availability of a novel iteration of the device [42]. In the lack of clear data about the benefit of CPDs to prevent clinical neurological events, despite a strong rationale and direct biological evidence, it has been postulated that available trials were underpowered to demonstrate a reduction of clinical events individually. In a meta-analysis including only evidence from randomized controlled trials, independently of the device used, CPDs were associated with a non-significant trend towards lower risk for death or stroke (ARR: 3.5%; NNT of 28) [52]. Another more recent meta-analysis also failed to show any clinical benefit (RR for stroke: 0.88, 95% CI 0.57 to 1.36, $p = 0.566$; RR for disabling stroke: 0.85,

95% CI 0.21 to 3.41, $p = 0.818$) and also no significant difference in terms of total lesion volume on MRI was evident (-74.94, 95% CI -174.31 to 24.4, $p = 0.139$) [20]. Notably, these analyses do not include the most recent (and largest) PROTECTED TAVR study. In terms of observational evidence, an analysis of the large Society of Thoracic Surgeons-American College of Cardiology Transcatheter Valve Therapy (STS-ACC TVT) Registry database encompassing over 120,000 patients also found no significant reduction in stroke with the use of CPD, although in a propensity-match analysis, CPD was associated with a significant reduction of in-hospital stroke (odds ratio, 0.82 [95% CI, 0.69–0.97]; absolute risk difference, -0.28% [95% CI, -0.52 to -0.03]) [53]. In summary, evidence that routine use of CPDs during TAVR is of clinical benefit is lacking. However, there is a strong biological rationale and abundant proof of safety and efficacy. Therefore, it is possible that CPD might be beneficial in selected, higher-risk populations and/or in particularly young patients when maximal precautions from adverse events are warranted. Table 2 summarizes the main characteristics and results of randomized controlled trials (RCTs) investigating CPDs in TAVR. Cost-effectiveness analyses were performed only for Sentinel, reporting a probability to be cost-effective ranging from 45 to 86% at 30 days [54] and 57.5% at 5 years [55].

Table 2. Main results of randomized controlled trials on cerebral protection devices in transcatheter aortic valve replacement.

RCT	Year	Sample Size	Prosthetic Valve	Endpoints	Results
DEFLECT III [56]	2015	TriGuard ($n = 46$) Controls ($n = 39$)	Balloon-expandable Self-expandable	- Safety endpoint: all-cause mortality, all stroke, life-threatening bleeding, acute kidney injury, and major vascular complications; - Efficacy endpoints: cerebral ischemic lesions on DW-MRI; neurocognitive deterioration.	- Strokes: CPD = 2, control = 2; - Safety endpoint: CPD 21.7% vs. control 30.8% ($p = 0.34$); - Efficacy endpoint: higher freedom from the ischemic lesion with CPD (46% ITT); lower new neurocognitive deterioration (CPD 3.1% vs. control 15.4%, $p = 0.16$).
EMBOL-X [57]	2015	Embol-x ($n = 14$) Controls ($n = 16$)	Balloon-expandable	- Efficacy endpoints: number of lesions on DW-MRI; lesion size.	- No strokes reported; - New lesion on DW-MRI: CPD 57% vs. control 69% ($p = 0.70$). - Smaller lesions with CPD ($p = 0.27$).
MISTRAL-C [58]	2016	Sentinel ($n = 32$) Controls ($n = 33$)	Balloon-expandable Self-expandable	- Primary endpoint: new cerebral lesions on DW-MRI; - Secondary endpoint: neurocognitive deterioration.	- Strokes: CPD = 1, control = 6; - New brain lesion: CPD 73% vs. control 87% ($p = 0.31$). - >10 new brain lesions: CPD 0% vs. control 20% ($p = 0.03$). - Smaller total lesion volume with CPD ($p = 0.057$); - Neurocognitive deterioration: CPD 4% vs. control 27% ($p = 0.017$).
CLEAN-TAVI [23]	2016	Claret Montage Dual Filter System ($n = 50$) Controls ($n = 50$)	Self-expandable	- Primary endpoint: new cerebral lesions on DW-MRI; - Secondary endpoints: difference in the volume of new lesions on DW-MRI; neurocognitive deterioration.	- Strokes: CPD = 5, control = 5; - N. of new lesions lower in the CPD group ($p < 0.001$); - The volume of new lesions is lower in the CPD group ($p = 0.001$). - Neurocognitive deterioration: no differences;
SENTINEL [43]	2017	Sentinel ($n = 123$) Controls ($n = 119$)	Balloon-expandable Self-expandable	- Safety endpoint: all-cause mortality, all stroke, acute kidney injury; - Efficacy endpoints: difference in the volume of new lesions on DW-MRI; neurocognitive deterioration.	- Stokes: CPD 5.6% vs. control 9.1% ($p = 0.25$); - Safety endpoint: CPD 7.3% vs. control 9.9% ($p = 0.41$). - Volume of new lesions: CPD 102.8 mm^3 vs. control 178 mm^3 ($p = 0.33$); - Neurocognitive deterioration: no differences.

Table 2. *Cont.*

RCT	Year	Sample Size	Prosthetic Valve	Endpoints	Results
REFLECT II [42]	2021	TriGuard 3 (*n* = 121) Controls (*n* = 58)	Balloon-expandable Self-expandable	- Safety endpoint: all-cause mortality, all stroke, life-threatening bleeding, acute kidney injury, major vascular complications, coronary artery obstruction, and valve-related dysfunction; - Efficacy endpoints: all-cause mortality or stroke; neurocognitive deterioration; freedom from new lesions on DW-MRI; the difference in the volume of new lesions on DW-MRI.	- Strokes: CPD 8.3% vs. control 5.3% (*p* = 0.57); - Safety endpoint: CPD 15.9% vs. control 7% (*p* = 0.11); - Efficacy endpoint: neurocognitive deterioration CPD 14.1% vs. control 7.6% (*p* = 0.18); new ischemic lesions CPD 85% vs. control 84.9% (*p* = 1); similar volume of new lesions (*p* = 0.405).
PROTECTED TAVR [51]	2022	Sentinel (*n* = 1501) Controls (*n* = 1499)	Balloon-expandable Self-expandable	- Primary endpoint: clinical stroke; - Secondary endpoints: disabling stroke, death, transient ischemic attack, delirium, major or minor vascular complications at the CPD access site, and acute kidney injury.	- Primary endpoint: CPD 2.3% vs. control 2.9% (*p* = 0.30); - Secondary endpoints: disabling stroke CPD 0.5% vs. control 1.3% (*p* < 0.05); death CPD 0.5% vs. control 0.3%; transient ischemic attack CPD 0.1% vs. control 0.1%.

4. Cerebral Protection in EP Labs

Electrophysiologic procedures have a non-negligible risk of stroke or systemic embolism, particularly those performed on the left side of the heart. Periprocedural stroke risk is estimated between 0.1 and 0.9% in patients undergoing catheter ablation (CA) of AF [59–62], between 0.8 and 1.8% in patients undergoing CA of VT [63,64], and 0.7–1.1% in patients undergoing LAAC [65,66]. Data about the benefits of CPDs in EP labs are still missing, and those available are mainly from retrospective studies. Nevertheless, LAAC remains the second procedure with the highest use of CPD reported in the literature after TAVR. LAA is the most common site of thrombus formation in patients with nonvalvular AF [67]. Oral anticoagulation (OAC) is used to prevent and treat AF-related thrombus. However, LAA thrombus has also been noted in patients who have received full therapeutic anticoagulation [68,69]. Therefore, OAC may fail to either prevent or resolve the thrombus. In this specific scenario, LAAC may be a potential option [70,71]. Major LAAC studies have excluded patients with LAA thrombosis due to the expected high risk of systemic embolization. Consequentially, the absence of data regarding the feasibility and safety of LAAC in the presence of LAA thrombus led to a nonclear indication of this procedure in the latest guidelines on LAAC [72,73]. It must be noted that AF patients with failure of OAC therapy, including those with stroke, transient ischemic attack (TIA), or multiple findings of LAAC thrombosis at transesophageal echocardiography have limited therapeutic chances and a very high risk of incurring ischemic events [74,75]. In recent years, some retrospective studies [24] and one multicenter registry [76] highlighted the feasibility and safety of this procedure using Amulet (St. Jude Medical) and Watchman (Boston Scientific) devices. In a study, LAAC was proposed in combination with OAC as an enhancement of antithrombotic therapy in AF patients incurred in stroke/systemic embolism despite OAC, reporting optimistic results in terms of feasibility and safety after 5 years of follow-up [77]. The use of CPD in this scenario may further reduce the risk of severe intraprocedural complications. However, the use of CPD in above cited studies has been reported in <30% of procedures. In the systematic review by Sharma et al. [24], 17 patients received cerebral protection with different devices. No strokes were reported, but vascular complications were not assessed. In the multicenter TRAPEUR registry, a CPD (Sentinel) was used in five patients [76]. Procedural success was achieved in all patients, with only one major bleeding and four minor vascular complications observed. There was no periprocedural peripheral embolic event identified. More recently, a few retrospective studies focused on exploring intraprocedural and short/medium effects of CPD use in LAAC with concomitant LAA thrombosis. In the largest multicenter European study, 27 patients from eight centers with AF and LAA thrombus underwent LAA closure and cerebral protection with the Sentinel device [78]. The procedural outcome was reached in 100% of patients with any complication reported. Another single-center study treated 21 patients using Sentinel and TriGuard 3, reporting a low rate of minor vascular complications (4%) and an absence of major complications [36]. The mean procedure time, including placement of the CPD, was 103 min. Compared to LAAC without LAA sludge/thrombosis, the procedure time was longer (103 vs. 60 min, as reported in PRAGUE 17) [79]. The mean hospitalization time was 2.9 ± 2.2 days. At a follow-up of 587 days, one TIA and two non-cardiovascular deaths were noted. Currently, there are no validated criteria to identify patients with LAA thrombosis and a high risk of embolization during LAAC. Moreover, unlike TAVR, studies on the use of CMR to identify possible subclinical cerebral injuries that led to the rupture of a part of the thrombus during the device placement are lacking. Overall, despite the absence of comparative studies between use vs. nonuse of CPD in LAAC with LAA thrombosis, data available so far highlighted the feasibility and safety of this procedure, associated with either intraprocedural low risk of thromboembolism or other major complications. VTs are life-threatening arrhythmias with higher prevalence in patients with structural heart diseases [80]. In patients with HF, half of the deaths are sudden due to life-threatening ventricular arrhythmias, including VTs [81]. Frequently, VT can be difficult to manage clinically, and implantable cardioverter defibrillators (ICDs) have been shown to effectively prevent sudden cardiac death due to ventricular arrhythmias, but not to prevent the recurrence of episodes of VT. Moreover, appropriate ICD shocks are associated with significant morbidity and increased rates of mortality [82]. CA is being increasingly performed as adjunctive therapy to prevent or reduce ICD therapies when antiarrhythmic drugs are ineffective or not desired. However, VT ablation is associated with a significant risk of complications, including cerebrovascular accidents due to embolic events. The incidence of stroke in patients undergoing VT ablation in the context of structural heart disease has been reported to be up to 2.7% [83]. The presence of intra-cardiac thrombus is an absolute contraindication to VT ablation due to the high risk of embolization during the procedure. The highest prevalence of LV thrombus is related to ischemic heart diseases, while an intracardiac thrombus is rarely found in dilated cardiomyopathy. Left ventricle ejection fraction (LVEF) <40% and left ventricle (LV) aneurysm are independent predictors of LV thrombus [84]. However, 58% of patients without pre-procedural evidence of LV thrombosis undergoing routine VT ablation procedures show new cerebral ischemic lesions on postprocedural cerebral MRI [63]. Although these embolic events were initially thought to be subclinical, current investigations showed they might have negative neurocognitive effects [85]. While a number of strategies have been developed to minimize the risk of procedure-related embolic events, including peri-procedure anticoagulation, use of irrigated ablation catheters, and selective use of retrograde-aortic access, the risk of brain emboli remains high [63]. Application of the CPD during CA of VT seems to be feasible and safe, and captured debris from an acute thrombosis was demonstrated in several studies despite sufficient ACT, while foreign material was found in 55% of filters [63]. Two small studies specifically investigated CPD in patients undergoing VT ablation. A study reported feasibility and safety in a series of 11 patients with ischemic heart disease using Sentinel [18]. Debris in the device was detected in all patients at the end of the procedure. The other study reported the use of Sentinel and TriGuard 3 in seven patients undergoing VT ablation of mixed etiology without complications [35]. In a single-center experience of using CPD in EP labs, nine patients (30%) underwent VT ablation [36]. Among those, five showed LAA thrombosis, three showed LV thrombosis or severe spontaneous echo contrast, and one had mobile thrombotic material in the aortic arch detected prior to the intervention. Table 3 summarizes the clinical characteristics and main results of the above-cited studies. Paradoxically, the use of CPD during AF ablation, the most frequent cause of ischemic stroke/systemic embolism worldwide, is currently limited to one case of a patient with evidence of severe left atrial smoke [86]. A database reported a periprocedural stroke rate of 0.4% during CA of AF, which is non-negligible considering the volume of procedures performed worldwide daily [87]. Other studies reported an even higher rate, ranging from 0.9 to 1.4% [88,89]. Generation of cerebral microembolisms (firstly: air or thrombus entry via sheaths; secondly: coagulum formation on the catheter itself or over-delivered ablation lesions; thirdly: gas bubble formation occurring during CA) was reported from CMR studies, probably resulting from the technical aspects of the procedure [90]. The modality of ablation, including catheter type, affects this risk. Both preclinical and clinical studies confirmed that the air forcing into the left atrium through the septal sheath during the introduction of a ring catheter is the main source of gaseous microembolisms [91–95]. A pilot randomized study of the use of Sentinel for cerebral protection during CA of AF is currently ongoing (ClinicalTrials.gov Identifier: NCT04685317).

Table 3. Available studies on cerebral protection device use in EP labs.

Studies	Study Type	Year	Procedure Type	Sample Size	Results
Heeger et al. [18]	Retrospective study	2018	VT ablation	Sentinel (*n* = 11)	– Procedural success: 100%; – No strokes reported; – No complications.
Sharma et al. [24]	Systematic review	2020	LAAC with LAA thrombosis	N = 58 CPD (not specified, *n* = 17)	– Procedural success: 100%; – Strokes: 1; – Device-related thromboses: 2.
Boccuzzi et al. [78]	Registry	2021	LAAC with LAA thrombosis	Sentinel (*n* = 27)	– Procedural success: 100%; – No strokes reported; – No complications.
Zachariah et al. [35]	Research letter	2022	VT ablation	Sentinel (*n* = 6) TriGuard 3 (*n* = 1)	– Procedural success: 100%; – No strokes reported; – No complications.
Trapeur [76]	Registry	2022	LAAC with LAA thrombosis	N = 53 Sentinel (*n* = 5)	– Procedural success: 100%; – No strokes reported; – Not reported CPD safety and efficacy.
Berg et al. [36]	Retrospective study	2023	LAAC with LAA thrombosis VT ablation	Sentinel (*n* = 14) TriGuard 3 (*n* = 21) Sentinel (*n* = 5) TriGuard 3 (*n* = 4)	– Procedural success: 100%; – No strokes reported; – Four minor vascular access complications.

5. Future Perspectives

CPDs have been used for the prevention of cerebral embolization in carotid stenting procedures or cardiac surgery for nearly two decades, have a proven safety profile, and have demonstrated clinically meaningful reduction in neurological events. Now, new devices have been developed for cardiac TA. So far, CPDs are designed as filters or deflectors, with reported similar efficacy and safety in cerebral protection. However, comparative studies among the devices are not yet available.

The use of CPDs in TAVR is a developing field that recognizes the likelihood that mechanical manipulation of interventional devices in the vasculature, as well as aortic valve and aortic annulus, may result in stroke and new ischemic lesions by dislodging pre-existing atherosclerotic and other debris. Future studies with a larger population and greater statistical power are needed to prove the real benefit of CPD in preventing significant clinical cerebrovascular events in this field. Particularly, studies focusing on younger populations undergoing TAVR will be of paramount importance.

New clinical scenarios of CPD applicability should also be investigated. As the complexity of both structural and coronary interventions is constantly growing, along with treating patients at higher ischemic risk, the use of CPD could be useful, mitigating the occurrence of cerebrovascular events. Patients undergoing protected percutaneous coronary intervention with the use of impeller or complex, high-risk, and indicated percutaneous coronary interventions (CHIP) are often at increased risk of embolic events and would benefit from the use of CPD. Transcatheter interventions on the mitral valve with severe mitral annular calcification (MAC) are another source of calcium emboli, with a possible risk of severe ischemic complications [96,97]. Future studies on these unexplored fields are needed to explore the possible benefits of CPS use in different clinical scenarios. However, due to a lack of data, it is still challenging for treating clinicians to determine whether to offer CPD to all patients routinely or to use these devices selectively in patients they feel are at high risk of procedural stroke. We do not currently have randomized data to inform which patients truly are at higher risk, and who might be expected to derive benefit from CPD. Pre-procedural assessment by CT angiography, which is already used to assess the aortic root anatomy and orientation, should also be systematically used to stratify patient risk of intraprocedural stroke and then to identify patients who may benefit from the use of a CPD [98,99]. The recent availability of CPD in EP labs allowed for the treatment of patients who, in principle, would have been excluded for high intraprocedural risk of stroke, such as LAAC and VT ablation with concomitant intracardiac thrombus. Any LAAC in the presence of a thrombus runs the risk of dislodgement and embolization. Therefore, modification of the procedure to minimize interventions within the LAA has to be considered [24]. Several alternative approaches have been described so far, such as minimum LAA contrast injection and catheter manipulation (no-touch technique), removal of the delivery sheath outside the LAA with careful advancement of partially opened devices, and placement of the delivery sheath in the proximal LAA with cautious advancement. Types of LAAC devices could potentially affect the feasibility of the procedure in presence of LAA thrombus. The risk of distal touching and embolization might be higher with umbrella-shaped devices like the Watchman, because the Watchman delivery sheath has to be advanced into the LAA until its marker aligns with the ostial plane of the LAA [100]. The deployment happens from the distal to the proximal direction. The newer Watchman FLX has several new features compared with the previous generations, which may make the procedure safer [101]. The Watchman FLX has a reduced device length and closed distal nitinol loops to allow safe navigation of the partially deployed device in the LAA. In addition, when fully deployed, the Watchman FLX has only one-half the depth compared with the Watchman. On the contrary, lobe and disc devices like Amulet, which have a short length, allow for a shallow deployment without having to engage the LAA distally, and potentially avoid any contact with the thrombus. Furthermore, the deployment happens from the proximal to distal direction, with a minor risk of disturbing a distally located LAA thrombus. Partial or complete retrieval and re-deployment may significantly increase the risk of thrombus dislodgement; therefore, meticulous planning and attention to detail must be paid, including device sizing. In VT ablation, intracardiac echocardiography was demonstrated to be helpful in avoiding thrombus contact during catheter manipulation [102]. As cited above, microembolism could derive from procedure-related technical aspects; therefore, the minimum number of transeptal punctures should be used. Thrombus formation can also occur during the procedure and be dislodged into the systemic circulation in the form of microemboli. Silent cerebral lesions due to the microemboli formation during CA of AF were largely confirmed in the past [90,103], but their causal role in the development of cognitive defects in short term was reported as transient or completely absence by some studies [95,104]. Instead, the long-term effects of cerebral microembolization during AF ablation have not investigated yet and, in any case, are hard to investigate due to several confounding factors; this might be the reason why, currently, there are no studies that propose the intraprocedural use of the CPD. Few studies investigated the embolic risk of the different CA techniques [90]. RF and cryoballoon are modalities used widely throughout the world. Transcranial Doppler monitoring studies show significant microembolic signals with any ablation modality. The number of signals appears much higher with nonirrigated RF compared with irrigated RF and appears lowest—but not negligible—with cryoablation [105]. a higher degree of blood damage, platelet activation, and thrombogenesis with RF ablation compared to cryoablation [106,107]. Several studies reported that the multielectrode-phased RF (PVAC) catheter led to a substantially higher rate of microthrombi formation [108–110]. Managing electrodes could reduce thromboembolic events with the PVAC [111,112]. Similarly, the new very high-power, short-duration ablation (vHPSD) involving high-power (up to 90 watts) RF ablation delivered over a short duration (as little as 4 s), reported a high rate of silent cerebral lesions, albeit with no clinical strokes or cognitive impairment [113]. Pulsed-field ablation (PFA) works by using electrical fields to induce the electroporation of cells. As different cell types have different electroporation thresholds, PFA brings significant safety advantages by minimizing damage to extracardiac structures such as the esophagus and phrenic nerve. One-year outcomes from the IMPULSE and PEFCAT I + II studies found that PFA was very safe, with only 1 TIA in 121 patients, and of the eighteen patients who underwent cranial MRI scanning post-PFA ablation, one (who had suffered a clinical TIA) showed an acute lesion, and another had a single silent cerebral lesion [114]. The MANIFEST-PF survey, including data on 1758 patients across 24 clinical centers, reported TIAs in two patients (0.11%) and stroke in seven patients (0.39%) [115].

6. Conclusions

TA has revolutionized the treatment of the most common heart diseases, but is not free from possible severe complications. Intraprocedural stroke is a well-documented and feared potential risk of TA, despite the technological advancements and operator experience. As most cases are procedure-related embolizations, CPDs have excellent potential to prevent acute embolism, and their employment has allowed them to carry out procedures previously not feasible due to high thromboembolic risk. Given the large number of procedures performed daily in either Cath labs or EP labs, universally accepted criteria to identify patients at high risk of intraprocedural thromboembolism in whom CPD could be useful are needed. Moreover, it should be noted that the efficacy of CPD on the reduction of cerebral events has not been proved with any type of device and further adequately powered RCTs are needed to establish the optimal role of CPD in TA.

Author Contributions: A.P., C.M., M.G. and A.M. wrote the original draft; I.G., M.B., L.G., S.V. and M.V. reviewed and edited the draft; G.C., M.C. and D.G.D.R. took care of visualization; J.O., P.M. and F.G. supervised the work. All authors have read and agreed to the published version of the manuscript.

Funding: This research received no external funding.

Institutional Review Board Statement: Not requested.

Informed Consent Statement: Not requested.

Data Availability Statement: Not requested.

Conflicts of Interest: The authors declare no conflict of interest.

References

1. Davidson, L.J.; Davidson, C.J. Transcatheter Treatment of Valvular Heart Disease. *JAMA* **2021**, *325*, 2480–2494. [CrossRef] [PubMed]
2. Latib, A.; Mustehsan, M.H.; Abraham, W.T.; Jorde, U.P.; Bartunek, J. Transcatheter interventions for heart failure. *EuroIntervention* **2023**, *18*, 1135–1149. [CrossRef] [PubMed]
3. Canfield, J.; Totary-Jain, H. 40 Years of Percutaneous Coronary Intervention: History and Future Directions. *J. Pers. Med.* **2018**, *8*, 33. [CrossRef] [PubMed]
4. Wolpert, C.; Pitschner, H.; Borggrefe, M. Evolution of ablation techniques: From WPW to complex arrhythmias. *Eur. Hear. J. Suppl.* **2007**, *9*, I116–I121. [CrossRef]
5. Giustino, G.; Dangas, G.D. Stroke prevention in valvular heart disease: From the procedure to long-term management. *EuroIntervention* **2015**, *14*, W26–W31. [CrossRef]
6. Carrena, O.; Young, R.; Tarrar, I.H.; Nelson, A.J.; Woidyla, D.; Wang, T.Y.; Mehta, R.H. Trends in the Incidence and Fatality of Peripercutaneous Coronary Intervention Stroke. *J. Am. Coll. Cardiol.* **2022**, *80*, 1772–1774. [CrossRef]
7. Kogan, E.V.; Sciria, C.T.; Liu, C.F.; Wong, S.C.; Bergman, G.; Ip, J.E.; Thomas, G.; Markowitz, S.M.; Lerman, B.B.; Kim, L.K.; et al. Early Stroke and Mortality after Percutaneous Left Atrial Appendage Occlusion in Patients with Atrial Fibrillation. *Stroke* **2023**, *54*, 947–954. [CrossRef]
8. Song, Z.-L.; Wu, S.-H.; Zhang, D.-L.; Jiang, W.-F.; Qin, M.; Liu, X. Clinical Safety and Efficacy of Ablation for Atrial Fibrillation Patients with a History of Stroke. *Front. Cardiovasc. Med.* **2021**, *8*, 630090. [CrossRef]
9. Ma, V.Y.; Chan, L.; Carruthers, K.J. Incidence, Prevalence, Costs, and Impact on Disability of Common Conditions Requiring Rehabilitation in the United States: Stroke, Spinal Cord Injury, Traumatic Brain Injury, Multiple Sclerosis, Osteoarthritis, Rheumatoid Arthritis, Limb Loss, and Back Pain. *Arch. Phys. Med. Rehabil.* **2014**, *95*, 986–995.e1. [CrossRef]
10. Lansky, A.J.; Brown, D.; Pena, C.; Pietras, C.G.; Parise, H.; Ng, V.G.; Meller, S.; Abrams, K.J.; Cleman, M.; Margolis, P.; et al. Neurologic Complications of Unprotected Transcatheter Aortic Valve Implantation (from the Neuro-TAVI Trial). *Am. J. Cardiol.* **2016**, *118*, 1519–1526. [CrossRef]
11. Vermeer, S.E.; Prins, N.D.; Heijer, T.D.; Hofman, A.; Koudstaal, P.J.; Breteler, M.M. Silent Brain Infarcts and the Risk of Dementia and Cognitive Decline. *N. Engl. J. Med.* **2003**, *348*, 1215–1222. [CrossRef]
12. Bokura, H.; Kobayashi, S.; Yamaguchi, S.; Iijima, K.; Nagai, A.; Toyoda, G.; Oguro, H.; Takahashi, K. Silent Brain Infarction and Subcortical White Matter Lesions Increase the Risk of Stroke and Mortality: A Prospective Cohort Study. *J. Stroke Cerebrovasc. Dis.* **2006**, *15*, 57–63. [CrossRef] [PubMed]
13. Maleki, K.; Mohammadi, R.; Hart, D.; Cotiga, D.; Farhat, N.; Steinberg, J.S. Intracardiac Ultrasound Detection of Thrombus on Transseptal Sheath: Incidence, Treatment, and Prevention. *J. Cardiovasc. Electrophysiol.* **2005**, *16*, 561–565. [CrossRef] [PubMed]

14. Mehta, R.I.; I Mehta, R.; E Solis, O.; Jahan, R.; Salamon, N.; Tobis, J.M.; Yong, W.H.; Vinters, H.V.; Fishbein, M.C. Hydrophilic polymer emboli: An under-recognized iatrogenic cause of ischemia and infarct. *Mod. Pathol.* **2010**, *23*, 921–930. [CrossRef] [PubMed]
15. Aldenhoff, Y.B.; Hanssen, J.H.; Knetsch, M.L.; Koole, L.H. Thrombus Formation at the Surface of Guide-Wire Models: Effects of Heparin-releasing or Heparin-exposing Surface Coatings. *J. Vasc. Interv. Radiol.* **2007**, *18*, 419–425. [CrossRef]
16. Frerker, C.; Schlüter, M.; Sanchez, O.D.; Reith, S.; Romero, M.E.; Ladich, E.; Schröder, J.; Schmidt, T.; Kreidel, F.; Joner, M.; et al. Cerebral Protection During MitraClip Implantation: Initial Experience at 2 Centers. *JACC Cardiovasc. Interv.* **2016**, *9*, 171–179. [CrossRef]
17. Feld, G.K.; Tiongson, J.; Oshodi, G. Particle formation and risk of embolization during transseptal catheterization: Comparison of standard transseptal needles and a new radiofrequency transseptal needle. *J. Interv. Card. Electrophysiol.* **2011**, *30*, 31–36. [CrossRef]
18. Heeger, C.; Metzner, A.; Schlüter, M.; Rillig, A.; Mathew, S.; Tilz, R.R.; Wohlmuth, P.; Romero, M.E.; Virmani, R.; Fink, T.; et al. Cerebral Protection During Catheter Ablation of Ventricular Tachycardia in Patients with Ischemic Heart Disease. *J. Am. Heart Assoc.* **2018**, *7*, e009005. [CrossRef]
19. Stachon, P.; Kaier, K.; Heidt, T.; Wolf, D.; Duerschmied, D.; Staudacher, D.; Zehender, M.; Bode, C.; Mühlen, C.v.Z. The Use and Outcomes of Cerebral Protection Devices for Patients Undergoing Transfemoral Transcatheter Aortic Valve Replacement in Clinical Practice. *JACC Cardiovasc. Interv.* **2021**, *14*, 161–168. [CrossRef]
20. Ahmad, Y.; Howard, J.P. Meta-Analysis of Usefulness of Cerebral Embolic Protection during Transcatheter Aortic Valve Implantation. *Am. J. Cardiol.* **2021**, *146*, 69–73. [CrossRef]
21. Zahid, S.; Ullah, W.; Uddin, M.F.; Rai, D.; Abbas, S.; Khan, M.U.; Hussein, A.; Salama, A.; Bandyopadhyay, D.; Bhaibhav, B.; et al. Cerebral Embolic Protection during Transcatheter Aortic Valve Implantation: Updated Systematic Review and Meta-Analysis. *Curr. Probl. Cardiol.* **2023**, *48*, 101127. [CrossRef] [PubMed]
22. Kaur, A.; Dhaliwal, A.; Sohal, S.; Kliger, C.; Velagapudi, P.; Basman, C.; Dominguez, A.C. TCT-327 Clinical and Radiographic Measures of Stroke-Related Outcomes with Cerebral Embolic Protection Devices during TAVR: A Meta-Analysis. *J. Am. Coll. Cardiol.* **2022**, *80*, B131. [CrossRef]
23. Haussig, S.; Mangner, N.; Dwyer, M.G.; Lehmkuhl, L.; Lücke, C.; Woitek, F.; Holzhey, D.M.; Mohr, F.W.; Gutberlet, M.; Zivadinov, R.; et al. Effect of a Cerebral Protection Device on Brain Lesions following Transcatheter Aortic Valve Implantation in Patients with Severe Aortic Stenosis: The CLEAN-TAVI Randomized Clinical Trial. *AMA* **2016**, *316*, 592–601. [CrossRef]
24. Sharma, S.P.; Cheng, J.; Turagam, M.K.; Gopinathannair, R.; Horton, R.; Lam, Y.-Y.; Tarantini, G.; D'Amico, G.; Rofastes, X.F.; Lange, M.; et al. Feasibility of Left Atrial Appendage Occlusion in Left Atrial Appendage Thrombus: A Systematic Review. *JACC Clin. Electrophysiol.* **2020**, *6*, 414–424. [CrossRef] [PubMed]
25. Agrawal, A.; Isogai, T.; Shekhar, S.; Kapadia, S. Cerebral Embolic Protection Devices: Current State of the Art. *US Cardiol. Rev.* **2023**, *17*, e02. [CrossRef]
26. Kang, G.; Lee, J.; Song, T.; Pantelic, M.; Reeser, N.; Keimig, T.; Nadig, J.; Villablanca, P.; Frisoli, T.; Eng, M.; et al. 3-Dimensional CT Planning for Cerebral Embolic Protection in Structural Interventions. *JACC Cardiovasc. Imaging* **2020**, *13*, 2673–2676. [CrossRef]
27. Cubero-Gallego, H.; Pascual, I.; Rozado, J.; Ayesta, A.; Hernandez-Vaquero, D.; Diaz, R.; Alperi, A.; Avanzas, P.; Moris, C. Cerebral protection devices for transcatheter aortic valve replacement. *Ann. Transl. Med.* **2019**, *7*, 584. [CrossRef]
28. Steinvil, A.; Benson, R.T.; Waksman, R.; Chhatriwalla, A.K.; Allen, K.B.; Saxon, J.T.; Cohen, D.J.; Aggarwal, S.; Hart, A.J.; Baron, S.J.; et al. Embolic Protection Devices in Transcatheter Aortic Valve Replacement. *Circ. Cardiovasc. Interv.* **2016**, *9*, e003287. [CrossRef]
29. Demir, O.M.; Iannopollo, G.; Mangieri, A.; Ancona, M.B.; Regazzoli, D.; Mitomo, S.; Colombo, A.; Weisz, G.; Latib, A. The Role of Cerebral Embolic Protection Devices During Transcatheter Aortic Valve Replacement. *Front. Cardiovasc. Med.* **2018**, *5*, 150. [CrossRef]
30. Rodés-Cabau, J.; Kahlert, P.; Neumann, F.-J.; Schymik, G.; Webb, J.G.; Amarenco, P.; Brott, T.; Garami, Z.; Gerosa, G.; Lefèvre, T.; et al. Feasibility and Exploratory Efficacy Evaluation of the Embrella Embolic Deflector System for the Prevention of Cerebral Emboli in Patients Undergoing Transcatheter Aortic Valve Replacement. *JACC Cardiovasc. Interv.* **2014**, *7*, 1146–1155. [CrossRef]
31. Nombela-Franco, L.; Armijo, G.; Tirado-Conte, G. Cerebral embolic protection devices during transcatheter aortic valve implantation: Clinical versus silent embolism. *J. Thorac. Dis.* **2018**, *10*, S3604–S3613. [CrossRef]
32. Gasior, T.; Mangner, N.; Bijoch, J.; Wojakowski, W. Cerebral embolic protection systems for transcatheter aortic valve replacement. *J. Interv. Cardiol.* **2018**, *31*, 891–898. [CrossRef] [PubMed]
33. Baumbach, A.; Mullen, M.; Brickman, A.M.; Aggarwal, S.K.; Pietras, C.G.; Forrest, J.K.; Hildick-Smith, D.; Meller, S.M.; Gambone, L.; den Heijer, P.; et al. Safety and performance of a novel embolic deflection device in patients undergoing transcatheter aortic valve replacement: Results from the DEFLECT I study. *EuroIntervention* **2015**, *11*, 75–84. [CrossRef] [PubMed]
34. Samim, M.; van der Worp, B.; Agostoni, P.; Hendrikse, J.; Budde, R.P.; Nijhoff, F.; Ramjankhan, F.; Doevendans, P.A.; Stella, P.R. TriGuard™ HDH embolic deflection device for cerebral protection during transcatheter aortic valve replacement. *Catheter. Cardiovasc. Interv.* **2017**, *89*, 470–477. [CrossRef]
35. Zachariah, D.; Limite, L.R.; Mazzone, P.; Marzi, A.; Radinovic, A.; Baratto, F.; Italia, L.; Ancona, F.; Paglino, G.; Della Bella, P. Use of Cerebral Protection Device in Patients Undergoing Ventricular Tachycardia Catheter Ablation. *JACC Clin. Electrophysiol.* **2022**, *8*, 528–530. [CrossRef] [PubMed]

36. Berg, J.; Preda, A.; Fierro, N.; Marzi, A.; Radinovic, A.; Della Bella, P.; Mazzone, P. A Referral Center Experience with Cerebral Protection Devices: Challenging Cardiac Thrombus in the EP Lab. *J. Clin. Med.* **2023**, *12*, 1549. [CrossRef]
37. Jagielak, D.; Targonski, R.; Ciecwierz, D. First-in-Human Use of the Next-generation ProtEmbo Cerebral Embolic Protection System During Transcatheter Aortic Valve-in-valve Implantation. *Interv. Cardiol. Rev. Res. Resour.* **2021**, *16*, 1–4. [CrossRef]
38. Jagielak, D.; Targonski, R.; Frerker, C.; Abdel-Wahab, M.; Wilde, J.; Werner, N.; Lauterbach, M.; Leick, J.; Grygier, M.; Misterski, M.; et al. Safety and performance of a novel cerebral embolic protection device for transcatheter aortic valve implantation: The PROTEMBO C Trial. *EuroIntervention* **2022**, *18*, 590–597. [CrossRef]
39. Vernikouskaya, I.; Rottbauer, W.; Gonska, B.; Rodewald, C.; Seeger, J.; Rasche, V.; Wöhrle, J. Image-guidance for transcatheter aortic valve implantation (TAVI) and cerebral embolic protection. *Int. J. Cardiol.* **2017**, *249*, 90–95. [CrossRef]
40. Giannopoulos, S.; Armstrong, E.J. WIRION™ embolic protection system for carotid artery stenting and lower extremity endovascular intervention. *Futur. Cardiol.* **2020**, *16*, 527–538. [CrossRef]
41. Latib, A.; Mangieri, A.; Vezzulli, P.; Spagnolo, P.; Sardanelli, F.; Fellegara, G.; Pagnesi, M.; Giannini, F.; Falini, A.; Gorla, R.; et al. First-in-Man Study Evaluating the Emblok Embolic Protection System During Transcatheter Aortic Valve Replacement. *JACC Cardiovasc. Interv.* **2020**, *13*, 860–868. [CrossRef]
42. Nazif, T.M.; Moses, J.; Sharma, R.; Dhoble, A.; Rovin, J.; Brown, D.; Horwitz, P.; Makkar, R.; Stoler, R.; Forrest, J.; et al. Randomized Evaluation of TriGuard 3 Cerebral Embolic Protection After Transcatheter Aortic Valve Replacement: REFLECT II. *JACC Cardiovasc. Interv.* **2021**, *14*, 515–527. [CrossRef]
43. Kapadia, S.R.; Kodali, S.; Makkar, R.; Mehran, R.; Lazar, R.M.; Zivadinov, R.; Dwyer, M.G.; Jilaihawi, H.; Virmani, R.; Anwaruddin, S.; et al. Protection Against Cerebral Embolism During Transcatheter Aortic Valve Replacement. *J. Am. Coll. Cardiol.* **2017**, *69*, 367–377. [CrossRef]
44. Mangieri, A.; Montalto, C.; Poletti, E.; Sticchi, A.; Crimi, G.; Giannini, F.; Latib, A.; Capodanno, D.; Colombo, A. Thrombotic Versus Bleeding Risk After Transcatheter Aortic Valve Replacement. *J. Am. Coll. Cardiol.* **2019**, *74*, 2088–2101. [CrossRef] [PubMed]
45. Ciobanu, A.-O.M.; Gherasim, L.M.; Vinereanu, D.M. Risk of Stroke After Transcatheter Aortic Valve Implantation: Epidemiology, Mechanism, and Management. *Am. J. Ther.* **2021**, *28*, e560–e572. [CrossRef] [PubMed]
46. Armijo, G.; Nombela-Franco, L.; Tirado-Conte, G. Cerebrovascular Events After Transcatheter Aortic Valve Implantation. *Front. Cardiovasc. Med.* **2018**, *5*, 104. [CrossRef] [PubMed]
47. Schmidt, T.; Leon, M.B.; Mehran, R.; Kuck, K.-H.; Alu, M.C.; Braumann, R.E.; Kodali, S.; Kapadia, S.R.; Linke, A.; Makkar, R.; et al. Debris Heterogeneity across Different Valve Types Captured by a Cerebral Protection System during Transcatheter Aortic Valve Replacement. *JACC Cardiovasc. Interv.* **2018**, *11*, 1262–1273. [CrossRef]
48. Leon, M.B.; Smith, C.R.; Mack, M.J.; Makkar, R.R.; Svensson, L.G.; Kodali, S.K.; Thourani, V.H.; Tuzcu, E.M.; Miller, D.C.; Herrmann, H.C.; et al. Transcatheter or Surgical Aortic-Valve Replacement in Intermediate-Risk Patients. *N. Engl. J. Med.* **2016**, *374*, 1609–1620. [CrossRef]
49. Vahanian, A.; Alfieri, O.; Andreotti, F.; Antunes, M.J.; Barón-Esquivias, G.; Baumgartner, H.; Borger, M.A.; Carrel, T.P.; De Bonis, M.; Evangelista, A.; et al. Guidelines on the management of valvular heart disease (version 2012): The Joint Task Force on the Management of Valvular Heart Disease of the European Society of Cardiology (ESC) and the European Association for Cardio-Thoracic Surgery (EACTS). *Eur. J. Cardiothorac. Surg.* **2012**, *42*, S1–S44. [CrossRef]
50. Otto, C.M.; Nishimura, R.A.; Bonow, R.O.; Carabello, B.A.; Erwin, J.P.; Gentile, F.; Jneid, H.; Krieger, E.V.; Mack, M.; McLeod, C.; et al. 2020 ACC/AHA Guideline for the Management of Patients with Valvular Heart Disease: Executive Summary: A Report of the American College of Cardiology/American Heart Association Joint Committee on Clinical Practice Guidelines. *Circulation* **2021**, *143*, e35–e71. [CrossRef]
51. Kapadia, S.R.; Makkar, R.; Leon, M.; Abdel-Wahab, M.; Waggoner, T.; Massberg, S.; Rottbauer, W.; Horr, S.; Sondergaard, L.; Karha, J.; et al. Cerebral Embolic Protection during Transcatheter Aortic-Valve Replacement. *N. Engl. J. Med.* **2022**, *387*, 1253–1263. [CrossRef]
52. Giustino, G.; Sorrentino, S.; Mehran, R.; Faggioni, M.; Dangas, G. Cerebral Embolic Protection During TAVR: A Clinical Event Meta-Analysis. *J. Am. Coll. Cardiol.* **2017**, *69*, 465–466. [CrossRef] [PubMed]
53. Butala, N.M.; Makkar, R.; Secemsky, E.A.; Gallup, D.; Marquis-Gravel, G.; Kosinski, A.S.; Vemulapalli, S.; Valle, J.A.; Bradley, S.M.; Chakravarty, T.; et al. Cerebral Embolic Protection and Outcomes of Transcatheter Aortic Valve Replacement: Results from the Transcatheter Valve Therapy Registry. *Circulation* **2021**, *143*, 2229–2240. [CrossRef] [PubMed]
54. Ferket, B.S.; Morey, J.R.; Gelijns, A.C.; Moskowitz, A.J.; Giustino, G. Abstract 156: Cost-Effectiveness Analysis of the Sentinel Cerebral Embolic Protection Device During Transcatheter Aortic Valve Replacement. *Circ. Cardiovasc. Qual. Outcomes* **2019**, *12*, A156. [CrossRef]
55. Alkhouli, M.; Ganz, M.; Mercaldi, K.; McGovern, A.; Griffiths, R.; Kapadia, S. TCT-305 Cost-Effectiveness of Cerebral Embolic Protection with the SENTINEL Device in Transcatheter Aortic Valve Replacement: A US Medicare Payer Perspective. *J. Am. Coll. Cardiol.* **2021**, *78*, B125. [CrossRef]
56. Lansky, A.J.; Schofer, J.; Tchetche, D.; Stella, P.; Pietras, C.G.; Parise, H.; Abrams, K.; Forrest, J.K.; Cleman, M.; Reinöhl, J.; et al. A prospective randomized evaluation of the TriGuard™ HDH embolic DEFLECTion device during transcatheter aortic valve implantation: Results from the DEFLECT III trial. *Eur. Hear. J.* **2015**, *36*, 2070–2078. [CrossRef]

57. Wendt, D.; Kleinbongard, P.; Knipp, S.; Al-Rashid, F.; Gedik, N.; El Chilali, K.; Schweter, S.; Schlamann, M.; Kahlert, P.; Neuhäuser, M.; et al. Intraaortic Protection from Embolization in Patients Undergoing Transaortic Transcatheter Aortic Valve Implantation. *Ann. Thorac. Surg.* **2015**, *100*, 686–691. [CrossRef]
58. Van Mieghem, N.M.; van Gils, L.; Ahmad, H.; van Kesteren, F.; van der Werf, H.W.; Brueren, G.; Storm, M.; Lenzen, M.; Daemen, J.; Heuvel, A.F.v.D.; et al. Filter-based cerebral embolic protection with transcatheter aortic valve implantation: The randomised MISTRAL-C trial. *EuroIntervention* **2016**, *12*, 499–507. [CrossRef]
59. Patel, D.; Bailey, S.M.; Furlan, A.J.; Ching, M.; Zachaib, J.; DI Biase, L.; Mohanty, P.; Horton, R.P.; Burkhardt, J.D.; Sanchez, J.E.; et al. Long-Term Functional and Neurocognitive Recovery in Patients Who Had an Acute Cerebrovascular Event Secondary to Catheter Ablation for Atrial Fibrillation. *J. Cardiovasc. Electrophysiol.* **2010**, *21*, 412–417. [CrossRef]
60. Cappato, R.; Calkins, H.; Chen, S.-A.; Davies, W.; Iesaka, Y.; Kalman, J.; Kim, Y.-H.; Klein, G.; Natale, A.; Packer, D.; et al. Updated Worldwide Survey on the Methods, Efficacy, and Safety of Catheter Ablation for Human Atrial Fibrillation. *Circ. Arrhythm. Electrophysiol.* **2010**, *3*, 32–38. [CrossRef]
61. Santangeli, P.; Di Biase, L.; Horton, R.; Burkhardt, J.D.; Sanchez, J.; Al-Ahmad, A.; Hongo, R.; Beheiry, S.; Bai, R.; Mohanty, P.; et al. Ablation of atrial fibrillation under therapeutic warfarin reduces periprocedural complications: Evidence from a meta-analysis. *Circ. Arrhythmia Electrophysiol.* **2012**, *5*, 302–311. [CrossRef] [PubMed]
62. Bohnen, M.; Stevenson, W.G.; Tedrow, U.B.; Michaud, G.F.; John, R.M.; Epstein, L.M.; Albert, C.M.; Koplan, B.A. Incidence and predictors of major complications from contemporary catheter ablation to treat cardiac arrhythmias. *Heart Rhythm* **2011**, *8*, 1661–1666. [CrossRef]
63. Whitman, I.R.; Gladstone, R.A.; Badhwar, N.; Hsia, H.H.; Lee, B.K.; Josephson, S.A.; Meisel, K.M.; Dillon, W.P.; Hess, C.P.; Gerstenfeld, E.P.; et al. Brain Emboli After Left Ventricular Endocardial Ablation. *Circulation* **2017**, *135*, 867–877. [CrossRef] [PubMed]
64. Kuck, K.-H.; Schaumann, A.; Eckardt, L.; Willems, S.; Ventura, R.; Delacrétaz, E.; Pitschner, H.-F.; Kautzner, J.; Schumacher, B.; Hansen, P.S. Catheter ablation of stable ventricular tachycardia before defibrillator implantation in patients with coronary heart disease (VTACH): A multicentre randomised controlled trial. *Lancet* **2010**, *375*, 31–40. [CrossRef] [PubMed]
65. Holmes, D.R.; Kar, S.; Price, M.J.; Whisenant, B.; Sievert, H.; Doshi, S.K.; Huber, K.; Reddy, V.Y. Prospective randomized evaluation of the Watchman Left Atrial Appendage Closure device in patients with atrial fibrillation versus long-term warfarin therapy: The PREVAIL trial. *J. Am. Coll. Cardiol.* **2014**, *64*, 1–12. [CrossRef] [PubMed]
66. Reddy, V.Y.; Sievert, H.; Halperin, J.; Doshi, S.K.; Buchbinder, M.; Neuzil, P.; Huber, K.; Whisenant, B.; Kar, S.; Swarup, V.; et al. Percutaneous left atrial appendage closure vs. warfarin for atrial fibrillation: A randomized clinical trial. *JAMA* **2014**, *312*, 1988–1998. [CrossRef]
67. Cresti, A.; García-Fernández, M.A.; De Sensi, F.; Miracapillo, G.; Picchi, A.; Scalese, M.; Severi, S. Prevalence of auricular thrombosis before atrial flutter cardioversion: A 17-year transoesophageal echocardiographic study. *EP Eur.* **2015**, *18*, 450–456. [CrossRef]
68. Scherr, D.; Dalal, D.; Chilukuri, K.; Dong, J.U.N.; Spragg, D.; Henrikson, C.A.; Nazarian, S.; Cheng, A.; Berger, R.D.; Abraham, T.P.; et al. Incidence and Predictors of Left Atrial Thrombus Prior to Catheter Ablation of Atrial Fibrillation. *J. Cardiovasc. Electrophysiol.* **2009**, *20*, 379–384. [CrossRef]
69. Fukuda, S.; Watanabe, H.; Shimada, K.; Aikawa, M.; Kono, Y.; Jissho, S.; Taguchi, H.; Umemura, J.; Yoshiyama, M.; Shiota, T.; et al. Left atrial thrombus and prognosis after anticoagulation therapy in patients with atrial fibrillation. *J. Cardiol.* **2011**, *58*, 266–277. [CrossRef]
70. Guarracini, F.; Bonvicini, E.; Preda, A.; Martin, M.; Muraglia, S.; Casagranda, G.; Mochen, M.; Coser, A.; Quintarelli, S.; Branzoli, S.; et al. Appropriate use criteria of left atrial appendage closure devices: Latest evidences. *Expert Rev. Med. Devices* **2023**, *20*, 493–503. [CrossRef]
71. Preda, A.; Baroni, M.; Varrenti, M.; Vargiu, S.; Carbonaro, M.; Giordano, F.; Gigli, L.; Mazzone, P. Left Atrial Appendage Occlusion in Patients with Failure of Antithrombotic Therapy: Good Vibes from Early Studies. *J. Clin. Med.* **2023**, *12*, 3859. [CrossRef]
72. Saw, J.; Holmes, D.R.; Cavalcante, J.L.; Freeman, J.V.; Goldsweig, A.M.; Kavinsky, C.J.; Moussa, I.D.; Munger, T.M.; Price, M.J.; Reisman, M.; et al. SCAI/HRS expert consensus statement on transcatheter left atrial appendage closure. *Heart Rhythm* **2023**, *20*, e1–e16. [CrossRef]
73. Glikson, M.; Wolff, R.; Hindricks, G.; Mandrola, J.; Camm, A.J.; Lip, G.Y.; Fauchier, L.; Betts, T.R.; Lewalter, T.; Saw, J.; et al. EHRA/EAPCI expert consensus statement on catheter-based left atrial appendage occlusion—An update. *EuroIntervention* **2020**, *15*, 1133–1180. [CrossRef] [PubMed]
74. Seiffge, D.J.; De Marchis, G.M.; Koga, M.; Paciaroni, M.; Wilson, D.; Cappellari, M.; Macha, K.; Tsivgoulis, G.; Ambler, G.; Arihiro, S.; et al. Ischemic Stroke despite Oral Anticoagulant Therapy in Patients with Atrial Fibrillation. *Ann. Neurol.* **2020**, *87*, 677–687. [CrossRef] [PubMed]
75. Lowe, B.S.; Kusunose, K.; Motoki, H.; Varr, B.; Shrestha, K.; Whitman, C.; Tang, W.H.W.; Thomas, J.D.; Klein, A.L. Prognostic Significance of Left Atrial Appendage "Sludge" in Patients with Atrial Fibrillation: A New Transesophageal Echocardiographic Thromboembolic Risk Factor. *J. Am. Soc. Echocardiogr.* **2014**, *27*, 1176–1183. [CrossRef]
76. Sebag, F.S.; Garot, P.; Galea, R.; De Backer, O.; Lepillier, A.; De Meesteer, A.; Hildick-Smith, D.; Armero, S.; Moubarak, G.; Ducrocq, G.; et al. Left atrial appendage closure for thrombus trapping: The international, multicentre TRAPEUR registry. *EuroIntervention* **2022**, *18*, 50–57. [CrossRef]

77. Margonato, D.; Preda, A.; Ingallina, G.; Rizza, V.; Fierro, N.; Radinovic, A.; Ancona, F.; Patti, G.; Agricola, E.; Della Bella, P.; et al. Left atrial appendage occlusion after thromboembolic events or left atrial appendage sludge during anticoagulation therapy: Is two better than one? Real-world experience from a tertiary care hospital. *J. Arrhythmia* **2023**, *39*, 395–404. [CrossRef] [PubMed]
78. Boccuzzi, G.G.; Montabone, A.; D'Ascenzo, F.; Colombo, F.; Ugo, F.; Muraglia, S.; De Backer, O.; Nombela-Franco, L.; Meincke, F.; Mazzone, P. Cerebral protection in left atrial appendage closure in the presence of appendage thrombosis. *Catheter. Cardiovasc. Interv.* **2021**, *97*, 511–515. [CrossRef] [PubMed]
79. Osmancik, P.; Herman, D.; Neuzil, P.; Hala, P.; Taborsky, M.; Kala, P.; Poloczek, M.; Stasek, J.; Haman, L.; Branny, M.; et al. Left Atrial Appendage Closure Versus Direct Oral Anticoagulants in High-Risk Patients with Atrial Fibrillation. *J. Am. Coll. Cardiol.* **2020**, *75*, 3122–3135. [CrossRef]
80. Lopez, E.M.; Malhotra, R. Ventricular Tachycardia in Structural Heart Disease. *J. Innov. Card. Rhythm Manag.* **2019**, *10*, 3762–3773. [CrossRef]
81. Santangeli, P.; Rame, J.E.; Birati, E.Y.; Marchlinski, F.E. Management of Ventricular Arrhythmias in Patients with Advanced Heart Failure. *J. Am. Coll. Cardiol.* **2017**, *69*, 1842–1860. [CrossRef] [PubMed]
82. Streitner, F.; Herrmann, T.; Kuschyk, J.; Lang, S.; Doesch, C.; Papavassiliu, T.; Streitner, I.; Veltmann, C.; Haghi, D.; Borggrefe, M. Impact of Shocks on Mortality in Patients with Ischemic or Dilated Cardiomyopathy and Defibrillators Implanted for Primary Prevention. *PLoS ONE* **2013**, *8*, e63911. [CrossRef] [PubMed]
83. Cronin, E.M.; Bogun, F.M.; Maury, P.; Peichl, P.; Chen, M.; Namboodiri, N.; Aguinaga, L.; Leite, L.R.; Al-Khatib, S.M.; Anter, E.; et al. 2019 HRS/EHRA/APHRS/LAHRS expert consensus statement on catheter ablation of ventricular arrhythmias. *Heart Rhythm* **2020**, *17*, e2–e154. [CrossRef] [PubMed]
84. Bonnin, T.; Roumegou, P.; Sridi, S.; Mahida, S.; Bustin, A.; Duchateau, J.; Tixier, R.; Derval, N.; Pambrun, T.; Chniti, G.; et al. Prevalence and risk factors of cardiac thrombus prior to ventricular tachycardia catheter ablation in structural heart disease. *Europace* **2023**, *25*, 487–495. [CrossRef] [PubMed]
85. Medi, C.; Evered, L.; Silbert, B.; Teh, A.; Halloran, K.; Morton, J.; Kistler, P.; Kalman, J. Subtle Post-Procedural Cognitive Dysfunction After Atrial Fibrillation Ablation. *J. Am. Coll. Cardiol.* **2013**, *62*, 531–539. [CrossRef] [PubMed]
86. Valeri, Y.; Russo, A.D.; Falanga, U.; Volpato, G.; Compagnucci, P.; Barbarossa, A.; Cipolletta, L.; Parisi, Q.; Casella, M.; Piva, T. First report of cerebral embolic protection system use during combined atrial fibrillation Pulse Field Ablation and left atrial appendage closure. *Authorea* **2022**. preprints. [CrossRef]
87. Noseworthy, P.A.; Kapa, S.; Madhavan, M.; Van Houten, H.; Haas, L.; McLeod, C.; Friedman, P.; Asirvatham, S.; Shah, N.; Packer, D. Abstract 16200: Risk of Stroke After Catheter Ablation or Cardioversion for Atrial Fibrillation: Results from a Large Administrative Database, 2008–2012. *Circulation* **2014**, *130*, A16200.
88. Di Biase, L.; Burkhardt, J.D.; Mohanty, P.; Sanchez, J.E.; Horton, R.; Gallinghouse, G.J.; Lakkireddy, D.; Verma, A.; Khaykin, Y.; Hongo, R.; et al. Periprocedural stroke and management of major bleeding complications in patients undergoing catheter ablation of atrial fibrillation: The impact of periprocedural therapeutic international normalized ratio. *Circulation* **2010**, *121*, 2550–2556. [CrossRef]
89. Scherr, D.; Sharma, K.; Dalal, D.; Spragg, D.; Chilukuri, K.; Cheng, A.; Dong, J.; Henrikson, C.A.; Nazarian, S.; Berger, R.D.; et al. Incidence and Predictors of Periprocedural Cerebrovascular Accident in Patients Undergoing Catheter Ablation of Atrial Fibrillation. *J. Cardiovasc. Electrophysiol.* **2009**, *20*, 1357–1363. [CrossRef]
90. Calvert, P.; Kollias, G.; Pürerfellner, H.; Narasimhan, C.; Osorio, J.; Lip, G.Y.H.; Gupta, D. Silent cerebral lesions following catheter ablation for atrial fibrillation: A state-of-the-art review. *EP Eur.* **2023**, *25*, euad151. [CrossRef]
91. Haines, D.E.; Stewart, M.T.; Ahlberg, S.; Barka, N.D.; Condie, C.; Fiedler, G.R.; Kirchhof, N.A.; Halimi, F.; Deneke, T. Microembolism and catheter ablation I: A comparison of irrigated radiofrequency and multielectrode-phased radiofrequency catheter ablation of pulmonary vein ostia. *Circ. Arrhythm. Electrophysiol.* **2013**, *6*, 16–22. [CrossRef] [PubMed]
92. Kiss, A.; Nagy-Baló, E.; Sándorfi, G.; Édes, I.; Csanádi, Z. Cerebral microembolization during atrial fibrillation ablation: Comparison of different single-shot ablation techniques. *Int. J. Cardiol.* **2014**, *174*, 276–281. [CrossRef] [PubMed]
93. Miyazaki, S.; Watanabe, T.; Kajiyama, T.; Iwasawa, J.; Ichijo, S.; Nakamura, H.; Taniguchi, H.; Hirao, K.; Iesaka, Y. Thromboembolic Risks of the Procedural Process in Second-Generation Cryoballoon Ablation Procedures. *Circ. Arrhythmia Electrophysiol.* **2017**, *10*, e005612. [CrossRef] [PubMed]
94. Takami, M.; Lehmann, H.I.; Parker, K.D.; Welker, K.M.; Johnson, S.B.; Packer, D.L. Effect of Left Atrial Ablation Process and Strategy on Microemboli Formation during Irrigated Radiofrequency Catheter Ablation in an In Vivo Model. *Circ. Arrhythm. Electrophysiol.* **2016**, *9*, e003226. [CrossRef]
95. Lasek-Bal, A.; Puz, P.; Wieczorek, J.; Nowak, S.; Wnuk-Wojnar, A.; Warsz-Wianecka, A.; Mizia-Stec, K. Cerebral microembolism during atrial fibrillation ablation can result from the technical aspects and mostly does not cause permanent neurological deficit. *Arch. Med. Sci.* **2020**, *16*, 1288–1294. [CrossRef]
96. Braemswig, T.B.; Kusserow, M.; Kruppa, J.; Reinthaler, M.; Erdur, H.; Fritsch, M.; Curio, J.; Alushi, B.; Villringer, K.; Galinovic, I.; et al. Cerebral embolisation during transcatheter edge-to-edge repair of the mitral valve with the MitraClip system: A prospective, observational study. *EuroIntervention* **2022**, *18*, e160–e168. [CrossRef]
97. Vella, C.; Preda, A.; Ferri, L.; Montorfano, M. Intravascular Coronary Lithotripsy for the Treatment of Iatrogenic Calcium Embolization: The "Block and Crack" Technique. In *Catheterization and Cardiovascular Interventions*; Wiley: Hoboken, NY, USA, 2023. [CrossRef]

98. Hecker, F.; Arsalan, M.; Walther, T. Managing Stroke During Transcatheter Aortic Valve Replacement. *Interv. Cardiol. Rev. Res. Resour.* **2017**, *12*, 25–30. [CrossRef]
99. Perry, T.E.; George, S.A.; Lee, B.; Wahr, J.; Randle, D.; Sigurðsson, G. A guide for pre-procedural imaging for transcatheter aortic valve replacement patients. *Perioper. Med.* **2020**, *9*, 36. [CrossRef]
100. Jalal, Z.; Iriart, X.; Dinet, M.L.; Selly, J.B.; Tafer, N.; Renou, P.; Sibon, I.; Thambo, J.B. Extending percutaneous left atrial appendage closure indications using the AMPLATZER™ Cardiac Plug device in patients with persistent left atrial appendage thrombus: The thrombus trapping technique. *Arch. Cardiovasc. Dis.* **2016**, *109*, 659–666. [CrossRef]
101. Tzikas, A.; Bergmann, M.W. Left atrial appendage closure: Patient, device and post-procedure drug selection. *EuroIntervention* **2016**, *12*, X48–X54. [CrossRef]
102. Peichl, P.; Wichterle, D.; Čihák, R.; Aldhoon, B.; Kautzner, J. Catheter Ablation of Ventricular Tachycardia in the Presence of an Old Endocavitary Thrombus Guided by Intracardiac Echocardiography. *Pacing Clin. Electrophysiol.* **2016**, *39*, 581–587. [CrossRef] [PubMed]
103. Haines, D.E.; Stewart, M.T.; Barka, N.D.; Kirchhof, N.; Lentz, L.R.; Reinking, N.M.; Urban, J.F.; Halimi, F.; Deneke, T.; Kanal, E.; et al. Microembolism and Catheter Ablation II. *Circ. Arrhythm. Electrophysiol.* **2013**, *6*, 23–30. [CrossRef] [PubMed]
104. Zhang, J.; Xia, S.-J.; Du, X.; Jiang, C.; Lai, Y.-W.; Wang, Y.-F.; Jia, Z.-X.; He, L.; Tang, R.-B.; Dong, J.-Z.; et al. Incidence and risk factors of post-operative cognitive decline after ablation for atrial fibrillation. *BMC Cardiovasc. Disord.* **2021**, *21*, 341. [CrossRef] [PubMed]
105. Sauren, L.D.; VAN Belle, Y.; DE Roy, L.; Pison, L.; LA Meir, M.; VAN DER Veen, F.H.; Crijns, H.J.; Jordaens, L.; Mess, W.H.; Maessen, J.G. Transcranial Measurement of Cerebral Microembolic Signals during Endocardial Pulmonary Vein Isolation: Comparison of Three Different Ablation Techniques. *J. Cardiovasc. Electrophysiol.* **2009**, *20*, 1102–1107. [CrossRef]
106. van Oeveren, W.; Crijns, H.J.G.M.; Korteling, B.J.; Wegereef, E.W.; Haan, H.; Tigchelaar, I.; Hoekstra, A. Blood damage, platelet and clotting activation during application of radiofrequency or cryoablation catheters: A comparative in vitro study. *J. Med Eng. Technol.* **1999**, *23*, 20–25. [CrossRef]
107. Neumann, T.; Kuniss, M.; Conradi, G.; Janin, S.; Berkowitsch, A.; Wojcik, M.; Rixe, J.; Erkapic, D.; Zaltsberg, S.; Rolf, A.; et al. MEDAFI-Trial (Micro-embolization during ablation of atrial fibrillation): Comparison of pulmonary vein isolation using cryoballoon technique vs. radiofrequency energy. *Europace* **2011**, *13*, 37–44. [CrossRef]
108. Siklódy, C.H.; Deneke, T.; Hocini, M.; Lehrmann, H.; Shin, D.-I.; Miyazaki, S.; Henschke, S.; Fluegel, P.; Schiebeling-Römer, J.; Bansmann, P.M.; et al. Incidence of Asymptomatic Intracranial Embolic Events After Pulmonary Vein Isolation: Comparison of Different Atrial Fibrillation Ablation Technologies in a Multicenter Study. *J. Am. Coll. Cardiol.* **2011**, *58*, 681–688. [CrossRef]
109. Gaita, F.; Leclercq, J.F.; Schumacher, B.; Scaglione, M.; Toso, E.; Halimi, F.; Schade, A.; Froehner, S.; Ziegler, V.; Sergi, D.; et al. Incidence of Silent Cerebral Thromboembolic Lesions After Atrial Fibrillation Ablation May Change According to Technology Used: Comparison of Irrigated Radiofrequency, Multipolar Nonirrigated Catheter and Cryoballoon. *J. Cardiovasc. Electrophysiol.* **2011**, *22*, 961–968. [CrossRef]
110. Wasmer, K.; Foraita, P.; Leitz, P.; Güner, F.; Pott, C.; Lange, P.; Eckardt, L.; Mönnig, G. Safety profile of multielectrode-phased radiofrequency pulmonary vein ablation catheter and irrigated radiofrequency catheter. *Europace* **2016**, *18*, 78–84. [CrossRef]
111. Wieczorek, M.; Hoeltgen, R.; Brueck, M. Does the number of simultaneously activated electrodes during phased RF multielectrode ablation of atrial fibrillation influence the incidence of silent cerebral microembolism? *Heart Rhythm* **2013**, *10*, 953–959. [CrossRef]
112. Zellerhoff, S.; Ritter, M.A.; Kochhäuser, S.; Dittrich, R.; Köbe, J.; Milberg, P.; Korsukewitz, C.; Dechering, D.G.; Pott, C.; Wasmer, K.; et al. Modified phased radiofrequency ablation of atrial fibrillation reduces the number of cerebral microembolic signals. *EP Eur.* **2013**, *16*, 341–346. [CrossRef] [PubMed]
113. Reddy, V.Y.; Grimaldi, M.; De Potter, T.; Vijgen, J.M.; Bulava, A.; Duytschaever, M.F.; Martinek, M.; Natale, A.; Knecht, S.; Neuzil, P.; et al. Pulmonary Vein Isolation with Very High Power, Short Duration, Temperature-Controlled Lesions: The QDOT-FAST Trial. *JACC Clin. Electrophysiol.* **2019**, *5*, 778–786. [CrossRef] [PubMed]
114. Reddy, V.Y.; Dukkipati, S.R.; Neuzil, P.; Anic, A.; Petru, J.; Funasako, M.; Cochet, H.; Minami, K.; Breskovic, T.; Sikiric, I.; et al. Pulsed Field Ablation of Paroxysmal Atrial Fibrillation: 1-Year Outcomes of IMPULSE, PEFCAT, and PEFCAT II. *JACC Clin. Electrophysiol.* **2021**, *7*, 614–627. [CrossRef] [PubMed]
115. Ekanem, E.; Reddy, V.Y.; Schmidt, B.; Reichlin, T.; Neven, K.; Metzner, A.; Hansen, J.; Blaauw, Y.; Maury, P.; Arentz, T.; et al. Multinational survey on the methods, efficacy, and safety on the post-approval clinical use of pulsed field ablation (MANIFEST-PF). *Europace* **2022**, *24*, 1256–1266. [CrossRef]

Disclaimer/Publisher's Note: The statements, opinions and data contained in all publications are solely those of the individual author(s) and contributor(s) and not of MDPI and/or the editor(s). MDPI and/or the editor(s) disclaim responsibility for any injury to people or property resulting from any ideas, methods, instructions or products referred to in the content.

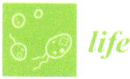

Article

Safety and Efficacy of an Innovative Everolimus-Coated Balloon in a Swine Coronary Artery Model

Christos S. Katsouras [1], Alexandros Tousis [2], Georgios Vasilagkos [2], Arsen Semertzioglou [3], Athanassios Vratimos [3], Ioanna Samara [1], Georgia Karanasiou [4], Vasileios S. Loukas [4], Grigorios Tsigkas [2], Dimitrios Fotiadis [4], Lampros K. Michalis [1], Periklis Davlouros [2] and Anargyros N. Moulas [5],*

[1] 2nd Department of Cardiology, University Hospital of Ioannina, University of Ioannina, 45110 Ioannina, Greece; cskats@yahoo.com (C.S.K.); ioan.samara31@gmail.com (I.S.); lamprosmihalis@gmail.com (L.K.M.)

[2] Department of Cardiology, University Hospital of Patras, 26504 Patras, Greece; alextousis21@gmail.com (A.T.); giorgosvasilagkos@gmail.com (G.V.); gregtsig@upatras.gr (G.T.); pdav@upatras.gr (P.D.)

[3] Rontis Hellas SA, 41500 Larissa, Greece; arsen.semertzioglou@rontis.com (A.S.); athanassios.vratimos@rontis.com (A.V.)

[4] Department of Biomedical Research, Institute of Molecular Biology and Biotechnology, Department of Materials Science and Engineering, Unit of Medical Technology and Intelligent Information Systems, University of Ioannina, 45110 Ioannina, Greece; g.karanasiou@gmail.com (G.K.); billloukas@gmail.com (V.S.L.); fotiadis@uoi.gr (D.F.)

[5] General Department, University of Thessaly, 41500 Larissa, Greece

* Correspondence: moulas@uth.gr; Tel.: +30-2410684361

Abstract: Background: Drug-coated balloons have been used as a non-stenting treatment in coronary and peripheral artery disease. Until recently, only sirolimus- and paclitaxel-coated balloons have been investigated in clinical trials. We evaluated the safety and efficacy of an innovative everolimus-coated balloon (ECB) in a swine coronary artery model. Methods: thirty-two swine coronary arteries were prepared through dilatation with a non-coated angioplasty balloon in a closed-chest model. During a period of 90 days, the following four groups (four animals per group, two coronary arteries per animal) were compared for safety and efficacy: A, Rontis ECB with 2.5 µg/mm^2 of drug per balloon surface; B, Rontis ECB with 7.5 µg/mm^2; C, Rontis Europa Ultra bare balloon; and D, Magic Touch, Concept Medical, sirolimus-coated balloon with a drug load of 1.3 µg/mm^2. Results: Differences in local biological effects (arterial reaction scores) and surface of intimal area (mm^2) were not statistically significant between the treatment groups. Numerically, group A showed the lowest intimal area and intimal mean thickness, while group B showed the lowest stenosis among all groups. Conclusions: ECB was safe and effective in a porcine coronary artery model. The dose of everolimus may play a role in the biocompatibility of the balloon.

Keywords: drug coated balloon; everolimus; coronary arteries; angioplasty; porcine model

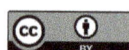

1. Introduction

The routine use of drug-eluting stents (DES) for percutaneous treatment of coronary disease has shown that DES are more effective in preventing restenosis than bare-metal stents [1]. However, in-stent-restenosis (ISR) remains a major complication even after new generation DES have been introduced into the market. Recent data has suggested that treatment of ISR may account for 5–10% of all percutaneous coronary procedures performed [2,3]. A third consecutive procedure in recurrent ISR involving a third DES implantation results in a further increase in the ISR rate [4]. An additional drawback of current DES is the need for dual antiplatelet therapy at least four months after angioplasty, whereas a significant proportion of patients must discontinue the administration of the second antiplatelet agent for non-cardiac reasons soon after the procedure.

Drug-coated balloons (DCBs) are endovascular balloons coated with a drug that is delivered to the target endothelial site during inflation and contact with the vascular tissue without leaving a permanent implant behind following the procedure [5]. Commercially available DCBs for coronary interventions use paclitaxel and sirolimus. Studies reported that DCBs are an alternative to DES for ISR [6,7]. Moreover, there is evidence that treatment of de novo coronary lesions with DCBs is associated with a similar risk of restenosis and a lower risk of target lesion thrombosis compared to DES in patients with specific anatomical or clinical characteristics [8]. Furthermore, DCBs offer the option for a shorter duration of double antiplatelet therapy, allowing their use in patients with a high risk for bleeding [8].

Everolimus is a synthetic immunosuppressant derived from a chemical modification of rapamycin that promotes cell cycle arrest in the late G1 phase. Everolimus was originally used in second-generation drug-eluting stents and, due to its proven safety and efficacy, was subsequently used in newer drug-eluting stents and bioresorbable stents [9].

Everolimus has not been tested in DCBs. Based on the fact that everolimus-eluting stents generally perform better than paclitaxel-eluting stents and, in some aspects, better than sirolimus-eluting stents [10,11], we hypothesized that an everolimus-coated balloon could perform better than existing DCBs. The primary scientific questions of this study were whether the developed everolimus balloon is safe and efficient in a swine coronary artery model and what the possible effects of the therapeutic dose of the drug are.

2. Materials and Methods

Sixteen female pigs (four animals in each of the four groups, as described below), 5–6 months of age, weighing between 50 and 55 kg, were used. The number of necessary samples was determined with power analysis [12]. The experiments were conducted at a licensed facility of the University Hospital of Patras (University of Patras, Patras, Greece). The facility was equipped with individual cages in climate-controlled rooms. The animals were given a minimum 24-h period for acclimatization after transportation to the facility and experimental procedures. Food was withheld 12 h prior to anesthesia. The test protocols were approved by the Animal Care and Use Board of Patras University Hospital's ethics committee and by the veterinary board of Western Greece's Provincial authorities. Additionally, the protocols complied with the medical research ethical principles of the Declaration of Helsinki, the ARRIVE guidelines, and the European Union legislation according to the principle of the 3Rs (Reduction, Refinement, Replacement), ensuring an adequate but low number of animals, improved experimental techniques, and living conditions such that the animals were kept to minimum pain or suffering [13,14].

2.1. Anesthesia and Intubation

All animal experiments were performed under general anesthesia (15 mg/kg intramuscular ketamine and 2 mg/kg xylazine) followed by endotracheal intubation (FiO_2:0.4). Continuous propofol infusion (1–1.4 mg/kg) was administered during anesthesia [15,16]. Pulse oximetry (via the animal's tail) and heart rate were monitored throughout the operation. Each animal was marked with their assigned number in both ears after anesthesia and prior to the procedure.

The right superficial femoral artery was chosen for arterial access under ultrasound guidance [17]. The Seldinger technique with a 21-gauge needle was used, a 6-Fr-10 cm radial artery sheath (Terumo Medical Corporation®, Shibuya, Japan) was inserted, and 100 U/kg heparin was administered intra-arterially. Intra-arterial blood pressure was monitored throughout the procedure. Dual antiplatelet therapy (aspirin 100 mg plus Clopidogrel 75 mg) was administrated to each animal daily for 2 days prior to the procedure and for 10 days afterward, followed by administration of Aspirin 100 mg daily for 80 days.

2.2. Coronary Artery Balloon Dilatation

Procedures were performed with a Philips Allura Flat-Panel Angiography Unit (Philips, Amsterdam, The Netherlands). All procedures were carried out by three experienced operators

(C.S.K., G.T., and P.D.). Engagement of the left and right coronary arteries was mainly achieved by the Amplatzer AR1® (Cook Medical®, Bloomington, IN, USA.) catheter and the Right Coronary Bypass® (RCB) catheter (Cordis Corporation®, Hialeah, FL, USA), respectively.

Four groups were compared: group A, Rontis everolimus-coated balloon 2.5 µg/mm^2 of drug per balloon surface; group B, Rontis everolimus-coated balloon 7.5 µg/mm^2; group C, Rontis Europa Ultra bare balloon; and group D: sirolimus-coated balloon with a dose of 1.3 µg/mm^2 (Magic Touch, Concept Medical, Gujarat, India). The test device (everolimus DCB) was a drug-coated angioplasty catheter based on the Europa Ultra coronary balloon catheter delivery platform (Rontis Hellas SA, Larissa, Greece). The balloon's surface was coated with a proprietary biocompatible excipient system and a therapeutic dose of the drug everolimus (2.5 or 7.5 µg drug per mm^2 of balloon surface). This formulation forms a homogenous film-like coating around the balloon that helps reduce drug wash-off when advancing the catheter and navigating through the blood vessels and promotes effective drug delivery into the vessel wall when the balloon is deployed at the target lesion site.

Initially, a coronary angiogram and an Optical Coherence Tomography Study (OCT, Dragonfly™ OPTIS™ Imaging Catheter, Abbott, IL, USA) were performed. Afterward, the vessel was prepared through dilatation with a standard, non-coated angioplasty balloon (Europa Ultra, 3.5 mm × 15 mm, Rontis Hellas SA, Larissa, Greece) with a balloon-to-artery diameter ratio of 1.1:1, aiming to cause intimal damage and trigger the onset of vascular repair in order to develop an atherosclerotic lesion (two coronary vessels per animal, one dilatation per vessel). The location of the target sites was specified by fluoroscopy of the radio-opaque markers on the balloon catheters in relation to other landmarks of vascular anatomy, such as the ostium of the treated artery, the left main (or other) bifurcation, diagonal and septal branches, marginal branches, and right artery branches. Usually, the area of interest was located a few millimeters distally or proximally to an arterial bifurcation. Data from the OCT were also used for verification of the lumen's diameter and as an additional landmark, e.g., the distance from the ostium or other marks. The best angiographic image was selected for use as a visual guide during the second phase of the experiment and was displayed alongside the working monitor.

Then, the angiographic table was locked, and, using the aforementioned angiographic image, the balloon catheters under investigation were deployed. Each pig received two balloon "treatments" in two corresponding arteries (one treatment per artery; either the Left Anterior Descending Artery (LAD), Right Coronary Artery (RCA), and/or Left Circumflex Artery (LCX)). The balloons (3.5 mm × 20 mm in all 4 groups) were inflated at the area of interest. The everolimus DCBs and bare balloons were inflated for 60 s at a pressure of 10 atm, while the sirolimus DCBs were inflated at 8 atm. Inflation pressure was applied in accordance with the specific compliance chart of each product, aiming to overinflate the balloon in order to reach a diameter 0.1–0.2 mm greater than the nominal luminal diameter. OCT was performed after the inflation in order to detect possible dissections or any other problems in the vasculature. Finally, the vascular status was assessed by coronary angiography. A vascular closure device (Angio-Seal 6F, Terumo Medical Corporation®, Shibuya, Japan) was used to seal the catheterization site, while an ultrasound verified the absence of local bleeding.

The study duration was 90 days. At the end of the study period, new angiography and OCT studies were performed on the treated vessels, and thereafter, the animals were sacrificed, and specific tissues (the target arterial sites and biopsies from specific internal organs, including the myocardium) were collected for histomorphometry and histopathological evaluation. A macroscopic (visual) investigation of the internal organs also took place, looking for any signs of systemic toxicity possibly associated with DCB deployment and drug/excipient wash-off. Data from OCT were collected for a parallel study aiming to develop an in silico simulation of the process and compare OCT data with data from histomorphometry. For the purposes of this study, data from the OCT were used only for verification of the lumen's diameter and as an additional landmark of the area of interest.

2.3. Histotechnology and Histomorphology by Image Analysis

A scoring system reference was used to assess the arterial wall reaction at the dilatation areas by recording endothelial cell loss, deposits of fibrin attached to the intima, tunica intima proliferation, tunica intima and/or media inflammation, focal or diffuse medial hypertrophy and fibrosis, lamina elastica rupture, smooth muscle proliferation in the intima, proteoglycan/collagen presence and distribution, arterial inflammation, medial smooth muscle cell (SMC) loss, the presence of markers suggesting a host reaction associated with the process (polymorphonuclear cells, lymphocytes, plasma cells, macrophages, giant cells, necrosis, fibrosis, peristrut hemorrhage/fibrin accumulation, neovascularization, fatty infiltrate), elastic lamina (EL) rupture (external EL rupture, internal EL rupture), and medial hypertrophy (focal, diffuse). A scoring system, adapted from ISO 10993-6:2016, was applied. A score from 0 to 4 for each parameter was applied according to the histological findings. Score differences between 0.0 to 2.9 were considered no or minimal host reaction, 3.0 to 8.9 slight host reaction, 9.0 to 15.0 moderate host reaction, and ≥ 15.1 severe host reaction compared to a reference material, as per ISO 10993-6:2016. Limited systemic effects were also evaluated.

Regarding the quantitative parameters analyzed by histopathology, each treatment site was transversally trimmed at five approximately equidistant levels of the artery segment, two End Segments (End 1 and End 2), two Middle-End Segments (Middle-End 1 and Middle-End 2) and one Middle Segment, then dehydrated, embedded in paraffin wax, sectioned at an approximate thickness of 2–4 μm, and stained with Hematoxylin and Eosin (HE) and Elastin Trichrome (ET) (Figure 1).

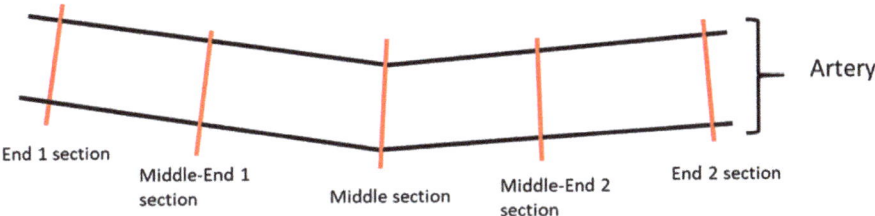

Figure 1. Illustrative image of the sectioning of the artery samples. Each treatment site was transversally trimmed at five approximately equidistant levels of the artery segment: two end sections, two middle-end sections, and one middle section.

All arterial segments were image scanned by an Olympus Slideview VS200 slide scanner using a VS-264C camera and 20× objective (Olympus Life Science, Hamburg, Germany). Quantitative evaluation was performed using Olympus imaging and image analysis software cellSens v1.18 (Olympus Life Science, Hamburg, Germany). The following parameters were measured on the two HE-stained end segments (End 1 and End 2) and three HE-stained middle segments (Middle-End 1, Middle, and Middle-End 2) for all arteries: area within external elastic lamina (EEL; μm^2), area within internal elastic lamina (IEL; μm^2), lumen (μm^2), intima (μm^2, calculation: IEL − Lumen), media (μm^2, calculation: EEL − IEL), stenosis [%, calculation: 100 − (100 × Lumen/IEL)], and intimal mean thickness (μm) (average value from 10 equidistant thickness measurements) (Figure 2).

Quantitative parameters were overall combined [either End segments (End 1 + End 2), Middle segments (Middle-End 1 + Middle + Middle-End 2), or all segments (End 1 + Middle-End 1 + Middle + Middle-End 2 + End 2)]. For intimal thickness, a mean value was calculated from ten measured values per vessel. These arithmetic mean values were used for further descriptive statistics.

Tissues from the spleen, liver, kidneys, lungs, and myocardium were also dehydrated, paraffin-embedded, sectioned at an approximate thickness of 2–4 μm, and stained with

Hematoxylin and Eosin (HE) in order to detect any signs of systemic toxicity occurring due to ECB application. All sections were QC under light microscopy.

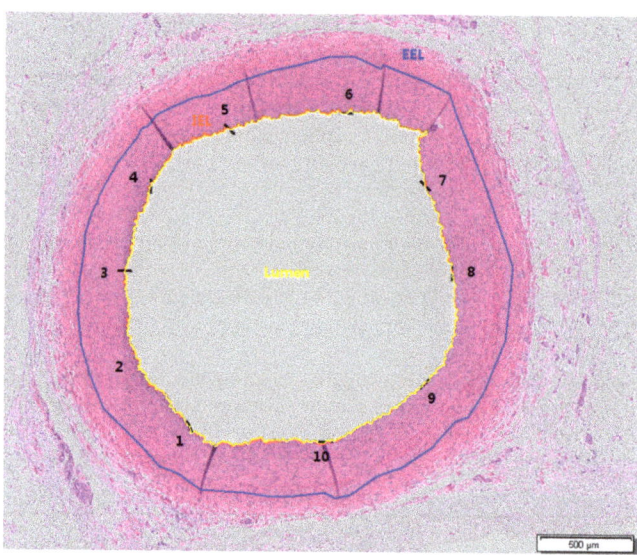

Figure 2. Exemplary image indicating the measured parameters in the examined artery segments. Animal 16, Middle-End 1 Segment, Artery RCA, group A, HE, and objective ×20. External elastic lamina (EEL) (blue color), internal elastic lamina (IEL) (red color), and lumen (in yellow). Intimal thickness measurements were performed at ten equidistant points (black color), and the average was calculated. The numbers (1–10) indicate the positions where thickness measurements were conducted.

2.4. Data Comparison and Statistical Analysis

The devices were compared for safety and efficacy. The primary safety endpoint was the absence of major adverse events (death or myocardial infarction) occurring immediately after the intervention and up to three months later. We also recorded any signs of coronary thrombus formation immediately after balloon inflation through angiography. Efficacy endpoints were based on the results of the histology and morphometry. The primary efficacy endpoint referred to the statistically significant comparison of neointimal formation ("intimal area" from the quantitative evaluation of histopathology) and arterial wall reaction score (from histology) between the test groups. Secondary endpoints involved an assessment of the area within the external elastic lamina, the area within the internal elastic lamina, lumen area, intima, media, lumen stenosis, and intimal mean thickness. Regarding systemic effects, findings from the spleen, liver, kidneys, lungs, and myocardium were also recorded. Statistical tests were performed using GraphPad Prism 9 (Graphpad Software, Boston, MA, USA). Descriptive statistics were used for the medial area, intimal area, stenosis, and intimal thickness. The Shapiro-Wilk test for normality was performed. When the data followed a normal distribution, the comparisons were performed with the unpaired Student's *t*-test. When data did not follow a normal distribution, the Mann-Whitney test was used (in all cases, p-values < 0.05 were considered statistically significant).

3. Results

The balloons were successfully dilated into the target arteries, and in all cases, no severe complications were detected during the procedure. No sustained or non-sustained ventricular tachycardias were noted, and no severe dissections were seen in the final angiography. No angiographic thrombus was detected. All closure devices were placed uneventfully.

One animal (group C, bare balloons) died; the pig did not wake up after the angioplasty procedure without an obvious cause identified by the veterinarian. All other animals (N = 15) survived the scheduled study period, and 30 "treated" coronary arteries were examined.

3.1. Systemic Reactions

Thrombosis within the myocardium or systemic organs was not detected. Porcine pleuropneumonia was observed in four animals, a very common condition in young pigs, which usually leads to chronic sequels, such as pleural fibrosis, often with adhesions to the pericardium. Within the kidneys, the presence of minimal focal chronic infarcts in two pigs was noted, one from Group A and one from Group D. There were no significant differences in incidence/severity among the treatments.

The histological evaluation of the LAD, RCA, and LCX myocardial irrigated areas revealed focal perivascular inflammatory infiltrate of small-sized arteries in animal no. P03 (grade 1, group A) and in animal no. P12 (grade 2, group B) of a medium-sized artery with medial hyperplasia. There were no associated changes in the adjacent pericardium, such as necrosis or degeneration. Other findings within LAD, RCA, and LCX myocardial irrigated areas, such as mixed cell inflammatory infiltrate or the presence of myotubes, could be associated with the balloon deployment, but there were no relevant differences in incidence or severity between groups.

3.2. Arteries at the Dilatation Site and Host Reaction

The arterial wall reaction at the deployment sites varied in degrees of severity and consisted of one or more of the following findings.

(a) Vascular wall findings: the endothelium lining often showed multifocal loss of endothelial cells. Occasionally, there were multifocal minimal to slight deposits of fibrin attached to the endothelial surface and increased intimal layer thickness due to smooth muscle proliferation and deposition of proteoglycan or collagen production;

(b) Arterial inflammation: the tunica intima and/or media from most of the samples presented with minor infiltrate of inflammatory cells;

(c) The tunica media appeared thickened by multifocal hypertrophy of the smooth muscle cells;

(d) The occasional presence of lamina elastica rupture, more predominantly in the internal lamina;

(e) Host reaction associated with the balloon treatment sites consisted of minimal to slight infiltrate in a small number of neutrophils (polymorphonuclear cells), lymphocytes, and/or macrophages.

Fibrosis at the treatment site was minimal in two samples (one from group A and one from group B) and moderate in one sample from group D, where fatty infiltrate was also observed.

Numerically, the least severe host reaction associated with the balloon expansion site was found in groups A and B, followed by groups C and D. However, differences ($\leq$1.4 points) were minor among the treatment groups and per ISO 10993-6:2016 definition (Table 1). Representative pathology images of treated artery segments, one for each treatment group, are shown in Figure 3.

When combining all sections together (End 1, End 2, Midddle-End 1, Middle, and Middle-End 2), group A showed the lowest intimal area and intimal mean thickness, and group B showed the lowest stenosis among all groups. However, Group C showed the lowest medial area. No statistically significant differences were observed between the groups, except for the medial area, for which groups A and B showed a statistically significantly higher medial area than group C (p = 0.0054 and p = 0.0031, respectively), as seen in Table 2 and Figure 4.

Table 1. Histology results at the balloon deployment sites. Average scores at the arterial balloon deployment sites.

	Group A	Group B	Group C	Group D
Number of animals	4	3	4	4
Total Sample number	26	30	29	34
Sum Host Reaction Score Total	51	53	74	76
Host Reaction Average Score associated with the balloon deployment site	2.0	1.8	2.6	2.2
Vascular wall findings	5.2	5.9	5.7	5.4
Artery Inflammation	1.4	1.3	1.4	1.2
Medial smooth muscle cell (SMC) loss	0.0	0.0	0.0	0.0
Medial smooth muscle cell replacement tissue	0.0	0.0	0.0	0.0
Medial hypertrophy	1.8	2.1	1.6	2.8
Lamina elastic rupture	0.6	0.9	1.0	0.7
TOTAL Arterial Reaction Average Score	11.0	11.9	12.2	12.4

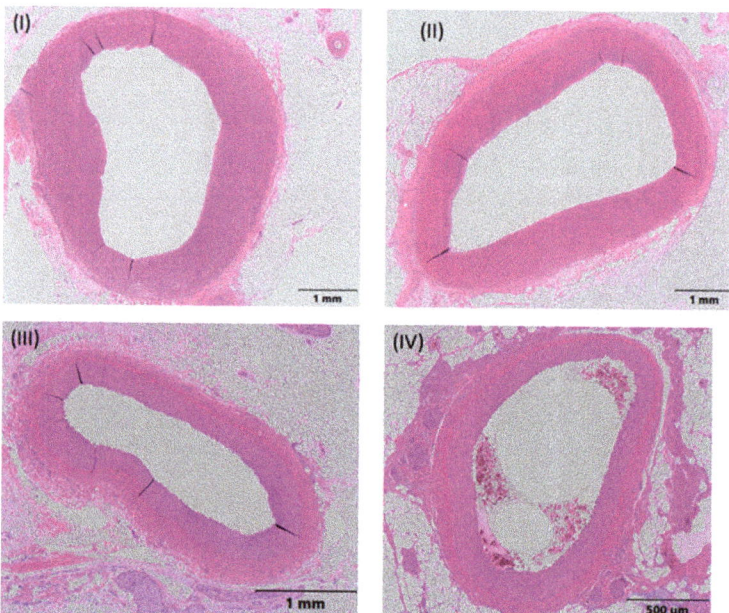

Figure 3. Representative pathology images of treated artery segments, one for each treatment group. The measurement parameters were the external elastic lamina (EEL), internal elastic lamina (IEL), lumen, intima, and media. Ten approximately equidistant measurements were used to measure the intimal thickness. (**I**) Animal 03, RCA, Middle-End 2, group A (everolimus-coated balloon 2.5 µg/mm^2), (**II**) Animal 04, LAD, Middle-End 1, group B (everolimus-coated balloon 7.5 µg/mm^2), (**III**) Animal 05, LCX, Middle-End 1, group C (uncoated (bare) balloon), and (**IV**) Animal 06, LAD-End 1, group D (sirolimus-coated balloon 1.3 µg/mm^2).

Table 2. The medial area, lumen area, intimal area, intimal mean thickness, and % stenosis (average (SD) with 95% confidence interval (CI)) in all treated arterial sections combined (End 1, End 2, Midddle-End 1, Middle, and Middle-End 2). * $p = 0.0054$, # $p = 0.0031$ comparison of groups with the respective symbol with group C.

	Group A	Group B	Group C	Group D
Lumen Area (mm^2)	3.23 (4.58) (1.38–5.08)	2.21 (2.38) (1.29–3.14)	1.64 (1.58) (1.03–2.25)	2.06 (2.82) (1.02–3.09)
Medial Area (mm^2)	4.39 (6.01) * (1.97–6.82)	3.25 (4.21) # (1.62–4.88)	1.68 (2.07) (0.87–2.48)	2.49 (3.71) (1.13–3.85)
Intimal Area (mm^2)	0.098 (0.113) (0.052–0.14)	0.138 (0.202) (0.06–2.16)	0.114 (0.189) (0.041–0.187)	0.114 (0.195) (0.042–0.185)
Stenosis (%)	7.97 (13.4) (2.58–13.37)	5.63 (5.29) (3.58–7.68)	6.41 (8.36) (3.17–9.66)	7.11 (13.12) (2.30–11.92)
Intimal Mean Thickness (μm)	15.06 (22.4)	17.72 (21.2)	17.1 (22.42)	17.36 (27.65)

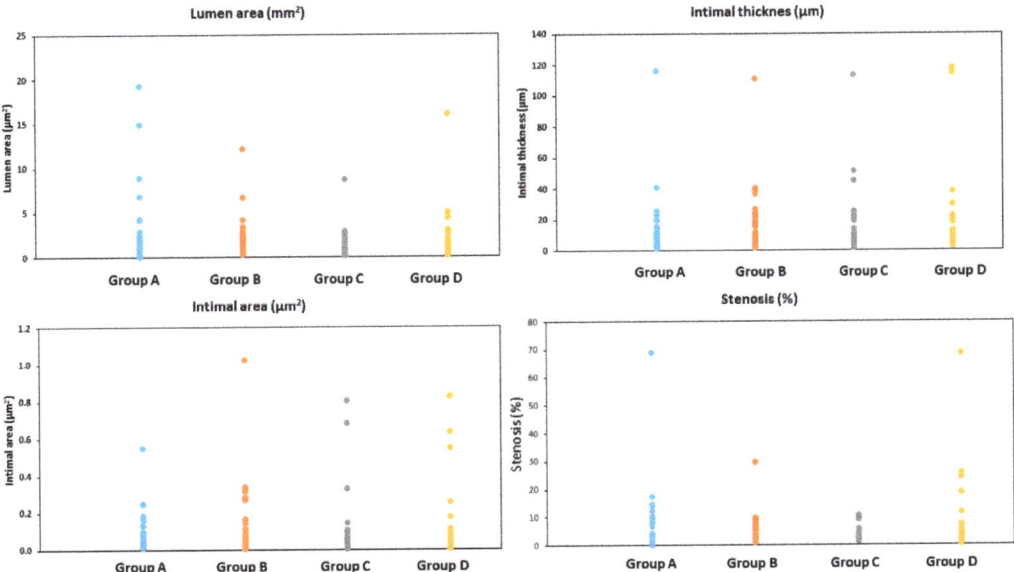

Figure 4. The lumen area, intimal mean thickness, intimal area, and % stenosis in all treated arterial sections combined (End 1, End 2, Midddle-End 1, Middle, and Middle-End 2). Group A = everolimus-coated balloon 2.5 μg/mm^2, group B = everolimus-coated balloon 7.5 μg/mm^2, group C = uncoated (bare) balloon, and group D = sirolimus-coated balloon 1.3 μg/mm^2.

In the Middle sections, group C showed the lowest medial area, intimal area, stenosis, and intimal mean thickness when compared to groups A, B, and D. Groups A and B showed a statistically significantly higher medial area than group C ($p = 0.0270$ and $p = 0.0160$, respectively) (Table 3).

In the End sections, group C showed the highest intimal area, stenosis, and intimal mean thickness when compared to groups A, B, and D. Group A showed the lowest intimal area, stenosis, and intimal mean thickness values among all groups. No statistically significant differences were observed between the groups, except for stenosis, for which group A showed a statistically significantly lower stenosis than group C ($p = 0.040$) (Table 4).

Other findings within the LAD, RCA, and LCX myocardial irrigated areas referring to mixed cell inflammatory infiltrate or the presence of myotubes could be associated with the balloon implantation, but there were no relevant differences in incidence or severity between treatments.

Table 3. The medial area, lumen area, intimal area, intimal mean thickness, and % stenosis (average (SD, 95% confidence interval)) in the middle sections combined (Midddle-End 1, Middle, and Middle-End 2).

	Group A	Group B	Group C	Group D
Lumen Area (mm^2)	1.71 (1.76) (0.73–2.68)	1.76 (1.48) (1.00–2.52)	1.47 (0.77) (1.07–1.86)	1.71 (1.30) (1.08–2.33)
Medial Area (mm^2)	2.61 (2.69) (1.13–4.10)	2.42 (1.91) (1.44–3.41)	1.31 (0.51) (1.05–1.57)	1.94 (2.09) (0.93–2.94)
Intimal Area (mm^2)	0.11 (0.14) (0.03–0.18)	0.14 (0.25) (0.06–0.19)	0.05 (0.03) (0.04–0.07)	0.13 (0.22) (0.02–0.23)
Stenosis (%)	11.01 (16.88) (1.67–20.35)	6.11 (6.58) (2.73–9.50)	3.97 (3.05) (2.41–5.54)	8.09 (15.67) (0.54–15.64)
Intimal Mean Thickness (μm)	19.2 (28.7) (1.7–20.4)	18.5 (25.7) (2.7–9.5)	10.0 (7.7) (2.4–5.5)	20.7 (34.1) (0.5–15.6)

Table 4. The medial area, lumen area, intimal area, intimal mean thickness, and % stenosis (average (SD) (95% confidence interval) in the end sections combined (End 1, End 2).

	Group A	Group B	Group C	Group D
Lumen Area (mm^2)	5.30 (6.31) (1.06–9.54)	2.91 (3.30) (0.69–5.12)	1.91 (2.39) (0.30–3.51)	2.60 (4.29) (0.00–5.32)
Medial Area (mm^2)	6.82 (8.30) (1.24–12.4)	4.53 (6.24) (0.33–8.72)	2.25 (3.26) (0.58–4.43)	3.37 (5.38) (0.00–6.78)
Intimal Area (mm^2)	0.09 (0.08) (0.04–0.13)	0.13 (0.12) (0.05–0.21)	0.21 (0.28) (0.03–0.4)	0.09 (0.15) (0.00–0.04)
Stenosis (%)	3.80 (3.83) (1.26–6.41)	4.87 (2.27) (3.34–6.39)	10.19 (12.17) (2.01–18.36)	5.57 (7.98) (0.49–10.64)
Intimal Mean Thickness (μm)	9.5 (6.3) (5.3–13.8)	16.5 (12.3) (8.2–24.8)	28.1 (32.3) (6.4–49.8)	12.1 (11.3) (4.9–19.3)

4. Discussion

In the current experimental study, we investigated whether or not the use of everolimus DCBs was safe and effective for the treatment of coronary arterial sites where an injury had been caused through the deployment of bare balloons using a swine model. We compared Rontis' everolimus DCBs (2 doses) with a non-coated balloon and a commercially available DCB. The results suggested that: (1) the devices were safe; (2) the test balloons created the least severe host reaction, although differences among all groups were not statistically significant; (3) their use was associated with minimal neointimal formation, especially at the ends of "injury" areas produced by plain balloons (less reaction with 2.5 μg/mm^2 balloon), although the differences were not statistically significant; and (4) the dose of everolimus may play a role in the biocompatibility of the device.

Everolimus, a semi-synthetic derivative of naturally occurring rapamycin with potent immunosuppressive and anti-proliferative effects, is one of the four mammalian targets of rapamycin (mTOR) inhibitors: sirolimus, everolimus, temsirolimus, and ridaforolimus [18,19]. These large molecules (molecular weight ~1000 kDa) inhibit the action of the mTOR protein kinase complex through the binding of the FK506 binding protein-12 (FKB12), which forms a ternary complex with mTOR [20].

Everolimus reduced neointimal proliferation in cultured human saphenous vein grafts [21]. Moreover, stent-mediated delivery of everolimus inhibited the formation of neointimal hyperplasia and neoatherosclerosis in porcine iliac arteries [22]. Everolimus eluting stents (EES) have been widely utilized in clinical practice in patients undergoing percutaneous coronary interventions. In a large randomized trial, the incidence of target lesion failure and stent thrombosis at 12 months post-intervention were similar in patients treated with either EES or sirolimus-eluting stents (both stents with durable polymers) [23]. However, at five years, the rates of target lesion revascularization, target vessel revascularization, recurrent myocardial infarction, and stent thrombosis were significantly lower in the EES group compared to the SES group [24]. Moreover, only the use of SES with a biodegradable polymer and/or ultrathin struts resulted in similar results to the use of EES with a durable polymer and thicker struts [25–27]. The causes for this "advantage" of everolimus are not clear. Minor differences in structure, systemic clearance, vessel wall levels of the drug, and the relative hydrophobicity of sirolimus may play a role [18,19].

DCBs have been used to treat ISR and de novo coronary disease with promising results. Different DCBs may result in differences in efficacy (late lumen loss) [28]. No everolimus DCB has been tested in experimental models (or in clinical practice). We investigated the results of a novel everolimus DCB in an experimental model of injury created by plain balloons in non-atherosclerotic swine coronary arteries. We tested two different doses of everolimus (2.5 or 7.5 µg drug per mm^2 of balloon surface). In the comparative evaluation (with a non-coated balloon and sirolimus DCB), differences were limited among the groups in total arterial reaction average score. Numerically, a lower score was found in groups with everolimus DCBs (both doses). There was no fibrosis at the treatment site in most cases (fibrosis was minimal in two samples and moderate in one). To the best of our knowledge, there are no similar studies for comparison. One study examined an everolimus-eluting bioresorbable vascular scaffold (Absorb) and the second-generation everolimus-eluting cobalt chromium XIENCE V stent in a porcine coronary artery model and found that inflammation was mild at six months in both groups. The inflammation score was greater at 12, 18, 30, and 36 months post-intervention in the Absorb and XIENCE groups. Both devices exhibited absent or minimal inflammation at 42 months [29]. In our DCB study, we provided data at only 90 days post-intervention. It is well known that increased inflammation has been correlated with a greater neointimal thickness and ISR in bare metal stents and DESs [30,31]. However, "continuous inflammation" is an important factor in the ISR, while the role of inflammation in restenosis after balloon angioplasty does not have the same significance as in ISR [32].

The intimal area was lower in everolimus-DCB groups, especially at the ends of "areas of interest". It is interesting that remodeling and neointima formation at the proximal reference segments significantly affect the restenotic process after successful plain balloon coronary angioplasty in humans [33]. The small differences among the groups may be due to the limited number of treated arteries and the observed large standard deviations for all groups and all parameters (data in Supplement). However, based on the results of both the intimal area and inflammatory response, we can assume the everolimus DCB is at least equivalent in safety and efficacy to the commercially available sirolimus-DCB. It is also interesting that we recorded small differences in the two groups of everolimus DCBs (2.5 or 7.5 µg drug per mm^2 of balloon surface). Histomorphometrically, the media area was greater in groups A and B compared to group C in the Mid-Segments (not in the End-Segments). However, groups A and B had a numerically larger EEL area, IEL area, and lumen area than group C in the same Mid-Areas. These results may be the consequences of positive remodeling after everolimus DCBs, as in an everolimus-eluting bioresorbable vascular scaffold [29], and, in combination with a lower intima area, indicate that the media area differences were not deemed to induce more stenosis in groups A and B.

Limitations

Our study has some limitations. First, vascular responses to the balloons in healthy (without atherosclerotic lesions) swine coronary arteries are likely different from those in diseased human arteries. Second, the observation period was three months. We do not know if we would have obtained the same results at different/additional time points after the procedure. Third, we performed the experiments on pigs weighing 50–55 kg, whereas the same animals, three months later, weighed more than 80 kg. Finally, despite all efforts to mark the "areas of interest" accurately, small divergences in balloon positioning between the first and second dilatation could not be excluded.

More than 25 years have passed since researchers started to examine local drug delivery for arteriosclerotic lesions [34]. During the last decade, the proportion of patients (and lesions) who underwent DCB coronary (or peripheral) angioplasty in catheterization laboratories has increased significantly [35]. Different drugs in DCB devices have not been tested in large, randomized, clinical head-to-head comparison studies despite the fact that experimental data suggest the absence of a class effect even within DCBs with the same drug but differences in excipients and catheter properties [36,37]. There is only clinical data from a study that evaluated two different paclitaxel DCBs for in-stent restenosis, a small study comparing paclitaxel- versus sirolimus-DCBs in de novo coronary lesions, and from indirect comparison between paclitaxel- and sirolimus-coated balloons exist [28,38,39]. Our experimental data showed that an everolimus-coated balloon device is feasible and at least equivalent in safety and efficacy to a commercially available sirolimus-coated balloon. We think that accumulated experimental and clinical data are necessary not only to promote the conduction of randomized clinical trials testing different drugs between different DCBs but also to better understand the "response to injury" cataract in atherosclerotic lesions, de novo, or within a previously placed stent. Maybe, in the end, every DCB device will find a different place on the self of the catheterization laboratory. We think that we are in the middle of the road. Obviously, further research is needed.

5. Conclusions

The present research is the first to investigate the safety and efficacy of an innovative everolimus DCB in an experimental model of swine coronary arteries. The use of an everolimus DCB is safe and effective with an acceptable degree of neointimal thickness 90 days post-intervention. The dose of everolimus may play a role in the biocompatibility of the balloon.

Author Contributions: Conceptualization, C.S.K., A.N.M., D.F. and G.T.; methodology L.K.M. and P.D.; investigation and experiments A.T., G.V., A.S., G.K., V.S.L., C.S.K., I.S., G.T., P.D. and A.V.; resources A.S. and A.V.; writing—original draft preparation, C.S.K., G.K., V.S.L., A.V. and I.S.; writing—review and editing, G.T., A.T., G.V., A.S., G.K., V.S.L., D.F., P.D., C.S.K., A.N.M. and L.K.M.; project administration A.N.M.; Supervision G.T., L.K.M., P.D., D.F. and C.S.K. All authors have read and agreed to the published version of the manuscript.

Funding: This research has been co-financed by the European Regional Development Fund of the European Union and Greek national funds through the Operational Program Competitiveness, Entrepreneurship, and Innovation under the call Research—Create—Innovate (project code: T2EDK-03677).

Institutional Review Board Statement: The experiments were approved by the animal care and use board of Patras University Hospital's ethics committee, as well as by the veterinary board of Western Greece's Provincial authorities, approval number PDE/DK/387789/1628/29-12-2021.

Informed Consent Statement: Not applicable.

Data Availability Statement: The data presented in this study are available on request from the corresponding author.

Conflicts of Interest: The authors declare no conflict of interest. The funders had no role in the design of the study, in the collection, analyses, or interpretation of data, in the writing of the manuscript, or in the decision to publish the results.

References

1. Stefanini, G.G.; Holmes, D.R., Jr. Drug-Eluting Coronary-Artery Stents. *N. Engl. J. Med.* **2013**, *368*, 254–265. [CrossRef] [PubMed]
2. Moussa, I.D.; Mohananey, D.; Saucedo, J.; Stone, G.W.; Yeh, R.W.; Kennedy, K.F.; Waksman, R.; Teirstein, P.; Moses, J.W.; Simonton, C. Trends and Outcomes of Restenosis After Coronary Stent Implantation in the United States. *J. Am. Coll. Cardiol.* **2020**, *76*, 1521–1531. [CrossRef] [PubMed]
3. Alfonso, F.; Kastrati, A. Clinical burden and implications of coronary interventions for in-stent restenosis. *EuroIntervention* **2021**, *17*, e355–e357. [CrossRef] [PubMed]
4. Theodoropoulos, K.; Mennuni, M.G.; Dangas, G.D.; Meelu, O.A.; Bansilal, S.; Baber, U.; Sartori, S.; Kovacic, J.C.; Moreno, P.R.; Sharma, S.K.; et al. Resistant in-stent restenosis in the drug eluting stent era. *Catheter. Cardiovasc. Interv.* **2016**, *88*, 777–785. [CrossRef]

5. Scheller, B.; Speck, U.; Abramjuk, C.; Bernhardt, U.; Böhm, M.; Nickenig, G. Paclitaxel Balloon Coating, a Novel Method for Prevention and Therapy of Restenosis. *Circulation* **2004**, *110*, 810–814. [CrossRef] [PubMed]
6. Unverdorben, M.; Vallbracht, C.; Cremers, B.; Heuer, H.; Hengstenberg, C.; Maikowski, C.; Werner, G.S.; Antoni, D.; Kleber, F.X.; Bocksch, W.; et al. Paclitaxel-Coated Balloon Catheter Versus Paclitaxel-Coated Stent for the Treatment of Coronary In-Stent Restenosis. *Circulation* **2009**, *119*, 2986–2994. [CrossRef] [PubMed]
7. Giacoppo, D.; Alfonso, F.; Xu, B.; Claessen, B.E.; Adriaenssens, T.; Jensen, C.; Pérez-Vizcayno, M.J.; Kang, D.-Y.; Degenhardt, R.; Pleva, L.; et al. Drug-Coated Balloon Angioplasty Versus Drug-Eluting Stent Implantation in Patients With Coronary Stent Restenosis. *J. Am. Coll. Cardiol.* **2020**, *75*, 2664–2678. [CrossRef] [PubMed]
8. Jeger, R.V.; Eccleshall, S.; Ahmad, W.A.W.; Ge, J.; Poerner, T.C.; Shin, E.-S.; Alfonso, F.; Latib, A.; Ong, P.J.; Rissanen, T.T.; et al. Drug-Coated Balloons for Coronary Artery Disease. *JACC Cardiovasc. Interv.* **2020**, *13*, 1391–1402. [CrossRef] [PubMed]
9. Piccolo, R.; Stefanini, G.G.; Franzone, A.; Spitzer, E.; Blöchlinger, S.; Heg, D.; Jüni, P.; Windecker, S. Safety and Efficacy of Resolute Zotarolimus-Eluting Stents Compared With Everolimus-Eluting Stents. *Circ. Cardiovasc. Interv.* **2015**, *8*, e002223. [CrossRef]
10. Meng, M.; Gao, B.; Wang, X.; Bai, Z.-G.; Sa, R.-N.; Ge, B. Long-term clinical outcomes of everolimus-eluting stent versus paclitaxel-eluting stent in patients undergoing percutaneous coronary interventions: A meta-analysis. *BMC Cardiovasc. Disord.* **2016**, *16*, 34. [CrossRef]
11. Park, K.W.; Kang, S.-H.; Velders, M.A.; Shin, D.-H.; Hahn, S.; Lim, W.-H.; Yang, H.-M.; Lee, H.-Y.; Van Boven, A.J.; Hofma, S.H.; et al. Safety and efficacy of everolimus- versus sirolimus-eluting stents: A systematic review and meta-analysis of 11 randomized trials. *Am. Hear. J.* **2013**, *165*, 241–250.e4. [CrossRef]
12. Charan, J.; Kantharia, N.D. How to calculate sample size in animal studies? *J. Pharmacol. Pharmacother.* **2013**, *4*, 303–306. [CrossRef] [PubMed]
13. du Sert, N.P.; Hurst, V.; Ahluwalia, A.; Alam, S.; Avey, M.T.; Baker, M.; Browne, W.J.; Clark, A.; Cuthill, I.C.; Dirnagl, U.; et al. The ARRIVE guidelines 2.0: Updated guidelines for reporting animal research. *PLoS Biol.* **2020**, *18*, e3000410. [CrossRef]
14. Directive 2010/63/EU of the European Parliament and of the Council of 22 September 2010 on the Protection of Animals Used for Scientific Purposes. OJ L 276/33. 2010.
15. Cicero, L.; Fazzotta, S.; Palumbo, V.D.; Cassata, G.; Monte, A.I.L. Anesthesia protocols in laboratory animals used for scientific purposes. *Acta Bio Medica Atenei Parm.* **2018**, *89*, 337–342. [CrossRef]
16. Smith, A.C.; Swindle, M.M. Anesthesia and Analgesia in Swine. In *Anesthesia and Analgesia in Laboratory Animals*; Academic Press: Cambridge, MA, USA, 2008; pp. 413–440. [CrossRef]
17. Tsigkas, G.; Vasilagkos, G.; Tousis, A.; Theofanis, M.; Apostolos, A.; Spyridonidis, I.; Goudas, L.; Karpetas, G.; Moulias, A.; Katsouras, C.S.; et al. Ultrasound-guided femoral approach for coronary angiography and interventions in the porcine model. *Sci. Rep.* **2022**, *12*, 1–7. [CrossRef]
18. Tedesco-Silva, H.; Saliba, F.; Barten, M.J.; De Simone, P.; Potena, L.; Gottlieb, J.; Gawai, A.; Bernhardt, P.; Pascual, J. An overview of the efficacy and safety of everolimus in adult solid organ transplant recipients. *Transplant. Rev.* **2021**, *36*, 100655. [CrossRef] [PubMed]
19. Arena, C.; Bizzoca, M.E.; Caponio, V.C.A.; Troiano, G.; Zhurakivska, K.; Leuci, S.; Muzio, L.L. Everolimus therapy and side-effects: A systematic review and meta-analysis. *Int. J. Oncol.* **2021**, *59*, 1–9. [CrossRef]
20. Meng, L.-H.; Zheng, X.S. Toward rapamycin analog (rapalog)-based precision cancer therapy. *Acta Pharmacol. Sin.* **2015**, *36*, 1163–1169. [CrossRef]
21. Semsroth, S.; Stigler, R.G.; Bernecker, O.Y.; Ruttmann-Ulmer, E.; Troppmair, J.; Macfelda, K.; Bonatti, J.O.; Laufer, G. Everolimus attenuates neointimal hyperplasia in cultured human saphenous vein grafts. *Eur. J. Cardio-Thoracic Surg.* **2009**, *35*, 515–520. [CrossRef] [PubMed]
22. Zhao, H.Q.; Nikanorov, A.; Virmani, R.; Schwartz, L.B. Inhibition of experimental neointimal hyperplasia and neoatherosclerosis by local, stent-mediated delivery of everolimus. *J. Vasc. Surg.* **2012**, *56*, 1680–1688. [CrossRef] [PubMed]
23. Park, K.W.; Chae, I.-H.; Lim, D.-S.; Han, K.-R.; Yang, H.-M.; Lee, H.-Y.; Kang, H.-J.; Koo, B.-K.; Ahn, T.; Yoon, J.-H.; et al. Everolimus-Eluting Versus Sirolimus-Eluting Stents in Patients Undergoing Percutaneous Coronary Intervention: The EXCELLENT (Efficacy of Xience/Promus Versus Cypher to Reduce Late Loss After Stenting) Randomized Trial. *J. Am. Coll. Cardiol.* **2011**, *58*, 1844–1854. [CrossRef]
24. Yano, H.; Horinaka, S.; Watahiki, M.; Watanabe, T.; Ishimitsu, T. Five-year outcomes after first- and second-generation drug-eluting stent implantation in all patients undergoing percutaneous coronary intervention. *J. Cardiol.* **2019**, *74*, 169–174. [CrossRef] [PubMed]
25. Kandzari, D.E.; Koolen, J.J.; Doros, G.; Garcia-Garcia, H.M.; Bennett, J.; Roguin, A.; Gharib, E.G.; Cutlip, D.E.; Waksman, R. Ultrathin Bioresorbable Polymer Sirolimus-Eluting Stents Versus Durable Polymer Everolimus-Eluting Stents. *JACC Cardiovasc. Interv.* **2022**, *15*, 1852–1860. [CrossRef] [PubMed]
26. Nakamura, M.; Kadota, K.; Nakagawa, Y.; Tanabe, K.; Ito, Y.; Amano, T.; Maekawa, Y.; Takahashi, A.; Shiode, N.; Otsuka, Y.; et al. Ultrathin, Biodegradable-Polymer Sirolimus-Eluting Stent vs Thin, Durable-Polymer Everolimus-Eluting Stent. *JACC Cardiovasc. Interv.* **2022**, *15*, 1324–1334. [CrossRef]

27. de Winter, R.J.; Katagiri, Y.; Asano, T.; Milewski, K.P.; Lurz, P.; Buszman, P.; Jessurun, G.A.J.; Koch, K.T.; Troquay, R.P.T.; Hamer, B.J.B.; et al. A sirolimus-eluting bioabsorbable polymer-coated stent (MiStent) versus an everolimus-eluting durable polymer stent (Xience) after percutaneous coronary intervention (DESSOLVE III): A randomised, single-blind, multicentre, non-inferiority, phase 3 trial. *Lancet* **2017**, *391*, 431–440. [CrossRef]
28. Ahmad, W.A.W.; Nuruddin, A.A.; Kader, M.A.S.A.; Ong, T.K.; Liew, H.B.; Ali, R.M.; Zuhdi, A.S.M.; Ismail, M.D.; Yusof, A.K.; Schwenke, C.; et al. Treatment of Coronary De Novo Lesions by a Sirolimus- or Paclitaxel-Coated Balloon. *JACC Cardiovasc. Interv.* **2022**, *15*, 770–779. [CrossRef]
29. Otsuka, F.; Pacheco, E.; Perkins, L.E.; Lane, J.P.; Wang, Q.; Kamberi, M.; Frie, M.; Wang, J.; Sakakura, K.; Yahagi, K.; et al. Long-Term Safety of an Everolimus-Eluting Bioresorbable Vascular Scaffold and the Cobalt-Chromium XIENCE V Stent in a Porcine Coronary Artery Model. *Circ. Cardiovasc. Interv.* **2014**, *7*, 330–342. [CrossRef] [PubMed]
30. Farb, A.; Weber, D.K.; Kolodgie, F.D.; Burke, A.P.; Virmani, R. Morphological Predictors of Restenosis After Coronary Stenting in Humans. *Circulation* **2002**, *105*, 2974–2980. [CrossRef] [PubMed]
31. Wilson, G.J.; Nakazawa, G.; Schwartz, R.S.; Huibregtse, B.; Poff, B.; Herbst, T.J.; Baim, D.S.; Virmani, R. Comparison of Inflammatory Response After Implantation of Sirolimus- and Paclitaxel-Eluting Stents in Porcine Coronary Arteries. *Circulation* **2009**, *120*, 141–149. [CrossRef] [PubMed]
32. Nakatani, M.; Takeyama, Y.; Shibata, M.; Yorozuya, M.; Suzuki, H.; Koba, S.; Katagiri, T. Mechanisms of restenosis after coronary intervention. *Cardiovasc. Pathol.* **2003**, *12*, 40–48. [CrossRef] [PubMed]
33. Hermans, W.R.; Foley, D.P.; Rensing, B.J.; Serruys, P.W. Morphologic changes during follow-up after successful percutaneous transluminal coronary balloon angioplasty: Quantitative angiographic analysis in 778 lesions—further evidence for the restenosis paradox. *Am. Hear. J.* **1994**, *127*, 483–494. [CrossRef] [PubMed]
34. Axel, D.I.; Kunert, W.; Göggelmann, C.; Oberhoff, M.; Herdeg, C.; Küttner, A.; Wild, D.H.; Brehm, B.R.; Riessen, R.; Köveker, G.; et al. Paclitaxel Inhibits Arterial Smooth Muscle Cell Proliferation and Migration In Vitro and In Vivo Using Local Drug Delivery. *Circulation* **1997**, *96*, 636–645. [CrossRef] [PubMed]
35. Muramatsu, T.; Kozuma, K.; Tanabe, K.; Morino, Y.; Ako, J.; Nakamura, S.; Yamaji, K.; Kohsaka, S.; Amano, T.; Kobayashi, Y.; et al. Clinical expert consensus document on drug-coated balloon for coronary artery disease from the Japanese Association of Cardiovascular Intervention and Therapeutics. *Cardiovasc. Interv. Ther.* **2023**, *38*, 166–176. [CrossRef] [PubMed]
36. Cremers, B.; Biedermann, M.; Mahnkopf, D.; Böhm, M.; Scheller, B. Comparison of two different paclitaxel-coated balloon catheters in the porcine coronary restenosis model. *Clin. Res. Cardiol.* **2009**, *98*, 325–330. [CrossRef] [PubMed]
37. Radke, P.; Joner, M.; Joost, A.; Byrne, R.; Hartwig, S.; Bayer, G.; Steigerwald, K.; Wittchow, E. Vascular effects of paclitaxel following drug-eluting balloon angioplasty in a porcine coronary model: The importance of excipients. *EuroIntervention* **2011**, *7*, 730–737. [CrossRef]
38. Liu, S.; Zhou, Y.; Shen, Z.; Chen, H.; Qiu, C.; Fu, G.; Li, H.; Yu, Z.; Zeng, Q.; Li, Z.; et al. A Randomized Comparison of 2 Different Drug-Coated Balloons for In-Stent Restenosis. *JACC Cardiovasc. Interv.* **2023**, *16*, 759–767. [CrossRef] [PubMed]
39. Cortese, B.; Caiazzo, G.; Di Palma, G.; De Rosa, S. Comparison Between Sirolimus- and Paclitaxel-Coated Balloon for Revascularization of Coronary Arteries: The SIRPAC (SIRolimus-PAClitaxel). *Cardiovasc. Revascularization Med.* **2021**, *28*, 1–6. [CrossRef]

Disclaimer/Publisher's Note: The statements, opinions and data contained in all publications are solely those of the individual author(s) and contributor(s) and not of MDPI and/or the editor(s). MDPI and/or the editor(s) disclaim responsibility for any injury to people or property resulting from any ideas, methods, instructions or products referred to in the content.

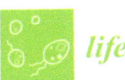

Article

The Relationship between Tricuspid Annular Longitudinal and Sphincter-Like Features of Its Function in Healthy Adults: Insights from the MAGYAR-Healthy Study

Attila Nemes *, Gergely Rácz, Árpád Kormányos, Zoltán Ruzsa, Alexandru Achim and Csaba Lengyel

Department of Medicine, Albert Szent-Györgyi Medical School, University of Szeged, H-6720 Szeged, Hungary; kormanyos.arpad@med.u-szeged.hu (Á.K.); zruzsa25@gmail.com (Z.R.); dr.alex.achim@gmail.com (A.A.); lecs@in1st.szote.u-szeged.hu (C.L.)
* Correspondence: nemes.attila@med.u-szeged.hu

Citation: Nemes, A.; Rácz, G.; Kormányos, Á.; Ruzsa, Z.; Achim, A.; Lengyel, C. The Relationship between Tricuspid Annular Longitudinal and Sphincter-Like Features of Its Function in Healthy Adults: Insights from the MAGYAR-Healthy Study. *Life* **2023**, *13*, 2079. https://doi.org/10.3390/life13102079

Academic Editors: Delia Mirela Tit and Cristiana Bustea

Received: 9 August 2023
Revised: 25 September 2023
Accepted: 28 September 2023
Published: 18 October 2023

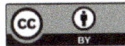

Copyright: © 2023 by the authors. Licensee MDPI, Basel, Switzerland. This article is an open access article distributed under the terms and conditions of the Creative Commons Attribution (CC BY) license (https://creativecommons.org/licenses/by/4.0/).

Abstract: Introduction. The tricuspid valve is an atrioventricular valve located on the right side of the heart, which consists of the fibrous tricuspid annulus (TA), three valvular leaflets and a supporting apparatus, the papillary muscles and the tendinous chords. The TA is an oval-shaped three-dimensional (3D) fibrous structure with a complex spatial movement during the cardiac cycle. Three-dimensional echocardiography (3DE) could help during "en-face" assessment of TA dimensions and related functional properties featuring its "sphincter-like" function. TA plane systolic excursion (TAPSE) is a displacement of the lateral edge of the TA toward the apex in systole measured in apical long-axis using M-mode echocardiography (MME). The aim of this study was to determine potential relationships between TA size and its "sphincter-like" and "longitudinal" functions in healthy adults with no functional tricuspid regurgitation. Methods. The present study consisted of 119 healthy patients (age: 34.6 ± 11.5 years, 70 men) who underwent routine echocardiography with M-mode-derived TAPSE measurement and 3DE. Two subgroups of healthy subjects were compared with each other. A total of 29 subjects with TAPSE between 17 and 21 mm were compared with 90 cases with TAPSE ≥ 22 mm. Results. Subjects with TAPSE of 17–21 mm had tendentiously dilated TA dimensions compared with subjects with TAPSE ≥ 22 mm. Significant differences could be detected in the end-systolic TA area (5.85 ± 1.90 cm^2 vs. 3.70 ± 1.22 cm^2, $p < 0.05$), leading to impaired TAFAC (24.8 ± 9.0% vs. 35.1 ± 9.1%, $p < 0.05$) in subjects with lower TAPSE (17–21 mm) compared with subjects with TAPSE ≥ 22 mm. TAPSE did not show correlations with any TA size or "sphincter-like" functional parameters as determined using 3DE. Conclusions. Three-dimensional echocardiography is capable of measuring TA dimensions and functional "sphincter-like" properties, which are associated with MME-derived TAPSE, suggesting a sensitive and harmonic TA function in healthy adults without functional tricuspid regurgitation.

Keywords: echocardiography; healthy; speckle tracking; three-dimensional; tricuspid annulus

1. Introduction

Evaluation of the right side of the heart has come to the forefront of scientific thinking in recent years. The reason for this is twofold: on the one hand, new therapeutic procedures have become clinically usable that can be used for many disorders affecting the right side of the heart (e.g., congenital heart disease, pulmonary hypertension, etc.). On the other hand, non-invasive examination options that are easy to learn and use and enable a detailed and extensive analysis have become widespread in routine clinics, e.g., three-dimensional echocardiography (3DE) [1–7].

The tricuspid valve (TV) is an atrioventricular valve located on the right side of the heart, which consists of the fibrotic tricuspid annulus (TA), three valvular leaflets and a supporting apparatus, the papillary muscles and the tendinous chords [1]. The TV is responsible for the one-way flow of blood from the right atrium (RA) to the right ventricle

(RV) without substantial regurgitation. While examining the TV was difficult in the past, new imaging options such as 3DE allow it to be examined in detail [4–11]. Therefore, every year, many studies are conducted focusing on the non-invasive evaluation of the TV.

Functional tricuspid regurgitation (FTR) is commonly a result of different cardiac diseases affecting the left heart with induced RV dilation and functional abnormalities, but it can be a result of a dilated RA and TA [1–3]. The TA is an oval-shaped three-dimensional (3D) fibrous structure with a complex spatial movement according to the heart cycle [1]. 3DE could help us understand the clinical implications of FTR, enabling "en-face" assessment of TA dimensions and related functional properties featuring its "sphincter-like" function [4–11]. However, the complexity of the TA function includes its longitudinal movement, which is well represented by its systolic excursion (TA plane systolic excursion, TAPSE), which can easily be determined via its M-mode-derived measurement [12–16]. A harmonic 3D movement of the TA could be theorized in healthy subjects before FTR develops. Therefore, due to limited quantitative information, the current study aimed to determine possible relationships between TA size and its "sphincter-like" and "longitudinal" functions in healthy adults without FTR.

2. Materials and Methods

Subjects: The present retrospective cohort study consisted of 154 healthy subjects who participated as a volunteer between 2011 and 2015, and the investigation was performed at our department. From this pool of healthy subjects, 35 individuals did not participate in this study due to image quality problems for 3DE measurements and/or M-mode assessment of TA plane systolic excursion (TAPSE). The remaining population was 119 subjects with a mean age of 30.1 ± 10.3 years (70 males). Their clinical parameters were within normal ranges, including weight (71.3 ± 12.3 kg), height (171.0 ± 10.2 cm), body surface area (1.84 ± 0.20 m^2), body mass index (22.9 ± 3.2 kg/m^2), systolic blood pressure (122.1 ± 4.6 mm Hg) and diastolic blood pressure (75.9 ± 4.1 mm Hg). An individual was considered healthy if they did not have acute or chronic illnesses in their medical history or showed ECG abnormality. Complete two-dimensional (2D) Doppler echocardiography was performed on all subjects and showed normal results. None of them were smokers or had a history of regular drug use. According to guidelines, TAPSE is considered to be normal if ≥ 17 mm, while the mean value of the TAPSE of healthy subjects was found approximately 21.5 mm in a recent study [12,13]. The group of healthy subjects was divided into 2 subgroups: subjects with TAPSE between 17 and 21 mm were compared with subjects with TAPSE ≥ 22 mm. All healthy volunteers underwent a complete M-mode, 2D Doppler echocardiographic and 3DE examination. This was a substudy of the Motion Analysis of the heart and Great vessels bY three-dimensionAl speckle-tRacking echocardiography in Healthy subjects (MAGYAR-Healthy) Study ("Magyar" means "Hungarian" in the Hungarian language). The study met the requirements of the Declaration of Helsinki (as revised in 2013 and the updated versions) and was approved by the Institutional and Regional Human Biomedical Research Committee of University of Szeged, Hungary, under the registration number 71/2011 and updated versions. All subjects provided informed consent.

M-mode and two-dimensional Doppler echocardiography: Two-dimensional Doppler echocardiographic examinations were performed in accordance with available professional guidelines and accepted practices. During the examinations, a Toshiba Artida™ echocardiography device was used, which could be connected to a PST-30BT (1–5 MHz) phased-array transducer. The person to be examined was asked to lie on their left side, and then, placing the transducer on the chest, measurements were taken from the typical sections from both the parasternal and apical directions. After performing left atrial and left ventricular measurements, the extent of any valvular regurgitation was determined using the continuous-wave Doppler method and visual estimation. Doppler echocardiography was used to exclude significant valvular stenosis as well. LV-EF was determined using Simpson's method. Representing systolic longitudinal motion of the TA, TAPSE was measured in apical long-axis as a displacement of the lateral edge of the TA toward the apex in systole (Figure 1) [12,17,18].

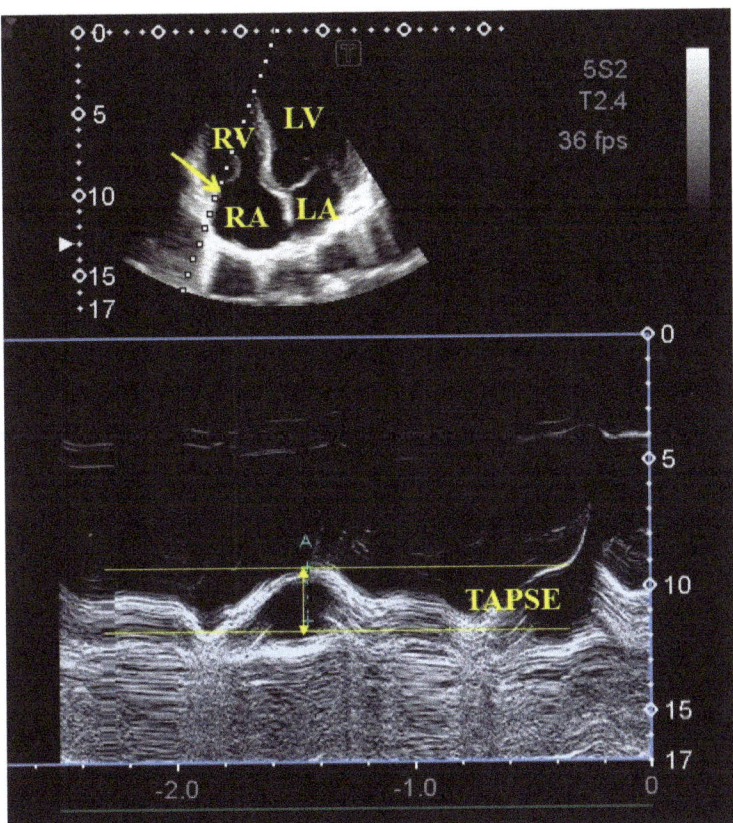

Figure 1. M-mode echocardiography-derived assessment of tricuspid annular plane systolic excursion (TAPSE) from apical four-chamber view. Abbreviations: LA = left atrium, LV = left ventricle, RA = right atrium, RV = right ventricle, TAPSE = tricuspid annular plane systolic excursion.

Three-dimensional echocardiography. The aforementioned Toshiba Artida™ cardiac ultrasound equipment attached to a PST-25SX matrix array transducer was used for 3DE examinations [5–7]. In accordance with our routines, pyramid-shaped 3D echocardiographic datasets were acquired from the apical window. Data were collected during six constant RR intervals seen on the ECG and during one breath hold, and an offline analysis was performed with the vendor-provided 3D Wall Motion-Tracking software (Ultra Extend, Toshiba Medical Systems, Tokyo, Japan, version 2.7) at a later date. Using the abovementioned 3D datasets, the software automatically selected apical two- (AP2CH) and four-chamber (AP4CH) views and 3 short-axis views at basal, midventricular and apical LV levels at end-diastole. Following the definition of the lateral and septal edges of the LV - mitral annulus and endocardial surface of the apical LV, a sequential analysis was conducted in order to create a 3D echocardiographic LV cast. Moreover, AP2CH and AP4CH views were helped to find the optimal TA level on the C7 short-axis view. Directly before tricuspid valve closure at end-diastole and directly before tricuspid valve opening at end-systole, the following TA morphological and functional parameters were calculated (Figure 2) [8,11,19].

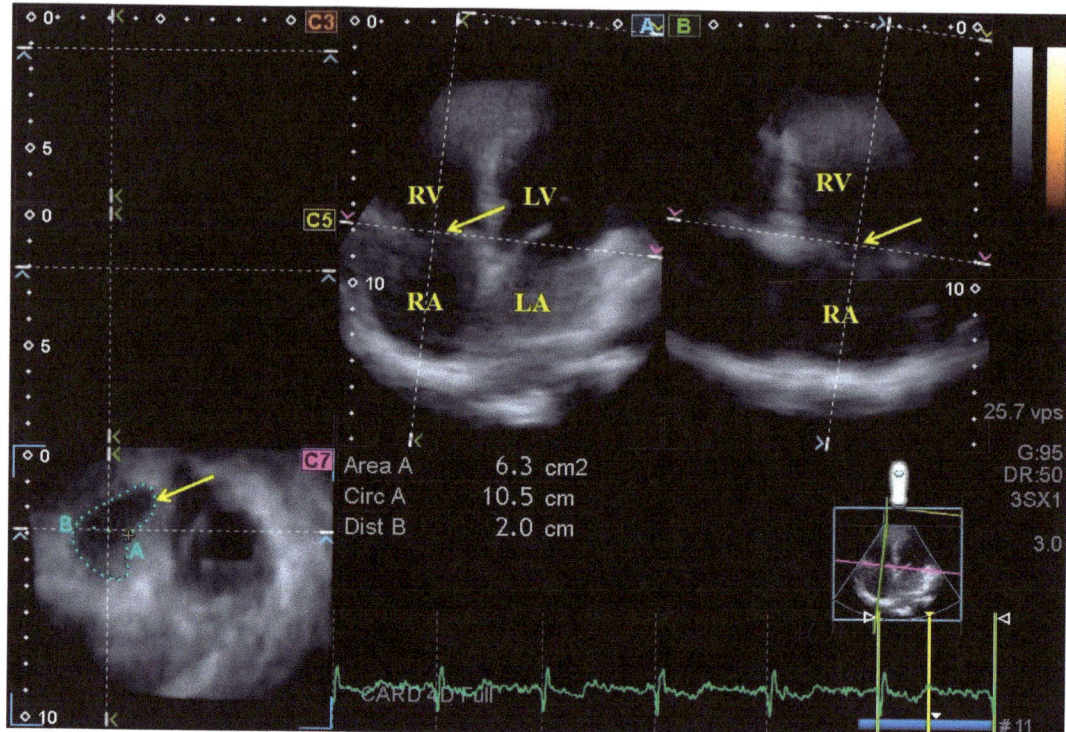

Figure 2. Assessment of the tricuspid annulus extracted from a three-dimensional full-volume dataset is presented: apical four-chamber view (**A**); apical two-chamber view (**B**); and a cross-sectional view at the level of the tricuspid annulus optimized in apical four- and two-chamber views (C7). The yellow arrow represents the tricuspid annular plane. Abbreviations: LA = left atrium, LV = left ventricle, RA = right atrium, RV = right ventricle, Area = TA area, Circ = TA perimeter, Dist = TA diameter.

2.1. Parameters Featuring TA Morphology

- TA diameter (TAD), evaluated by drawing a perpendicular line from the peak of TA curvature to the middle of the straight TA border;
- TA area (TAA), evaluated via planimetry;
- TA perimeter (TAP), evaluated via planimetry.

2.2. Parameters Featuring TA Function

- TA fractional shortening (TAFS), defined as ([end-diastolic TAD − end-systolic TAD]/end diastolic TAD) × 100;
- TA fractional area change (TAFAC), defined as ([end-diastolic TAA − end-systolic TAA]/end-diastolic TAA) × 100.

2.3. Statistical Analysis

Continuous data were presented as average ± standard deviation (SD), while categorical data were demonstrated as n (%). Statistical significance was considered to be present when $p < 0.05$. Levene's test was accomplished for assessing homogeneity of variances, while the Shapiro–Wilks test was used to test whether variables were normally distributed. Student's t-test was used for normally distributed datasets, while the Mann–Whitney–Wilcoxon test was performed for non-normally distributed datasets. Pearson's coefficients were measured to characterize correlations between variables. SPSS software (SPSS Inc., Chicago, IL, USA) was used for the statistical analyses.

3. Results

Demographic data. Two subgroups of healthy subjects were compared with each other: 29 subjects with TAPSE between 17 and 21 mm (average age: 27.2 ± 6.4 years, 16 men) were compared to 90 subjects with TAPSE ≥ 22 mm (average age: 30.0 ± 11.1 years, 33 men).

M-mode and two-dimensional Doppler echocardiography. In Table 1, the routine echocardiographic data of healthy subjects are presented. None of the subjects showed larger than grade 1 valvular insufficiency or significant valvular stenosis in any valve. No routine echocardiographic data differed between the subgroups.

Table 1. Two-dimensional Doppler echocardiographic data of healthy subjects.

Parameters	Subjects (n = 119)	TAPSE 17–21 mm (n = 29)	TAPSE ≥22 mm (n = 90)
LA diameter (mm)	36.9 ± 3.3	37.2 ± 3.4	36.8 ± 3.2
LV end-diastolic diameter (mm)	48.1 ± 3.6	47.8 ± 3.8	48.3 ± 3.6
LV end-diastolic volume (mL)	105.8 ± 24.0	100.4 ± 28.1	107.7 ± 22.2
LV end-systolic diameter (mm)	32.4 ± 3.5	31.9 ± 3.2	32.6 ± 3.6
LV end-systolic volume (mL)	38.3 ± 9.6	36.9 ± 9.0	38.9 ± 9.8
Interventricular septum (mm)	9.1 ± 1.2	8.9 ± 1.2	9.2 ± 1.2
LV posterior wall (mm)	9.3 ± 1.4	9.4 ± 1.6	9.3 ± 1.4
LV ejection fraction (%)	64.5 ± 4.3	64.9 ± 3.3	64.3 ± 4.6

Abbreviations: LA = left atrial, LV = left ventricular, TAPSE = tricuspid annular plane systolic excursion.

Three-dimensional echocardiography. Three-dimensional echocardiography-derived LV volumes, mass and EF together with TA dimensions and functional properties are presented in Tables 2 and 3. LV volumetric parameters did not differ between the subgroups. Subjects with TAPSE between 17 and 21 mm had tendentiously dilated TA dimensions as compared with subjects with TAPSE ≥ 22 mm. A significant difference was detected in the end-systolic TA area, leading to impaired TAFAC in subjects with lower TAPSE (17–21 mm).

Table 2. Comparison of three-dimensional-echocardiography-derived left ventricular parameters in healthy subjects.

Data	Subjects (n = 119)	TAPSE 17–21 mm (n = 29)	TAPSE ≥22 mm (n = 90)
LV-EDV (mL)	85.8 ± 20.8	82.4 ± 23.8	87.0 ± 19.7
LV-ESV (mL)	36.1 ± 10.2	34.4 ± 12.2	36.7 ± 9.4
LV-EF (%)	58.0 ± 5.7	58.8 ± 6.6	57.7 ± 5.4
LV mass (g)	164 ± 32	161 ± 28	165 ± 33

Abbreviations: LV = left ventricular, EDV = end-diastolic volume, ESV = end-systolic volume, EF = ejection fraction.

Table 3. Comparison of three-dimensional-echocardiography-derived tricuspid annular morphological and functional parameters in healthy subjects.

Data	Subjects (n = 119)	TAPSE 17–21 mm (n = 29)	TAPSE ≥22 mm (n = 90)
	Tricuspid annular dimensions		
TAD-D (cm)	2.55 ± 1.91	2.43 ± 0.40	2.10 ± 2.19
TAA-D (cm^2)	7.53 ± 1.66	7.70 ± 1.91	5.70 ± 1.58
TAP-D (cm)	10.57 ± 1.18	10.63 ± 1.22	9.30 ± 1.17
TAD-S (cm)	1.84 ± 0.29	1.90 ± 0.40	1.70 ± 0.25
TAA-S (cm^2)	5.41 ± 1.43	5.85 ± 1.90	3.70 ± 1.22 *
TAP-S (cm)	9.11 ± 1.11	9.32 ± 1.30	7.70 ± 1.05

Table 3. Cont.

Data	Subjects (n = 119)	TAPSE 17–21 mm (n = 29)	TAPSE ≥22 mm (n = 90)
	Tricuspid annular "sphincter-like" functional parameters		
TAFAC (%)	28.1 ± 9.2	24.8 ± 9.0	35.1 ± 9.1 *
TAFS (%)	23.0 ± 10.9	21.8 ± 10.2	19.1 ± 11.1
	Tricuspid annular longitudinal functional parameter		
TAPSE (mm)	23.8 ± 2.9	20.2 ± 0.9	23.0 ± 2.3 *

Abbreviations: TAA-D = end-diastolic tricuspid annular area, TAA-S = end-systolic tricuspid annular area, TAD-D = end-diastolic tricuspid annular diameter, TAD-S = end-systolic tricuspid annular diameter, TAFAC = tricuspid annular fractional area change, TAFS = tricuspid annular fractional shortening, TAP-D = end-diastolic tricuspid annular perimeter, TAP-S = end-systolic tricuspid annular perimeter, TAPSE = tricuspid annular plane systolic excursion. * $p < 0.05$ vs. TAPSE 17–21 mm.

Correlations. TAPSE did not show correlations with any TA sizes or "sphincter-like" functional properties as assessed using 3DE.

Feasibility of TA measurements using 3DE and M-mode echocardiography. This study comprised 154 healthy adults, but due to insufficient image quality, 35 cases had to be excluded. Therefore, the overall feasibility was 77.3%.

Reproducibility data of 3DE-derived TA assessments. The mean ± SD of the differences in values measured by two examiners proved to be 0.03 ± 0.20 cm and 0.02 ± 0.39 cm for end-diastolic and end-systolic TAD, 0.03 ± 0.70 cm^2 and −0.04 ± 0.69 cm^2 for end-diastolic and end-systolic TAA and −0.10 ± 0.61 cm and 0.05 ± 0.60 cm for end-diastolic and end-systolic TAP with a correlation coefficient of 0.96, 0.96, 0.97, 0.96, 0.96 and 0.96 ($p < 0.0001$ for all), respectively (interobserver agreement). Similarly, the mean ± SD of the differences in values measured two times by the same observer was 0.02 ± 0.21 cm and −0.03 ± 0.17 cm for end-diastolic and end-systolic TAD, −0.02 ± 1.18 cm^2 and −0.03 ± 0.38 cm^2 for end-diastolic and end-systolic TAA and −0.04 ± 0.73 cm and 0.07 ± 0.58 cm for end-diastolic and end-systolic TAP with a correlation coefficient of 0.95, 0.96, 0.95, 0.96, 0.96 and 0.97 ($p < 0.0001$ for all), respectively (intraobserver agreement).

4. Discussion

In recent decades, there has been a huge development in cardiovascular imaging due to the technological advances characterizing this period. In addition to magnetic resonance imaging and computer tomography becoming accessible and important imaging methods in cardiology, new echocardiographic methods have emerged and become part of the daily routine. Two-dimensional speckle-tracking echocardiography (2D-STE) is a widely used method for the quantitative characterization of wall movements using strain parameters. Its advantage lies in its simplicity, and it is an option available in most modern devices. The prognostic value of LV global longitudinal strain calculated with 2D-STE has been confirmed [17]. Despite the above facts, it is theoretically not optimal, since it only measures in a given plane and therefore does not take into account regional differences [20]. Three-dimensional echocardiography is used to examine the heart and its cavities in 3D using virtually created 3D models that take into account the cardiac cycle. Three-dimensional speckle-tracking echocardiography (3D-STE) combines the advantages of these two methods. While it allows the heart to be seen in 3D, with the help of the digitally acquired 3D echocardiographic "echocloud", it can measure not only the strain values, but also the rotational parameters at the same time as volumetric measurements. These advantages make 3D-STE the most modern echocardiographic method that is currently available, even though it has some limitations (e.g., problems with image quality) [4–12,17]. Despite the above advantages, 3D-STE is still not as widespread as 2D-STE or volumetric 3DE. Recent scientific findings have shown that 3DE is capable of measuring changes in annular size and calculating the functional parameters of the atrioventricular valves, taking into account the cardiac cycle. These functional parameters only characterize the sphincter-like function of the mitral or tricuspid valve calculated from changes in size (2D-projected diameter and area) of the given valve [8–11]. However, these valves are formations with a spatial complex structure, having spatial movement. Longitudinal spatial displacement is also present in the case of these valves, being characterized by a well-known and commonly used parameter called TAPSE [12].

Owing to the advantages of 3DE detailed above, this method is suitable for performing physiological studies by calculating several parameters at the same time using a digitally acquired 3DE database. In our present study, the LV volumes and the LV-EF were determined during 3DE along with the annular data of TV and the TAFAC and TAFS parameters characterizing the sphincter-like function of TA. Moreover, TAPSE was measured at the same time as the 3DE [4–11,20].

In a healthy person, the TA is a saddle-shaped dynamic structure, the expansion of which is accompanied by a change in its shape; as a result, it becomes more circular and planar [1]. In the event of backflow through the TV during systole, tricuspid regurgitation is present. Tricuspid regurgitation is organic in origin only in 10–15% of cases; most patients have FTR due to a distorted RV, papillary muscle/chordae or TA, with structurally normal leaflets [1–3]. FTR is mostly due to LV dysfunction, aortic or mitral valve disease or pulmonary vascular or interstitial disorders and is accompanied by consequent pulmonary hypertension [20,21]. FTR is considered to be "classical" or ventricular if it is secondary to TA enlargement and tethering of the leaflets and is associated with RV dilation/dysfunction. Previously, if there was no pulmonary hypertension or left heart disorder, FTR was considered to be idiopathic tricuspid regurgitation, which is closely associated with age and atrial fibrillation (AF). Recently, a new concept has been introduced, the so-called atrial FTR. This can be seen in the presence of AF, when RA enlargement and dysfunction lead to the dilation of the TA, leaflet malcoaptation and loss of TA sphincter-like function. Apparently, in these cases, RA dilation plays a greater role in TA dilation and FTR than the RV [3,19,21,22].

Evaluation of TAPSE is a well-known, old-fashioned, simple M-mode echocardiographic method with a significant prognostic value. It is easy to reproduce as a one-plane measurement of TA function in a longitudinal direction featuring its longitudinal displacement [12]. TAPSE is often used as an echocardiographic measurement of RV systolic function and a surrogate of the RV strain as well. TAPSE correlates with and predicts RV-EF [14]. TAPSE < 17 mm proved to have acceptable specificity in separating pathological conditions from healthy subjects [12,15], while its mean value was 21.7 ± 2.8 mm, according to a recent study, which is a lower value than previously described [12,13]. Abnormal TAPSE can be detected in pulmonary hypertension, RV ischemia, heart failure and congenital heart diseases [12,13,15].

Normal reference values for TA derived from 2D echocardiography and cardiac magnetic resonance imaging are available [23,24]. However, 3DE is the method of choice for non-invasive TA assessments as well [8–10,25–29]. Although this method is not widely used, mitral and tricuspid annuli could be easily assessed "en-face" following plane optimizations on AP2CH and AP4CH views with planimetry with respect to the cardiac cycle [4–11]. TAFAC and TAFS are quantitative features of TA's "sphincter-like" function during the cardiac cycle [25,26].

Non-invasive cardiovascular imaging technologies, including echocardiography, are developing rapidly in the XXIst century, allowing more detailed non-invasive morphologic and functional analysis of not only of the atria and the ventricles, but the valves as well. Moreover, these imaging techniques have become part of the daily routine of cardiologists. Three-dimensional echocardiography is a good example of this enormous technological advancement, allowing detailed analysis of cardiac mechanics [4–7]. However, a better understanding of the methods revealed some previously unknown problems. One such problem is that LV volumes measured with 2D echocardiography and those determined with 3DE are not interchangeable [30,31]. Our own presented results highlight this problem as well, since the LV volumes measured with different methods are different; the LV-EDV values measured with 3DE are lower. As a consequence, LV-EF is lower as well [30,31].

However, 3DE is reliable in determining LV-EF [31]. Based on international recommendations, the cut-off value for LV-EF determined using 2D echocardiography is ≥55% [17], while based on literature data, the cut-off value is around 47–55%, as measured using 3DE and considering age and gender [31]. Our results, presented herein, are in accordance with these facts.

In the present study, 3DE-derived TA dimensions and TAFAC were demonstrated to be associated with TAPSE assessed via M-mode echocardiography in healthy subjects without FTR. Lower TAPSE was associated with lower TAFAC, which was related to more dilated end-systolic TAA. However, direct correlations between TA functional features could not be demonstrated. This result suggests a relationship between echocardiographic TA dimensions and TA features for "sphincter-like" (TAFAC) and "longitudinal" (TAPSE) functions. These results could suggest sensitive and harmonic cooperative "sphincter-like" and "longitudinal" TA functions in healthy adults before FTR develops. However, other studies are required to confirm the presented results and to demonstrate abnormalities in the "sphincter-like" (TAFAC) and "longitudinal" (TAPSE) properties of TA function in different disorders with FTR.

5. Limitations

The following limitations arose during assessments:

- Although the TA has a characteristic spatial saddle shape, only its 2D-projected image was analyzed [1,2].
- The image quality of echocardiographic analysis is an important issue, still being worse in the case of 3DE than in the case of 2D echocardiography, which should be taken into account when interpreting the findings. 3DE has several technical difficulties, including lower frame rate and larger transducer size, which can significantly affect image quality. Nevertheless, considering both the advantages and disadvantages, the clinical role of 3DE is unquestionable [5–7].
- Three-dimensional echocardiography-derived image quality is also highly dependent on stitching and motion artifacts [5–7].
- This study did not compare 2D echocardiography versus 3DE in the measurement of TA.
- Three-dimensional echocardiography-derived chamber quantifications of atria and ventricles were also not performed in this study.
- Validation of our 3DE results using other imaging methods could have further strengthened the significance of our scientific findings. Similar studies may be the subject of clinical trials in the future.
- STE-derived featuring of the TA function was not purposed either.
- As FTR was assessed visually, using a more advanced quantification technique would have strengthened our findings [1–3].
- Healthy subjects were involved in this study. However, neither special laboratory tests nor imaging testing were performed to completely exclude disorders in the early stages.

6. Conclusions

Three-dimensional echocardiography is capable of measuring the TA's dimensions and functional "sphincter-like" properties, which are associated with TAPSE, suggesting a sensitive and harmonic TA function in healthy adults without FTR.

Author Contributions: Conceptualization, A.N.; Methodology, Á.K., G.R., Z.R. and A.A.; Software, Á.K.; Resources, C.L.; Data Curation, Á.K.; Writing—A.N., Á.K. and C.L. All authors have read and agreed to the published version of the manuscript.

Funding: This research received no external funding.

Institutional Review Board Statement: The authors are accountable for all aspects of the work in ensuring that questions related to the accuracy or integrity of any part of the work are appropriately investigated and resolved. This study was conducted in accordance with the Declaration of Helsinki (as revised in 2013). This study was approved by the Institutional and Regional Human Biomedical Research Committee of University of Szeged (Hungary) (no. 71/2011 and updated versions).

Informed Consent Statement: Informed consent was given by all subjects.

Data Availability Statement: The manuscript has not been published elsewhere.

Conflicts of Interest: The authors declare no conflict of interest.

References

1. Putthapiban, P.; Amini, M.R.; Abudayyeh, I. Anatomy of the Tricuspid Valve and Pathophysiology of Tricuspid Regurgitation. *Interv. Cardiol. Clin.* **2022**, *11*, 1–9. [CrossRef]
2. Tadic, M.; Cuspidi, C.; Morris, D.A.; Rottbauer, W. Functional tricuspid regurgitation, related right heart remodeling, and available treatment options: Good news for patients with heart failure? *Heart Fail. Rev.* **2022**, *27*, 1301–1312. [CrossRef]
3. Badano, L.P.; Muraru, D.; Enriquez-Sarano, M. Assessment of functional tricuspid regurgitation. *Eur. Heart J.* **2013**, *34*, 1875–1885. [CrossRef]
4. Franke, A.; Kuhl, H.P. Second-generation real-time 3D echocardiography: A revolutionary new technology. *MedicaMundi* **2003**, *47*, 34.
5. Nemes, A.; Kalapos, A.; Domsik, P.; Forster, T. Three-dimensional speckle-tracking echocardiography—A further step in non-invasive three-dimensional cardiac imaging. *Orv. Hetil.* **2012**, *153*, 1570–1577. [CrossRef]
6. Ammar, K.A.; Paterick, T.E.; Khanderia, B.K.; Jan, M.F.; Kramer, C.; Umland, M.M.; Tercius, A.J.; Baratta, L.; Tajik, A.J. Myocardial mechanics: Understanding and applying three-dimensional speckle tracking echocardiography in clinical practice. *Echocardiography* **2012**, *29*, 861–872. [CrossRef]
7. Urbano-Moral, J.A.; Patel, A.R.; Maron, M.S.; Arias-Godinez, J.A.; Pandian, N.G. Three-dimensional speckle-tracking echocardiography: Methodological aspects and clinical potential. *Echocardiography* **2012**, *29*, 997–1010. [CrossRef]
8. Nemes, A.; Kormányos, Á.; Rácz, G.; Ruzsa, Z.; Ambrus, N.; Lengyel, C. Normal reference values of tricuspid annular dimensions and functional properties in healthy adults using three-dimensional speckle-tracking echocardiography (insights from the MAGYAR-Healthy Study). *Quant. Imaging Med. Surg.* **2023**, *13*, 121–132. [CrossRef]
9. Volpato, V.; Mor-Avi, V.; Veronesi, F.; Addetia, K.; Yamat, M.; Weinert, L.; Genovese, D.; Tamborini, G.; Pepi, M.; Lang, R.M. Three-dimensional echocardiography investigation of the mechanisms of tricuspid annular dilatation. *Int. J. Cardiovasc. Imaging.* **2020**, *36*, 33–43. [CrossRef]
10. Bieliauskienė, G.; Kažukauskienė, I.; Kramena, R.; Zorinas, A.; Mainelis, A.; Zakarkaitė, D. Three-dimensional analysis of the tricuspid annular geometry in healthy subjects and in patients with different grades of functional tricuspid regurgitation. *Cardiovasc. Ultrasound.* **2023**, *21*, 17. [CrossRef]
11. Nemes, A.; Rácz, G.; Kormányos, Á. Tricuspid Annular Abnormalities in Isolated Left Ventricular Non-compaction-Insights From the Three-dimensional Speckle-Tracking Echocardiographic MAGYAR-Path Study. *Front. Cardiovasc. Med.* **2022**, *9*, 694616. [CrossRef] [PubMed]
12. Rudski, L.G.; Lai, W.W.; Afilalo, J.; Hua, L.; Handschumacher, M.D.; Chandrasekaran, K.; Solomon, S.D.; Louie, E.K.; Schiller, N.B. Guidelines for the echocardiographic assessment of the right heart in adults: A report from the American Society of Echocardiography endorsed by the European Association of Echocardiography, a registered branch of the European Society of Cardiology, and the Canadian Society of Echocardiography. *J. Am. Soc. Echocardiogr.* **2010**, *23*, 685–713. [PubMed]
13. Nel, S.; Nihoyannopoulos, P.; Libhaber, E.; Essop, M.R.; Dos Santos, C.F.; Matioda, H.; Waterworth, C.; Grinter, S.; Meel, R.; Peters, F. Echocardiographic Indices of the Left and Right Heart in a Normal Black African Population. *J. Am. Soc. Echocardiogr.* **2020**, *33*, 358–367. [CrossRef]
14. Sato, T.; Tsujino, I.; Ohira, H.; Oyama-Manabe, N.; Yamada, A.; Ito, Y.M.; Goto, C.; Watanabe, T.; Sakaue, S.; Nishimura, M. Validation study on the accuracy of echocardiographic measurements of right ventricular systolic function in pulmonary hypertension. *J. Am. Soc. Echocardiogr.* **2012**, *25*, 280–286. [CrossRef]
15. Tamborini, G.; Pepi, M.; Galli, C.A.; Maltagliati, A.; Celeste, F.; Muratori, M.; Rezvanieh, S.; Veglia, F. Feasibility and accuracy of a routine echocardiographic assessment of right ventricular function. *Int. J. Cardiol.* **2007**, *115*, 86–89. [CrossRef]
16. Ghio, S.; Recusani, F.; Klersy, C.; Sebastiani, R.; Laudisa, M.L.; Campana, C.; Gavazzi, A.; Tavazzi, L. Prognostic usefulness of the tricuspid annular plane systolic excursion in patients with congestive heart failure secondary to idiopathic or ischemic dilated cardiomyopathy. *Am. J. Cardiol.* **2000**, *85*, 837–884. [CrossRef]
17. Lang, R.M.; Badano, L.P.; Mor-Avi, V.; Afilalo, J.; Armstrong, A.; Ernande, L.; Flaskampf, F.A.; Foster, E.; Goldstein, S.A.; Kuznetsova, T.; et al. Recommendations for cardiac chamber quantification by echocardiography in adults: An update from the American Society of Echocardiography and the European Association of Cardiovascular Imaging. *J. Am. Soc. Echocardiogr.* **2015**, *28*, 1–39.e14. [CrossRef]
18. Lancellotti, P.; Tribouilloy, C.; Hagendorff, A.; Popescu, B.A.; Edvardsen, T.; Pierard, L.A.; Badano, L.; Zamorano, J.L. Scientific Document Committee of the European Association of Cardiovascular Imaging. Recommendations for the echocardiographic assessment of native valvular regurgitation: An executive summary from the European Association of Cardiovascular Imaging. *Eur. Heart J. Cardiovasc. Imaging* **2013**, *14*, 611–644. [CrossRef]

19. Nemes, A.; Kormányos, Á.; Ruzsa, Z.; Achim, A.; Ambrus, N.; Lengyel, C. Three-Dimensional Speckle-Tracking Echocardiography-Derived Tricuspid Annular Dimensions and Right Atrial Strains in Healthy Adults-Is There a Relationship? (Insights from the MAGYAR-Healthy Study). *J. Clin. Med.* **2023**, *12*, 4240. [CrossRef]
20. Gual-Capllonch, F.; Cediel, G.; Ferrer, E.; Teis, A.; Juncà, G.; Vallejo, N.; López-Ayerbe, J.; Bayes-Genis, A. Sex-Related Differences in the Mechanism of Functional Tricuspid Regurgitation. *Heart Lung Circ.* **2021**, *30*, e16–e22. [CrossRef]
21. Florescu, D.R.; Muraru, D.; Volpato, V.; Gavazzoni, M.; Caravita, S.; Tomaselli, M.; Ciampi, P.; Florescu, C.; Bălșeanu, T.A.; Parati, G.; et al. Atrial Functional Tricuspid Regurgitation as a Distinct Pathophysiological and Clinical Entity: No Idiopathic Tricuspid Regurgitation Anymore. *J. Clin. Med.* **2022**, *11*, 382. [CrossRef] [PubMed]
22. Muraru, D.; Addetia, K.; Guta, A.C.; Ochoa-Jimenez, R.C.; Genovese, D.; Veronesi, F.; Basso, C.; Iliceto, S.; Badano, L.P.; Lang, R.M. Right atrial volume is a major determinant of tricuspid annulus area in functional tricuspid regurgitation: A three-dimensional echocardiography study. *Eur. Heart J. Cardiovasc. Imaging* **2021**, *22*, 660–669. [CrossRef] [PubMed]
23. Dwivedi, G.; Mahadevan, G.; Jimenez, D.; Frenneaux, M.; Steeds, R.P. Reference values for mitral and tricuspid annular dimensions using two-dimensional echocardiography. *Echo. Res. Pract.* **2014**, *1*, 43–50. [CrossRef] [PubMed]
24. Zhan, Y.; Debs, D.; Khan, M.A.; Nguyen, D.T.; Graviss, E.A.; Shah, D.J. Normal Reference Values and Reproducibility of Tricuspid Annulus Dimensions Using Cardiovascular Magnetic Resonance. *Am. J. Cardiol.* **2019**, *124*, 594–598. [CrossRef]
25. Anwar, A.M.; Soliman, O.I.; Nemes, A.; van Geuns, R.J.M.; Geleijnse, M.L.; ten Cate, F.J. Value of assessment of tricuspid annulus: Real-time three-dimensional echocardiography and magnetic resonance imaging. *Int. J. Cardiovasc. Imaging* **2007**, *23*, 701–705. [CrossRef]
26. Anwar, A.M.; Geleijnse, M.L.; Soliman, O.I.; McGhie, J.S.; Frowijn, R.; Nemes, A.; van den Bosch, A.E.; Galema, T.W.; ten Cate, F.J. Assessment of normal tricuspid valve anatomy in adults by real-time three-dimensional echocardiography. *Int. J. Cardiovasc. Imaging* **2007**, *23*, 717–724. [CrossRef]
27. Muraru, D.; Gavazzoni, M.; Heilbron, F.; Mihalcea, D.J.; Guta, A.C.; Radu, N.; Muscogiuri, G.; Tomaselli, M.; Sironi, S.; Parati, G.; et al. Reference ranges of tricuspid annulus geometry in healthy adults using a dedicated three-dimensional echocardiography software package. *Front. Cardiovasc. Med.* **2022**, *9*, 1011931. [CrossRef]
28. Addetia, K.; Muraru, D.; Veronesi, F.; Jenei, C.; Cavalli, G.; Besser, S.A.; Mor-Avi, V.; Lang, R.M.; Badano, L.P. 3-Dimensional Echocardiographic Analysis of the Tricuspid Annulus Provides New Insights Into Tricuspid Valve Geometry and Dynamics. *JACC Cardiovasc. Imaging* **2019**, *12*, 401–412. [CrossRef]
29. Muraru, D.; Hahn, R.T.; Soliman, O.I.; Faletra, F.F.; Basso, C.; Badano, L.P. 3-Dimensional Echocardiography in Imaging the Tricuspid Valve. *JACC Cardiovasc. Imaging* **2019**, *12*, 500–515. [CrossRef]
30. Kleijn, S.A.; Aly, M.F.A.; Terwee, C.B.; van Rossum, A.C.; Kamp, O. Reliability of left ventricular volumes and function measurements using three-dimensional speckle tracking echocardiography. *Eur. Heart J. Cardiovasc. Imaging* **2012**, *13*, 159–168. [CrossRef]
31. Wood, P.W.; Choy, J.B.; Nanda, N.C.; Becher, H. Left ventricular ejection fraction and volumes: It depends on the imaging method. *Echocardiography* **2014**, *31*, 87–100. [CrossRef] [PubMed]

Disclaimer/Publisher's Note: The statements, opinions and data contained in all publications are solely those of the individual author(s) and contributor(s) and not of MDPI and/or the editor(s). MDPI and/or the editor(s) disclaim responsibility for any injury to people or property resulting from any ideas, methods, instructions or products referred to in the content.

Review

The Rare Condition of Left Ventricular Non-Compaction and Reverse Remodeling

Cristiana Bustea [1], Alexa Florina Bungau [1,2,*], Delia Mirela Tit [2,3,*], Diana Carina Iovanovici [2], Mirela Marioara Toma [2], Simona Gabriela Bungau [2,3], Andrei-Flavius Radu [1,2], Tapan Behl [4], Adrian Cote [5] and Elena Emilia Babes [6]

1. Department of Preclinical Disciplines, Faculty of Medicine and Pharmacy, University of Oradea, 410073 Oradea, Romania; cristianabustea@yahoo.com
2. Doctoral School of Biomedical Sciences, University of Oradea, 410087 Oradea, Romania; diana_iovanovici@yahoo.com (D.C.I.); mire.toma@yahoo.com (M.M.T.); sbungau@uoradea.ro (S.G.B.); andreiflavius.radu@gmail.com (A.-F.R.)
3. Department of Pharmacy, Faculty of Medicine and Pharmacy, University of Oradea, 410028 Oradea, Romania
4. School of Health Sciences & Technology, University of Petroleum and Energy Studies, Bidholi, Dehradun 248007, India; tapanbehl31@gmail.com
5. Department of Surgical Disciplines, Faculty of Medicine and Pharmacy, University of Oradea, 410073 Oradea, Romania; adrian.cote@didactic.uoradea.ro
6. Department of Medical Disciplines, Faculty of Medicine and Pharmacy, University of Oradea, 410073 Oradea, Romania; babes.emilia@gmail.com
* Correspondence: pradaalexaflorina@gmail.com (A.F.B.); mirela_tit@yahoo.com (D.M.T.)

Abstract: Left ventricular non-compaction (LVNC) is a rare disease defined by morphological criteria, consisting of a two-layered ventricular wall, a thin compacted epicardial layer, and a thick hyper-trabeculated myocardium layer with deep recesses. Controversies still exist regarding whether it is a distinct cardiomyopathy (CM) or a morphological trait of different conditions. This review analyzes data from the literature regarding diagnosis, treatment, and prognosis in LVNC and the current knowledge regarding reverse remodeling in this form of CM. Furthermore, for clear exemplification, we report a case of a 41-year-old male who presented symptoms of heart failure (HF). LVNC CM was suspected at the time of transthoracic echocardiography and was subsequently confirmed upon cardiac magnetic resonance imaging. A favorable remodeling and clinical outcome were registered after including an angiotensin receptor neprilysin inhibitor in the HF treatment. LVNC remains a heterogenous CM, and although a favorable outcome is not commonly encountered, some patients respond well to therapy.

Keywords: left ventricular non-compaction; heart failure; reverse remodeling; cardiomyopathy; cardiac magnetic resonance imaging; angiotensin receptor neprilysin inhibitor; ARNI therapy

1. Introduction

Left ventricular non-compaction (LVNC), also known as spongiform cardiomyopathy (CM), is a rare heart muscle disease that is due to the failure of myocardial compaction in the first trimester of fetal development. The ventricular wall in LVNC has two layers: a thick, hyper-trabeculated myocardium layer and a thin, compacted epicardial layer. After conducting autopsy research on a newborn with the congenital abnormalities of a coronary ventricular fistula and aortic atresia, Bellet and Gouley published the first description of LVNC in 1932. Isolated non-compaction CM was first described in an echocardiographic study performed by Engberding and Bender in 1984 [1].

There are controversies regarding whether LVNC is a distinct CM or a phenotypic manifestation of various cardiomyopathies [2]. The criteria for diagnosis are mainly based on the morphological changes detected in non-invasive imaging. The most commonly used diagnostic methods are echocardiography, cardiac magnetic resonance (CMR), and computed tomography [3]. Although the American Heart Association classifies LVNC as a main genetic CM [4], the pattern of non-compaction of the LV can be observed in several clinical situations. A persistent area of debate is the differentiation from normal LV trabeculation or the relationship with cardiomyopathies such as dilated or hypertrophic cardiomyopathy, which may share the same genetic basis.

The genetic pattern and clinical presentation are variable. The clinical picture is heterogeneous, but the main manifestations consist of heart failure (HF), thromboembolic events, and ventricular arrhythmias. Regarding genetic transmission, LVNC is usually autosomal dominant, but an autosomal recessive X-linked or mitochondrial inheritance type may be present [5]. LVNC may appear isolated or in association with other cardiac pathologies, and some cases appear in patients with neuromuscular diseases [3] or in patients with metabolic abnormalities [5–7]. Because it is currently uncertain whether LVNC is a distinct condition or a morphological characteristic that is influenced by other cardiomyopathies, the European Society of Cardiology's group of specialists on pericardial and myocardial illness includes it in the undefined cardiomyopathies category [8].

The therapeutic approach in LVNC is not well studied. For LVNC with reduced ejection fraction, therapeutic strategies were extrapolated from patients with dilated CM. The current guideline recommendation should be followed for HF treatment in LVNC. Previous reports have shown that some cases of LVNC and LV systolic dysfunction can develop reverse remodeling after optimal therapy [9–12]. Reverse remodeling in LVNC is associated with improved outcomes.

The purpose of the present study is to expose the therapeutic and diagnostic challenges of this rare disease. HF represents the most common presentation in LVNC, and there are no specific studies or recommendations for HF treatment in this type of patient. The novelty presented by the case that is provided as an example is the important improvement achieved after the optimization of HF treatment by adding angiotensin receptor neprilysin inhibitor (ARNI) to the therapy; this phenomenon has only been described in a few cases in the literature. For this study, published data from 1984 to 2023 on the topic were searched in the most known databases using the keywords mentioned at the beginning of the present paper.

2. Epidemiology and Pathogenesis

LVNC is a rare disease with a prevalence that is difficult to estimate, as the criteria for diagnosis are not uniformly defined. The current data report a prevalence of 0.01–0.3% in the adult population, with male predominance [13,14].

The myocardium presents intertrabecular recesses and a trabeculated structure during the formation of the heart. During the first trimester of pregnancy, the ventricular muscles undergo compaction to form a solid myocardial layer, and the intertrabecular recesses become the coronary arteries. Early impaired LV compaction during embryonal endomyocardial morphogenesis will result in the development of a compacted epicardial stratum and an endocardial stratum with pronounced trabeculae and profound intertrabecular recesses that connect to the LV cavity. Recently, some other opinions have emerged; Jensen et al. suggested that hyper-trabeculation in LVNC may result from the compacted myocardium growing into the ventricular lumen in a trabecular fashion [15]. Ventricular non-compaction is most commonly located at the apex of the heart due to the fact that the compaction process not only progresses from the epicardium to the endocardium, but also from the base toward the apex of the heart [16]. More than 80% of patients have the apical, mid-inferior, mid-lateral, and mid-anterior wall segments involved [3,17].

Right ventricle involvement may also be present during hyper-trabeculation, dilatation, and dysfunction [18]. A differential diagnosis between a pathologically non-compacted myocardium and increased trabeculations representing a normal variant depends on the existence of a thinner compacted myocardial wall in LVNC and a normal thickness of the compacted myocardial layer in the normal variant [13].

LVNC is usually associated with systolic dysfunction and a reduced ejection fraction. Hypokinesia of the compacted and non-compacted layers and the asynchronous contraction between the compacted and non-compacted myocardial layers will determine systolic dysfunction. Although epicardial coronary arteries are normal, subendocardial hypoperfusion may be present due to a discrepancy between the cardiac mass and the amount of capillaries and microcirculatory dysfunction. Progressive fibrosis determined by ischemia will depress LV systolic function and favor ventricular arrhythmias. Ventricular compliance is also affected by trabeculations, resulting in diastolic impairment. Hyper-trabeculations determine irregular relaxation, constrictive filling, and diastolic dysfunction [17,19].

3. Etiology

Regarding etiology, the most common form of LVNC is sporadic; however, it can also be familial, having autosomal dominant inheritance [18]. LVNC's existence has been associated with several genes, including more frequent sarcomere genes (82%) [20]. Genes that encode cellular signaling networks, such as sarcomere proteins, and ion channels that have been associated with LVNC are implied as well in dilated and hypertrophic CM [18]. LVNC may appear in association with other cardiomyopathies, including dilated CM, restrictive CM, hypertrophic CM, congenital heart diseases (Ebstein disease), or arrhythmogenic right ventricular CM [21]. LVNC can also be found to be associated with Barth syndrome, neuromuscular diseases, or metabolic diseases [5].

LV dysfunction is more common in genetic cases rather than in sporadic cases, and this is usually an indicator of a worse outcome [20]. The genes *MYBPC3*, *MYH7*, and *TTN* are the ones that are most often involved [21]. A genetic variant of *MYH7* seems to be associated with biventricular disease and a restrictive filling pattern of diastolic dysfunction [22]; alternatively, it is associated with a significant systolic dysfunction that is associated with a dilated phenotype [23] needing urgent transplant. Genetic testing has a good genetic yield and is useful for prognostic estimation, as patients without underlying an genetic cause have a better outcome [24].

When LVNC is identified, family screening may be beneficial in the evaluation of familial cases. First-degree relatives should be assessed as they can be affected in 13–50% of cases [5]. For family members with LVNC or trabeculations, close surveillance is recommended [25].

4. Clinical Presentation

The clinical presentation and morphological expression of LVNC are highly variable. Due to challenges in the diagnosis, according to the French LVNC records, there is a mean diagnosis delay of 6.43 ± 3 years, and 32% of patients are diagnosed with this impairment after 5 years or later [26].

The average age of patients (at diagnosis) might range from 37 ± 17 years [24] to 45 ± 17 years [27]; the majority of patients are symptomatic at the moment of diagnosis. HF is the main presentation form in up to 62% [17,25] of instances, and 98% of black people are affected [28]. Nearly 50% of subjects are in New York Heart Association (NYHA) classes III–IV at presentation. Aside from HF, thromboembolic events and arrhythmias are common clinical manifestations. Embolic events are the results of thrombus formation in the non-compacted myocardium deep clefts between trabeculations and are described in 5–38% of patients [17].

Arrhythmias are frequent in LVNC. Ventricular tachycardia occurs in 38–47% of cases because of a substrate that typically involves the non-compacted mid-apical LV segments. Ventricular tachycardia and fibrillation are more common in patients with severely reduced systolic function. Over 25% of cases have been reported for atrial fibrillation. Complete heart block and paroxysmal supraventricular tachycardia may also appear [17]. WPW syndrome was observed in 1.5% of cases [3]. QTc prolongation is observed in over 50% of patients, and early repolarization abnormalities are common [17].

5. Diagnostic Approach

The diagnosis is based on imagistic methods, with echocardiography and CMR imaging being the most used. Although the first echocardiographic diagnosis was published more than 30 years ago, there are still no generally accepted diagnostic criteria [3].

5.1. Echocardiography

The echocardiographic criteria proposed by Jenni are the most widely accepted and were confirmed in our patient. The parasternal short-axis view supports LVNC when the non-compacted layer/compacted layer end systolic ratio is bigger than two. The absence of other abnormalities of the heart and the presence of a color flow Doppler in the deep intertrabecular recesses are additional criteria for diagnosis [29].

Other echocardiographic criteria are those used by Chin et al., who defined LVNC as the proportion of compacted/compacted + non-compacted myocardium < 0.5 at end-diastole in the parasternal short-axis perspective of the apex and in the apical views for the LV free wall [30]. Stollberg's echocardiographic definition for LVNC is the presence of trabeculations (>3 trabeculae) seen in one imaging plane and apically extending from the LV wall towards the papillary muscle in end-diastole, synchronously moving with the compacted myocardium [31]. Only 30% of patients fulfill all three criteria. Other echocardiographic techniques are recommended for challenging cases. Speckle tracking echocardiography is useful in borderline cases because in LVNC, the LV twist is affected. Speckle tracking can identify the direction of the basal and apical rotations. Dalen et al. presented this abnormal rotation pattern in patients with LVNC, which was characterized by LV solid body rotation, with basal and apical rotation oriented in the same direction and almost no LV twist [32]. A reduced global longitudinal strain is a sensitive sign of systolic dysfunction [11]. Three-dimensional echocardiography analysis can evaluate the extent of the non-compacted layer and contribute to the diagnosis of patients with LVNC. Additional contrast in echocardiography is useful, according to the European Association of Cardiovascular Imaging's recommendations [33], and can better delineate endocardial borders, trabeculations, and the perfused intertrabecular recesses [34].

LV systolic dysfunction is common but not mandatory in subjects suffering from LVNC. The gravity of the disease is associated with LV dysfunction severity. The degree of LV dysfunction was found to be associated with the extent of myocardial non-compaction by some authors [35]. The amount of damaged segments and the ratio of non-compacted/compacted myocardium appear to be the main predictors of LV systolic malfunction, while left ventricular ejection fraction (LVEF) remains an important predictor of mortality [36]. In contradiction with these results, an Italian study on 238 consecutive patients with LVNC revealed that the amount of non-compacted segments does not appear to have a connection to ventricular dysfunction [37].

Another study that compared patients with isolated forms of LVNC to patients with dilated CM and prominent trabeculations revealed that the end-diastolic volume index and LV sphericity index were considerably lower in individuals with isolated LVNC; however, the patients had more trabeculated segments, a higher non-compacted/compacted myocardium ratio, and a significantly higher LVEF. The stroke volume index, cardiac output, and cardiac index were similar in patients with isolated forms of LVNC and those with dilated CM. The ratio of non-compacted to compacted myocardium and the amount of trabeculated segments were directly correlated with LV end-diastolic volume index and inversely correlated with LVEF in subjects with isolated forms of LVNC. The amount of non-compacted segments and the non-compacted/compacted myocardium ratio were not significantly correlated with the LV end-diastolic volume index or with LVEF in patients with dilated CM [38].

It seems that the systolic dysfunction of the LV is closely correlated with the location and severity of the abnormal myocardial segments and the electro-mechanical activation of these areas; it is less correlated with the number or ratio of non-compacted/compacted myocardium [39,40]. Mitral annulus enlargement and mitral regurgitation were similar in the LVNC and dilated CM patients, and there was no correlation between the number of non-compacted segments and mitral annulus diameter or area [41].

5.2. Cardiac Magnetic Resonance

Although currently, the diagnosis gold standard is echocardiography, in many cases, it is necessary to perform a multimodal imagistic evaluation (echocardiography and CMR). CMR imaging is superior for identifying non-compacted myocardium and trabeculations, particularly at end-diastole [42], and it allows for a non-invasive tissue evaluation, quantification of the extent of non-compacted myocardium, and detection of segmental non-compaction in any area of the LV wall. Coexistent right ventricular non-compaction can be better identified using CMR, and delayed enhancement imaging can visualize myocardial fibrotic areas that correlate with the severity of LV dysfunction [43] and may represent the substrate for potentially lethal arrhythmias, modifying the treatment of these patients by the preventive insertion of an internal cardioverter defibrillator [44].

Jacquier et al.'s criteria define LVNC based on the magnitude of the trabeculated mass. A specific and sensitive sign for the CMR identification of LVNC is a non-compacted mass that represents more than 20% of the global LV mass at end-diastole [45]. The CMR criteria of Peterson et al. for diagnosis are a non-compacted/compacted myocardium ratio > 2.3 in a long-axis end-diastolic image in at least two consecutive segments [42]. Nucifora et al. observed that in patients with LVNC, trabeculations are predominantly located on the apex, anterolateral, and inferolateral walls; systolic dysfunction of the LV was encountered in half of the cases, and more than half of the patients had mid-wall late gadolinium enhancement (LGE) [18].

In a multicentric prospective study, Andreini et al. [46] found that LV dilatation, systolic dysfunction, and late gadolinium enhancement are independent predictors of poor outcome. Although the degree of trabeculation did not have a significant prognostic impact, it seems that LV trabeculation is correlated with reduced myocardial deformation indexes [13]. Native T1 mapping can detect diffuse myocardial fibrosis earlier than LGE [47].

Dodd et al. [48] found a higher grade of delayed myocardial enhancement during CMR processing in patients with more advanced disease progression. In a retrospective study on 75 patients with LVNC that were evaluated with a CMR examination, echocardiography, and subsequent clinical follow-up, it was observed that mitral regurgitation was frequent in LVNC with LV dysfunction. In patients with severe MR, the LV remodeling was worse, and the coexistence of LGE was associated with a poorer outcome. Both fibrosis and moderate–severe mitral regurgitation are related to the occurrence and development of myocardial maladaptive remodeling, and they have a combined effect in worsening the outcome [49]. Recent studies have revealed the role of LGE findings in risk stratification. Although LGE seems to be less frequent in LVNC compared with other cardiomyopathies [50], it was reported in many studies to be an important predictor of major cardiac events, with added prognostic implications over LVEF [43,46,51,52]. Myocardial fibrosis detected by LGE may be a consequence of coronary microvascular dysfunction and decreased coronary flow reserve; it can be followed using adverse remodeling and severe HF, but it is also associated with severe arrhythmias and adverse outcomes [53,54]. A systematic review conducted by Grigoratos et al. [55], which included four studies, further confirmed that the presence of LGE in LVNC was associated with multiple adverse outcomes, including cardiac death. On the other hand, a negative LGE and preserved LVEF were the factors that were associated with a good prognosis.

These findings sustain the use of CMR in the routine assessment of patients with LVNC. LGE for the detection of fibrosis should be part of the evaluation and may influence treatment decision guidance with respect to the risk of sudden cardiac death [56].

The pattern of LGE provides supplementary information. A multicenter study that evaluated the prognostic role of LGE in LVNC observed an increased risk of major cardiac events when the size of the LGE exceeded 7.5%, was ring-like, had many segments, and involved the free wall [57].

It is obvious that patients with LVNC and a positive LGE have more maladaptive LV remodeling and a higher incidence of adverse cardiovascular events; the absence of LGE is associated with LV reverse remodeling and a good prognosis, especially if LVEF is preserved.

5.3. Computed Tomography

Contrast-enhanced computed tomography can describe the abnormal architecture of the non-compacted LV wall and assess ventricular function. The spatial resolution of cardiac computed tomography for the identification of LVNC is good and permits visualization of the coronary arteries and great vessels; also, it is able to exclude coronary artery disease in subjects that present a low likelihood of ischemic heart impairment [58,59].

LVNC may manifest alone as a morphological phenotype, can be linked to LV systolic dysfunction and dilation, or can be associated with LV hypertrophy. In MOGE(S) nosology, pure LVNC (MLVNC) and LVNC with LV hypertrophy (MLVNC-H), and LV dilatation and dysfunction (MLVNC-D) are distinguished [60].

6. Therapeutic Approach

There is no specific therapy for LVNC, as treatment is targeted at clinical manifestations: HF, arrhythmias, and systemic embolism prevention.

6.1. Treatment of Heart Failure and Evidence for Reverse Remodeling Therapies

Patients with HF should be managed according to the current guidelines [61]. During the progression of HF, there is an increased stimulation of the cytokine and neurohormonal structures with the consequence of an increased alteration of myocytes, myocyte loss, alterations in the extracellular matrix, and changes in LV chamber geometry. Treatments that can reverse this remodeling will determine a functional improvement [62].

ARNI therapy in patients with LVNC is reported in a limited number of cases [63,64]. Sacubitril/Valsartan therapy in an individual with LVNC was linked to an amelioration of the clinical and echocardiographic markers, as reported by Bonatto et al. This patient with LVNC presented HF and underwent standard medical treatment in accordance with the guidelines for 18 months; however, there was not an enhancement in the patient's clinical or echocardiographic markers. A considerable modification of the NYHA class (from III to I) along with considerable ventricular reverse remodeling followed the commencement of sacubitril/valsartan medication [63]. Another recent case study was reported concerning a patient with a dilated subtype of LVNC who had a spectacular improvement in LV systolic and diastolic function and important LV reverse remodeling with ARNI therapy [65]. PROVE HF (prospective investigation of ventricular remodeling, symptom relief, and biomarkers throughout Entresto therapy for HF) and EVALUATE HF (study comparing the effects of sacubitril/valsartan and enalapril on aortic stiffness in individuals with mild to moderate HF and a low ejection fraction) showed that ARNI-treated patients experienced positive LV remodeling, which was accompanied by a drop in NT-proBNP levels and clinical improvement; however, LVNC patients were not included in these investigations [66,67]. Furthermore, even in a short-term evaluation, ARNI appears to ameliorate LV size and hypertrophy more than angiotensin-converting enzyme inhibitors/angiotensin receptor inhibitors, as concluded in a recent meta-analysis on patients with HF and reduced ejection fraction [68].

The underlying mechanism of reverse remodeling remains partially unclear. The simultaneous inhibition of neprilysin and of the renin angiotensin aldosterone system using sacubitril/valsartan will result in a more effective neurohormonal modulation. By inhibiting neprilysin, an enzyme has a role in the degradation of natriuretic peptides in circulation, and all of the favorable effects of the circulating natriuretic peptides will be preserved. Vasoconstrictors angiotensin II and endothelin-1 are additionally divided by neprilysin, but the harmful effects of angiotensin II on the vascular system and heart are inhibited by valsartan [69]. Neprilysin inhibition may also influence the circulating levels of other peptides, which may additionally contribute to favorable effects of sacubitril/valsartan. Moreover, neprilysin cleaves apelin [70], and as a consequence of ARNI therapy, the level of apelin may increase, promoting angiotensin-converting enzyme 2 expression, stimulating the formation of vasodilating substrates, and antagonizing angiotensin II [71].

Beyond the impact on the renin–angiotensin–aldosterone system and the natriuretic peptide system, sacubitril/valsartan is reported to reverse cardiac remodeling. In the PROVE-HF trial, improved markers of cardiac function, volume decrease, and a reduction in the circulating levels of NT-proBNP were reported in subjects with HF with decreased ejection fraction that underwent treatment using sacubitril/valsartan [66]. Reverse LV remodeling with substantially enhanced ventricular volume overflow and dimension parameters, which subsequently determined the increase of LVEF, was reported in multiple other studies [72,73].

The cellular and molecular mechanisms of reverse remodeling in sacubitril/valsartan therapy are complex and still not completely understood. Sacubitril/Valsartan enhances myocardial calcium homeostasis, which helps promoting heart function [74] and may modulate proteins such as cysteine-rich protein 3 and titin, which participate in force transmission within the sarcomere [75].

Sacubitril/Valsartan affect cardiac structure and have an antihypertrophic effect that is not correlated with a blood pressure reduction. There are multiple mechanisms involved in the protective antihypertrophic effect. The two drugs act in synergy to prevent cardiomyocyte cell death and matrix remodeling. The combination of drugs blocks the activation of extracellular signal-regulated kinase that has an essential function in the pathogenesis of cardiac hypertrophy, and the combination also inhibits the angiotensin II receptor pathway. The molecular processes of the remodeling action of ARNI were described in a recent report. Valsartan inhibits proteins from the guanine nucleotide-binding complex, and sacubitril improves myocardial contractility and reduces myocardial cell death and hypertrophy [76]. In addition, sacubitril/valsartan suppresses several other signaling routes that are engaged in matrix remodeling, cardiac fibrosis, and apoptosis.

By blocking the TGF-1/Smad3 and Wnt/β-catenin signaling pathways, sacubitril/valsartan reduces cardiac fibrosis. Other signaling pathways such as the phosphatidylinositol 3-kinase/protein kinase B/glycogen synthase kinase-3β (PI3K/Akt/GSK-3β) and hypoxia-induced mitogenic actor (HIMF)-IL-6 may be influenced by sacubitril/valsartan, but further investigations are required to define them. These networks are involved in controlling cardiac fibrosis [77].

Mitochondrial energy production is increased by sacubitril/valsartan, leading to improved myocardial contractility via a SIRT3-dependent pathway. The effects of sacubitril/valsartan on nuclear respiratory factor-1 (NRF-1), nuclear respiratory factor-2, and mitochondrial transcription factor A needs further investigations [78].

Sacubitril/Valsartan antihypertrophic benefits are generally attributed to its potential to lessen extreme oxidative stress and inflammatory responses, which eventually slow down the remodeling process. Further investigations are required regarding the substance modulating actions on nuclear factor erythroid 2-related factor 2 (Nrf2)/antioxidant responsive element (Nrf2/ARE) signaling route, as well as how the substance acts on Kelch-like ECH-associated protein 1 (Keap1) [69]. In HF models, sacubitril/valsartan reduced the production of oxidative products, intracellular reactive oxygen species (ROS) such as inflammatory factors (IL-1β, interleukins IL-6, and TNF-α), and malondialdehyde [79]. In HF patients, a reduced oxidative stress and inflammation was revealed during therapy with sacubitril/valsartan [80,81].

Furthermore, there are some data suggesting that sacubitril/valsartan determines the better LV remodeling and outcome in subjects suffering from non-ischemic HF compared with those with ischemic HF [82,83].

Favorable remodeling, the improvement of systolic function, and the reduction of LV end-diastolic dimensions in LVNC after optimal therapy with medication or devices with known reverse remodeling potential were observed in a few studies and case reports (Table 1).

Table 1. Left ventricular reverse remodeling studies and case reports in LVNC.

Type of Study/ No. of Patients	LVNC Phenotype/ Associated Diseases	Treatment	Reverse Remodeling Main Findings	Ref.
Case study	Dilated Hypothyroidism	ARNI	LVEF increased by 29%, reduction of LV end-diastolic diameter by 7 mm	[63]
Case study	Dilated	ARNI beta-blockers diuretics, aldosterone antagonists	LVEF increased from 24% to 51% in 16 months, LV cavity decreased, diastolic function improved E/e' decreased from >15 to 10–14; the ratio of non-compacted/compacted myocardium decreased	[65]
Retrospective/ 51		3 betablockers 15 ACEi/ARB 33 dual therapies	88% had an improvement in LVEF by 16 ± 12% LV shortening fraction improved by 8 ± 9%	[12]
Prospective/ 23		ACEi and/or ARB and beta-blockers in addition to diuretics	39% had an absolute increase in LVEF > 10% at 6 months Regression of LVHT area showed significant correlations with the changes in LVEF	[39]
Prospective/ 20			60% responders vs. 28% with DCM	[43]
Prospective/11	Dilated		All patients were responders Phase standard deviation was reduced from $89.5'' \pm 14.2''$ to $63.7'' \pm 20.5''$	[84]
Prospective/15		CRT	LVEF increased from 27.6 ± 5.5 to 39.1 ± 7.0% ($p < 0.01$) LV volumes did not change significantly	[85]
Systematic review/70			50% responders LVEF increased from 8 to 36% NYHA class improved	[86]
Case study		Carvedilol, lisinopril, furosemide	LVEF increased from 15–20% to 55% and LVEDV decreased from 210 mL to 145 mL at 1 year	[44]
Case study	Dilated Polyneuropathy	Biventricular pacemaker system	LV function improved, LV size decreased, LVHT could not be longer detected	[10]
Case study	Dilated/ Severe aortic regurgitation	Aortic valve replacement	Regression of LV dimensions and improvement of LVEF	[9]
Case study		Standard HF treatment ICD-CRT	LVEF increased from 18 to 51%, morphologic features of LVNC become less clear	[45]
Case study	Dilated	ACEi, beta-blockers, diuretics, aldosterone antagonists	LVEF increased from 19 to 47%, LV end-diastolic diameter decreased from 70 mm to 61 mm, resolution of non-compacted appearance	[46]
Case study		ICD-CRT	LVEF increased from <20% to 60% with almost complete resolution of LVHT	[47]

LVEF, left ventricular ejection fraction; ARNI, angiotensin receptor neprilysininhibitor; ACEi, angiotensin converting enzyme inhibitor; ARB, angiotensin receptor blocker; CRT, cardiac resynchronization therapy; LVHT, left ventricle hyper trabeculation; LVEDV, left ventricular end-diastolic volume; DCM, dilated cardiomyopathy; ICD-CRT, internal cardioverter defibrillator-cardiac resynchronization therapy; HF, heart failure.

Therapy with at least one medication, such as beta-blockers, ACE inhibitors, or angiotensin receptor blockers, had a favorable effect in many young patients with the LVNC dilated phenotype, as evaluated in a retrospective study. There was a significant increase in the ejection fraction and shortening fraction ($p < 0.0001$) and a decrease in the LV end-diastolic dimensions ($p < 0.05$). Early diagnosis and medical treatment of LVNC can produce favorable LV remodeling [12]. Therapeutic approaches for patients with echocardiographic criteria for LVNC and reduced EF according to current HF guidelines resulted in several cases of the regression of LV hyper-trabeculations and an improvement in LV systolic function, which are associated with a better prognosis [87].

Bertini et al. concluded that the impact of cardiac resynchronization treatment on LV reverse remodeling in LVNC individuals and dilated CM are greater than in patients with dilated CM. By using standard and contrast echocardiography techniques, the authors observed a better response and greater LV reverse remodeling in those with a greater region of non-compaction. The amount of LVNC segments had a trend towards reduction compared with the baseline ($p = 0.067$), and patients with more trabeculated segments at baseline (>4) were more likely to be responders or super-responders ($p = 0.003$) [86].

Mechanical desynchrony is common in patients with LVNC, is independent from QRS width, and is correlated with the impaired electrical endocardial activation associated with the abnormal myocardium, which could justify an extended indication of biventricular pacing in this population. When analyzing the response to cardiac resynchronization therapy for individuals with LVNC as opposed to those with other cardiomyopathies by using gated-SPECT myocardial perfusion imaging, it was observed that cardiac resynchronization therapy contributes to an important improvement in patients with non-compaction myocardium. Desynchrony was assessed by determining the phase standard deviation, and patients with LVNC with more important desynchrony at baseline had the most significant improvement in intraventricular synchronism. The living standard improved in all patients, but non-ischemic subjects with and without LVNC had the most important improvements in LVEF and LV volume reduction [84].

Another study revealed that cardiac resynchronization therapy can improve the ejection fraction ($p < 0.01$), morphology, and mechanical desynchrony in LVNC patients. This study evaluated LV remodeling and mechanical synchronicity before/after 6 months of cardiac resynchronization therapy in LVNC patients. The LV reaction was established as a $\geq 15\%$ reduction in the LV end-systolic volume. A percentage of 33.3% responded to cardiac resynchronization therapy, and they were super-responders (reduction in LVESV > 30%). All three desynchronies (inter-ventricular, radial intra-ventricular, and longitudinal) and both the non-compacted to compacted myocardium ratio and quantity of non-compacted segments decreased (for all $p < 0.05$) [85].

In a systematic review of the literature that included 14 studies, the authors concluded that cardiac resynchronization therapy can provide beneficial effects, improving clinical status and LVEF in LVNC patients with HF. A more important LV reverse remodeling was observed in cardiac resynchronization therapy responders, and this therapy is able to improve the performance of LVNC segments [86].

Indications for CRT in LVNC remain the same as in other cardiomyopathies: symptomatic HF patients, despite optimal medical treatment and in sinus rhythm, have an LVEF $\leq 35\%$ and QRS duration ≥ 150 ms (class I level of evidence A) or between 130 and 149 ms (class IIa level of evidence B), mainly with a left bundle branch block morphology [88]. In addition, left bundle branch block is a frequent anomaly in LVNC that is reported in 41.7% of patients, as observed by Akhbour et al. [89]. A slightly higher incidence of left bundle branch block and a greater mean QRS width (although not statistically significant) are registered in this population compared with other cardiomyopathies [84].

Lin et al. reported a patient with a positive response to standard HF therapy, which is rarely encountered in patients with documented LVNC [90]. Stöllberger et al. reported the regression of LV hyper-trabeculation after improvement of LV systolic function with biventricular pacing. A compensatory mechanism of the failing heart was suggested as the etiology of LV hyper-trabeculation in this patient [10]. Cortez-Dias et al. described a case of a young black male with LVNC, severe LV systolic dysfunction, and severe aortic regurgitation who had a family history, possibly indicating a hereditary disorder; his case had an excellent evolution after aortic valve replacement [9]. Eurlings et al. presented a case of isolated LVNC treated with medical therapy and internal cardioverter defibrillator implantation that became less clear after 6 months of treatment [91], and another case was described by Luckie et al. using the resolution of echocardiographic features of LVNC in 18 months after standard medical therapy [92].

Vinardell et al. described the case of a woman with isolated LVNC who was managed by a guidelines-determined medical treatment, implantation of an internal cardioverter defibrillator, and resynchronization treatment; her complications resolved 2 years after the initial diagnosis with a normalization of LV volumes and ejection fraction and an almost complete resolution of the previously noted trabeculations. The authors concluded that non-compaction CM can either have a dynamic course or may be reversible, or that current morphologic criteria may occasionally misclassify a transient CM as non-compaction [93].

A non-compaction that is sometimes a partially reversible phenotype can be observed in athletes, pregnant women, and chronic HF patients, probably as an adaptive reaction to ventricular overload [94]. It is an area of debate whether a hyper-trabeculated LV without symptoms, LV dysfunction, or a family history of LVNC can be viewed as the initial stage of CM. Zemrak et al. followed up on 2742 asymptomatic subjects without known cardiovascular disease (CVD) that fulfilled the CMR criteria of LVNC at baseline for 10 years and observed that this morphological change appeared to be benign and was not linked with the deterioration of LV volumes or function over time [95]. LVNC includes a very large range, ranging from entirely morphological features with good a prognosis to a real muscular disorder with a possible adverse outcome [34].

6.2. Arrhythmias and Systemic Embolism Prevention

Anticoagulants are recommended in patients with LVEF $\leq$ 40%, atrial fibrillation, intracardiac thrombi, or previous embolic events [58]. Patients with malignant ventricular tachyarrhythmia necessitate the implantation an internal defibrillator as a supplementary measure to prevent sudden cardiac death. Radiofrequency ablation may be considered. Subjects with LVNC, CM, and an ejection fraction $\leq$ 35% have an indication for the insertion of an internal cardioverter defibrillator as an essential measure against unexpected cardiac death [96]. Finally, in subjects that do not respond to medical therapy, cardiac transplantation is an option, although it is rarely used in this condition.

7. Prognosis

In 2020, Aung et al. revealed in a meta-analysis that, when compared with dilated CM, LVNC patients have almost comparable risks of CV or death from all causes, ventricular arrhythmia, and thromboembolic complications [21,97]. Prognosis is mainly determined by the severity of LV systolic dysfunction; a low LVEF is the most significant indicator of an unfavorable result [21,97]. A recent study found that, as a group, compared with the general population, individuals with LVNC had worse overall survival rates, but those having a maintained LVEF and localized apical non-compaction responded better. Greater overall mortality was substantially correlated with the mid-non-compaction extent or basal non-compaction extent [98].

A recently published, large, multicenter French prospective registry found that, when comparing the results of 98 subjects having LVNC vs. 65 patients having dilated cardiomyopathy, an obvious trend toward poorer prognosis in LVNC vs. dilated CM was present for the studied patients with LV dysfunction. Although CV mortality was similar between LVNC and dilated CM, HF and/or rhythmic events (to a lesser degree) were more frequent in patients with LVNC, while embolic events occurred at the same rate [99].

Another recent retrospective multicentric study that included 200 patients with LVNC was aimed at evaluating the prognosis of different forms of LVNC. The subtype of dilated LVNC had the worst outcome, and independent factors for prognosis were age, LVEF < 50%, and ventricular tachycardia/fibrillation [100].

Long-term survival trials are warranted to assess the impact of different therapeutic strategies in individuals with LVNC [99]. Nevertheless, reverse remodeling, as in our patient, is associated with a better prognosis and lower mortality [101]. There is a wide spectrum of manifestations in LVNC, ranging from a strictly morphological perspective without hemodynamic impairment to a severe muscular disorder that is linked to a bad prognosis. The severity and mortality of LVNC in youth may be increased, as suggested by the current knowledge, particularly for those who present ventricular dysfunction within the first year of life [34].

8. Case Presentation

To clarify all aspects in the best way, our research exemplifies the situation of a 41-year-old male who had HF symptoms. LVNC CM was suspected at the time of transthoracic echocardiography and was subsequently confirmed during CMR processing. ARNI therapy was initiated, and the patient was prospectively observed for more than 12 months. Favorable remodeling and clinical outcomes were registered after including ARNI into the HF treatment. LVNC remains a heterogeneous CM, and although a favorable outcome is not commonly encountered, some patients respond well to therapy. The clinical presentation, paraclinical diagnosis, treatment strategy, and evolution are described. The patient filled out an informed consent form, and the study was carried out in conformity with the Declaration of Helsinki.

A 41-year-old male was hospitalized in February 2021 to the Cardiology Clinical Department of the Clinical County Emergency Hospital Oradea, Romania, with dyspnea at minimal exertion, dry cough, and fatigue. Symptoms occurred in the last 6 months and gradually worsened. On admission, he was already on a treatment that was initiated 3 months before, which used angiotensin converting enzyme (ACE) inhibitors (ramipril 5 mg/day), loop diuretics (furosemide 40 mg/day), mineral receptor antagonist (MRA) (spironolactone 50 mg/day), and beta-blockers (carvedilol 25 mg/day); however, his symptoms persisted. No family history of CM was present. On physical examination, we found a pulmonary stasis at the bases of the lungs, orthopnea, SO_2 = 93% on ambient air, a blood pressure of 130/80 mmHg, an AV = 100 beats/min, an S3 and S4 gallop, and a systolic murmur grade of III/VI in the LV area.

Initial evaluation of the patient included twelve-lead electrocardiogram (ECG) and transthoracic echocardiography techniques. The ECG (performed with EDAN SE 1201, Edan Instruments Inc., Shangai International Holding Corp. GmBH (Europe) Hamburg, Gemany) showed the sinus rhythm, a heart rate of 90 beats/min, diffuse ST-T changes, T negative waves in inferior and lateral leads, and a flattened T wave in the rest of the leads (Figure 1, own archive of the last author).

Transthoracic echocardiography (Figure 2, own archive of the last author), performed using VIVID E 95 (GE Vingmed Ultrasound AS, Horten, Norway), showed a moderately dilated LV with a morphologic image of a two-layered myocardium, which had trabeculations at the apex and in the mid-area of both the lateral anterior/inferior walls (Figure 2a,b). The ratio between the non-compacted/compacted myocardium at end systole in the short-axis perspective was 2.1. Color flow was present in the profound intertrabecular recesses (Figure 2c).

The contraction of the LV was severely altered, and diffuse hypokinesia was present, which was accentuated at the trabeculated area level. The left atrium (LA) was severely dilated. A spontaneous contrast was present in the LA and LV. Moderate mitral regurgitation due to LV dilatation was present. Compared with the biplane Simpson method baseline, the LVEF was reduced, and the LV end systolic and end-diastolic volumes were increased (Table 1). A tissue Doppler revealed decreased velocities at the level of the septal and lateral annulus. Examination of the LV diastolic function revealed a restrictive filling pattern of mitral diastolic inflow with an E/e' ratio = 15. The LVEF and global longitudinal strain were lower in the speckle tracking echocardiography results (35% and −9.2%). The characteristic of a decreased LV twist motion of 2.6 (determined using the difference between the peak rotation at the level of base and the apex in the short-axis view) for LVNC was found. The right ventricle had increased apical trabeculations but normal fractional area variations and a tricuspid annular plane systolic excursion (difficult to differentiate from the normal variant in the highly trabeculated right ventricle). The tricuspid regurgitation was medium, the inferior vena cava was dilated with diminished inspiratory collapse, and the systolic pressure in the pulmonary artery was 60 mmHg. A transthoracic echocardiographic examination was strongly suggestive of a LVNC CM with a dilation of the LV and a depressed ejection fraction. The morpho-functional phenotype for our patient according to the MOGE(S) system for cardiomyopathies is M LVNC-D, LVNC with LV dilatation, and dysfunction. Holter ECG (BTL-08 Holter H600, BTL Industries Ltd., Cleveland, United Kingdom) monitoring for 24 h showed ventricular premature beats at a percentage of 3%. Laboratory tests revealed an elevated NT-proBNP level (Table 2).

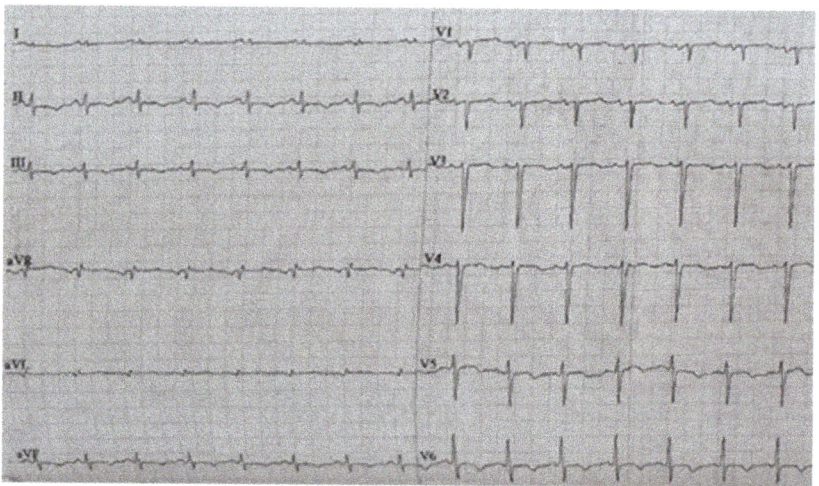

Figure 1. Twelve lead ECG.

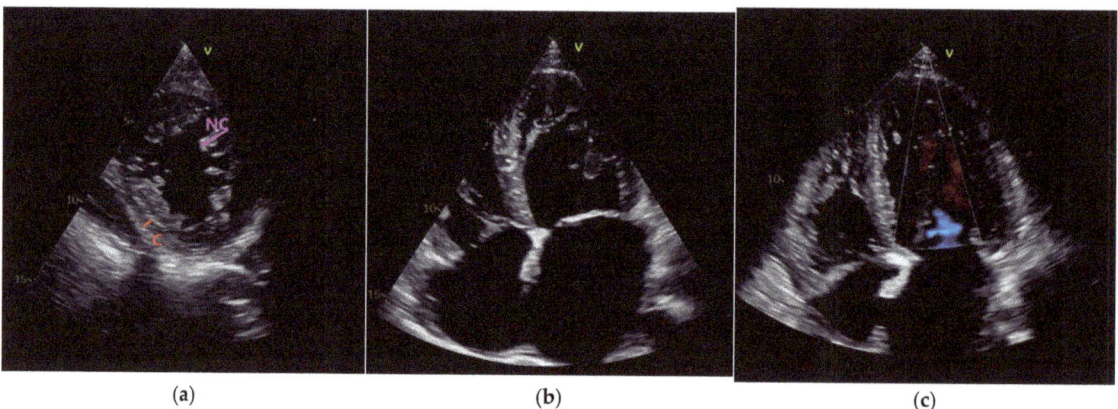

Figure 2. (a) Transthoracic echocardiography. Parasternal short-axis view. Non-compacted–NC/Compacted-C ratio > 2; (b) Apical 4 chamber view. Trabeculations at the apex and lateral wall of the LV, dilated left atrium. (c) Transthoracic echocardiography. Color flow in the intertrabecular recesses.

Table 2. Evolution of echocardiographic parameters and NT-proBNP level.

Parameters	Baseline	6 Months	12 Months
LVEDV (mL)	202	177	152
LVESV (mL)	133	92	72
LVEF (%)	35	48	54
LAVI (mL/m^2)	61	45	35
Mitral regurgitation	Moderate	Moderate	Mild
NT-proBNP (pg/mL)	5200	1102	420

LVEDV, left ventricular end-diastolic volume; LVESV, left ventricular end-systolic volume; LVEF, left ventricular ejection fraction; LAVI, left atrial volume index; NT-proBNP, N-terminal Pro B-type natriuretic peptide.

A coronarography showed normal epicardial coronary arteries and excluded the ischemic etiology of HF. Genetic tests were not available for our patient. The patient was scheduled for a CMR evaluation and a further clarification of the diagnosis. HF treatment was administered in accordance with the ESC guidelines. ACE inhibitors were replaced after a washout period of 36 h with ARNI- sacubitril/valsartan at 100 mg/day, which was titrated to 200 mg/day after 2 weeks and an increased dosage of up to 400 mg/day after another month. Loop diuretics, MRA, and betablockers were continued, and anticoagulants were also associated. SGLT-2 inhibitors were not prescribed because at that time, they were not available in our hospital and were not sustained on free prescription by the healthcare system. There was a significant clinical improvement at 6 months after discharge; the patient was in the NYHA class I, and no symptoms were present. CMR processing was performed (using Siemens Magnetom_Essenza 1.5 T., Siemens Shenzen Magnetic Resonance LTD, Shenzen, China) at this time, and it confirmed the diagnosis of LVNC by identifying trabeculations that were located at the apex and medial levels of the anterior and lateral walls of the LV. The ratio between the non-compacted and compacted layers was 2.3 during diastole at the level of the lateral wall, fulfilling the Petersen criteria for diagnosis (Figure 3, own archive of the last author).

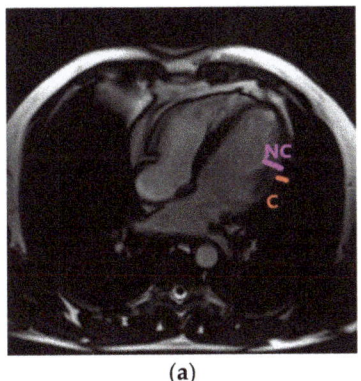 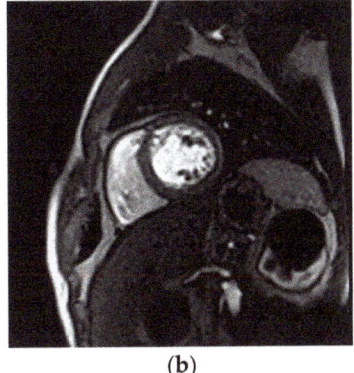

(a) (b)

Figure 3. Cardiac magnetic resonance. (a) Left ventricular non-compaction in four chamber view. NC, non-compacted; C, compacted LV wall. (b) Left ventricular non-compaction in short-axis view.

The LV was dilated, but significant reverse remodeling was observed at the time of echocardiography and CMR. LV and LA volumes were diminished compared with the initial evaluation, but contractility and LVEF were significantly improved. LGE was not detected in the CMR. After one year, the patient was free of symptoms, and a further improvement was observed at the time of echocardiography regarding the ejection fraction and left heart volumes (Table 1); however, increased trabeculations persisted. Figure 4 describes an algorithm used for the diagnosis of LVNC and illustrates the evolution of several parameters after treatment initiation. The clinical, biological, and echocardiographic elements showed a significant improvement, especially after 12 months of treatment.

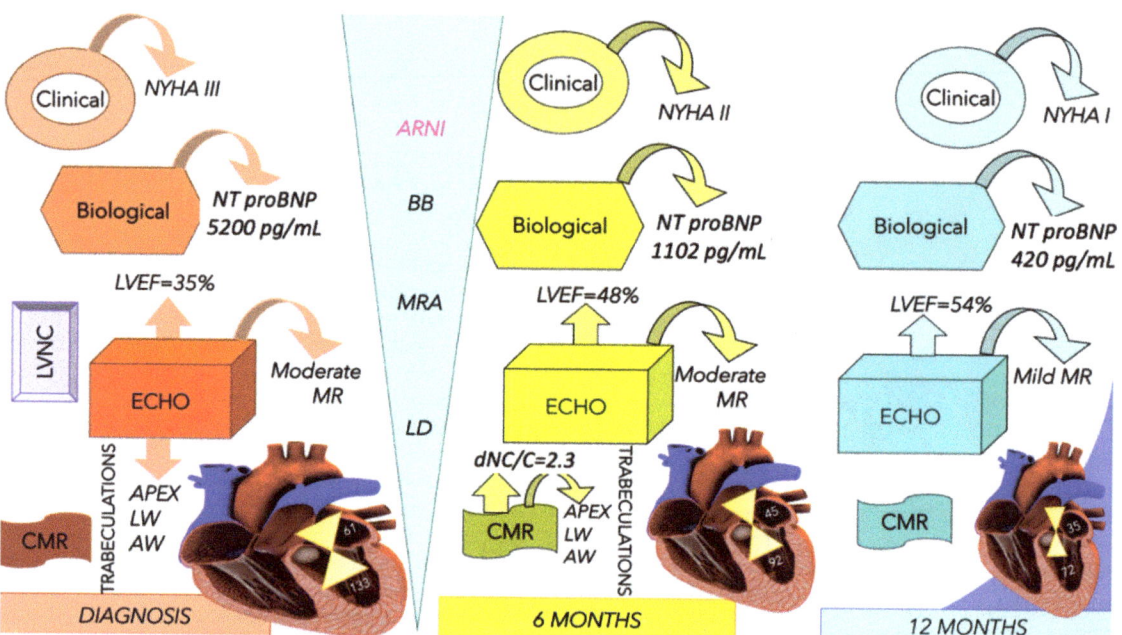

Figure 4. Elements of diagnosis for left ventricle non-compaction and the evolution of the presented case after therapy initiation. The numbers from the heart diagram illustrate the values of the indexed left atrial volume (mL/m^2) and end-systolic volume of the left ventricle (mL); there is an improvement of the mentioned parameters after treatment initiation, and the clinical and biological elements expressed the same evolution. ARNI, angiotensin receptor neprilysin receptor; AW, anterior wall; BB, beta-blockers; CMR, cardiac magnetic resonance imaging; ECHO, echocardiography; LD, loop diuretics; LVEF, left ventricle ejection fraction; LVNC, left ventricle non-compaction; LW, lateral wall; MR, mitral regurgitation; MRA, mineralocorticoid receptor antagonists; dNC/C, diastolicnon-compacted/compacted ratio; NT-proBNP, N-terminal pro-b type natriuretic peptide; NYHA, New York Heart Association.

Although it is not common, a favorable response, namely reverse cardiac remodeling, and clinical improvement, was observed after optimization of the treatment by adding ARNI to HF therapy.

The prognosis for LVNC is unpredictable due to the disorder's significant heterogeneity. The important reverse remodeling observed in this patient was one of the main reasons that determined us to report the case. A similar improvement was observed after introduction of ARNI therapy in a few other LVNC case reports [63,65].

It is known that ARNI therapy that is initiated as early as possible can lead to greater cardiac reverse remodeling benefit in HF patients, having a reduced ejection fraction vs. angiotensin receptor blockers or angiotensin-converting enzyme suppressors. A recent systematic study that included a large number of patients with HF with reduced EF revealed that ARNI treatment was linked to an amelioration of the EF (+5.11%, 95% CI 4.06 to 6.16) and LV dimensions compared with patients who followed a treatment with angiotensin receptor blockers or angiotensin-converting enzyme suppressors [68].

The impressive reverse remodeling appeared in the context of an up-titration of the drug to the dose of 400 mg as recommended by the guidelines [102].

However, the magnitude of reverse remodeling is variable across patients. Several characteristics that were present in our patient were identified as predictors of reverse remodeling in various studies in patients with HF and reduced EF and in patients with LVNC. The etiology and duration of HF are factors that can influence outcome. The increase in LVEF is more important in patients with non-ischemic or new-onset HF ($\leq$12 months) [103,104]. In an early and reversible stage of the disease, sacubitril/valsartan can prevent global cardiac remodeling, and this was sustained by the results of the PIONEER-HF trial (Comparison of Sacubitril/Valsartan Versus Enalapril on Effect on NT-proBNP in Patients Stabilized From an Acute Heart Failure Episode) [105].

The absence of a left bundle branch block is another independent predictor of reverse remodeling in cohort studies in patients with HF with reduced EF [106]. LV contractions are dyssynchronous, and inefficient, functional mitral regurgitation and reduced stroke volume are encountered in patients with left bundle branch blocks. The absence of myocardial fibrosis, as assessed using LGE CMR, in our patient is also correlated with reverse remodeling and a good prognosis [55,107]. Furthermore, an important decrease in NT-proBNP level is associated with greater improvements in the LVEF and a more important reduction of LV volumes [102]. Additionally, a younger age and a sinus rhythm identify a subgroup of patients with a more likely reverse LV remodeling [104]. All of these features that are associated with reverse remodeling were present in our patient.

9. Conclusions

The availability of high-resolution imaging techniques and the current awareness of the disease contribute to the increased number of patients that have been diagnosed lately with this CM. The diagnosis of LVNC is based on multimodality imaging investigations that combine echocardiography and CMR, but the diagnostic criteria are still not uniformly defined. There is a need for a consensus on the diagnostic criteria to avoid under- and over-diagnosis. To prevent overdiagnosis, it is still difficult to distinguish the LVNC phenotype from that of the healthy heart. Additionally, the phenotypes of other cardiomyopathies have a similar genetic profile overlap, which therefore represents another significant issue. Evidence supporting the treatment strategies in LVNC is limited, and no specific guidelines are available. Prospective trials to assess the management, therapeutic approach, and outcomes in this disease are warranted, but due to the low prevalence of this form of CM, this will present a real challenge.

Defining the CM etiology is important in all new-onset HF patients for the close monitoring and prevention of further complications or in the case that some specific treatment is attainable. Although irreversible LV dysfunction is more common in LVNC cardiomyopathies, the presented case highlights that the optimization of HF therapy is associated with significant reverse cardiac remodeling and important clinical improvement in some patients.

Author Contributions: All authors have equal contribution compared with the first author. All authors have read and agreed to the published version of the manuscript.

Funding: The APC was funded by the University of Oradea, Oradea, Romania.

Institutional Review Board Statement: Not applicable.

Informed Consent Statement: Informed consent was obtained from the subject involved in the study.

Data Availability Statement: Data are contained within the article.

Acknowledgments: The authors would like to thank the University of Oradea for supporting the payment of the invoice through an internal project.

Conflicts of Interest: The authors declare no conflict of interest.

References

1. Engberding, R.; Bender, F. Identification of a rare congenital anomaly of the myocardium by twodimensional echocardiography: Persistence of isolated myocardial sinusoids. *Am. J. Cardiol.* **1984**, *53*, 1733–1734. [CrossRef]
2. Minamisawa, M.; Koyama, J.; Ikeda, U. Left ventricular noncompaction cardiomyopathy: Recent update on genetics, usefulness of biomarkers, and speckle imaging. *J. Cardiol.* **2019**, *73*, 95–96. [CrossRef] [PubMed]
3. Gerecke, B.J.; Engberding, R. Noncompaction Cardiomyopathy—History and Current Knowledge for Clinical Practice. *J. Clin. Med.* **2021**, *10*, 2457. [CrossRef] [PubMed]
4. Maron, B.J.; Towbin, J.A.; Thiene, G.; Antzelevitch, C.; Corrado, D.; Arnett, D.; Moss, A.J.; Seidman, C.E.; Young, J.B. Contemporary Definitions and Classification of the Cardiomyopathies. *Circulation* **2006**, *113*, 1807–1816. [CrossRef]
5. Towbin, J.A.; Jefferies, J.L. Cardiomyopathies due to left ventricular noncompaction, mitochondrial and storage diseases, and inborn errors of metabolism. *Circ. Res.* **2017**, *121*, 838–854. [CrossRef] [PubMed]
6. Vesa, C.M.; Bungau, S.G. Novel Molecules in Diabetes Mellitus, Dyslipidemia and Cardiovascular Disease. *Int. J. Mol. Sci.* **2023**, *24*, 4029. [CrossRef]
7. Iorga, R.A.; Bacalbasa, N.; Carsote, M.; Bratu, O.G.; Stanescu, A.M.A.; Bungau, S.; Pantis, C.; Diaconu, C.C. Metabolic and cardiovascular benefits of GLP-1 agonists, besides the hypoglycemic effect. *Exp. Med.* **2020**, *20*, 2396–2400. [CrossRef]
8. Elliott, P.; Andersson, B.; Arbustini, E.; Bilinska, Z.; Cecchi, F.; Charron, P.; Dubourg, O.; Kühl, U.; Maisch, B.; McKenna, W.J.; et al. Classification of the cardiomyopathies: A position statement from the european society of cardiology working group on myocardial and pericardial diseases. *Eur. Heart J.* **2007**, *29*, 270–276. [CrossRef]
9. Cortez-Dias, N.; Varela, M.G.; Sargento, L.; Brito, D.; Almeida, A.; Cerqueira, R.; Lança, V.; Fernandes, A.R.; Tavares, P.; Pereira, R.A. Left ventricular non-compaction: A new mutation predisposing to reverse remodeling? *Rev. Port. De Cardiol. Orgao Da Soc. Port. De Cardiol.=Port. J. Cardiol. Off. J. Port. Soc. Cardiol.* **2009**, *28*, 185–194.
10. Stöllberger, C.; Keller, H.; Finsterer, J. Disappearance of left ventricular hypertrabeculation/noncompaction after biventricular pacing in a patient with polyneuropathy. *J. Card. Fail.* **2007**, *13*, 211–214. [CrossRef]
11. Wong, P.H.; Fung, J.W. Regression of non-compaction in left ventricular non-compaction cardiomyopathy by cardiac contractility modulation. *Int. J. Cardiol.* **2012**, *154*, e50–e51. [CrossRef] [PubMed]
12. Parent, J.J.; Towbin, J.A.; Jefferies, J.L. Medical therapy leads to favorable remodeling in left ventricular non-compaction cardiomyopathy: Dilated phenotype. *Pediatr. Cardiol.* **2016**, *37*, 674–677. [CrossRef] [PubMed]
13. Negri, F.; De Luca, A.; Fabris, E.; Korcova, R.; Cernetti, C.; Grigoratos, C.; Aquaro, G.D.; Nucifora, G.; Camici, P.G.; Sinagra, G. Left ventricular noncompaction, morphological, and clinical features for an integrated diagnosis. *Heart Fail. Rev.* **2019**, *24*, 315–323. [CrossRef] [PubMed]
14. Wengrofsky, P.; Armenia, C.; Oleszak, F.; Kupferstein, E.; Rednam, C.; Mitre, C.A.; McFarlane, S.I. Left ventricular trabeculation and noncompaction cardiomyopathy: A review. *EC Clin. Exp. Anat.* **2019**, *2*, 267.
15. Jensen, B.; van der Wal, A.C.; Moorman, A.F.; Christoffels, V.M. Excessive trabeculations in noncompaction do not have the embryonic identity. *Int. J. Cardiol.* **2017**, *227*, 325–330. [CrossRef] [PubMed]
16. Șerban, R.C.; Lupu, S.; Pintilie, I.; Scridon, A.; Dobreanu, D. Left ventricular noncompaction in a highly arrhythmogenic, apparently structurally normal heart. *Rom. J. Cardiol.* **2015**, *25*.
17. Weiford, B.C.; Subbarao, V.D.; Mulhern, K.M. Noncompaction of the ventricular myocardium. *Circulation* **2004**, *109*, 2965–2971. [CrossRef]
18. Nucifora, G.; Aquaro, G.D.; Masci, P.G.; Pingitore, A.; Lombardi, M. Magnetic resonance assessment of prevalence and correlates of right ventricular abnormalities in isolated left ventricular noncompaction. *Am. J. Cardiol.* **2014**, *113*, 142–146. [CrossRef]
19. Toader, D.; Paraschiv, A.; Tudorașcu, P.; Tudorașcu, D.; Bataiosu, C.; Balșeanu, A. Left ventricular noncompaction—A rare cause of triad: Heart failure, ventricular arrhythmias, and systemic embolic events: A case report. *J. Med. Case Rep.* **2021**, *15*, 316. [CrossRef]
20. Oechslin, E.; Jenni, R. Left ventricular noncompaction: From physiologic remodeling to noncompaction cardiomyopathy. *J. Am. Coll. Cardiol.* **2018**, *71*, 723–726. [CrossRef]
21. van Waning, J.I.; Caliskan, K.; Hoedemaekers, Y.M.; van Spaendonck-Zwarts, K.Y.; Baas, A.F.; Boekholdt, S.M.; van Melle, J.P.; Teske, A.J.; Asselbergs, F.W.; Backx, A.P. Genetics, clinical features, and long-term outcome of noncompaction cardiomyopathy. *J. Am. Coll. Cardiol.* **2018**, *71*, 711–722. [CrossRef] [PubMed]
22. Miura, F.; Shimada, J.; Kitagawa, Y.; Otani, K.; Sato, T.; Toki, T.; Takahashi, T.; Yonesaka, S.; Mizukami, H.; Ito, E. MYH7 mutation identified by next-generation sequencing in three infant siblings with bi-ventricular noncompaction presenting with restrictive hemodynamics: A report of three siblings with a severe phenotype and poor prognosis. *J. Cardiol. Cases* **2019**, *19*, 140–143. [CrossRef] [PubMed]
23. Rodriguez-Fanjul, J.; Tubio-Gómez, S.; Carretero Bellón, J.M.; Bautista-Rodríguez, C.; Sanchez-de-Toledo, J. Neonatal non-compacted cardiomyopathy: Predictors of poor outcome. *Pediatr. Cardiol.* **2020**, *41*, 175–180. [CrossRef] [PubMed]
24. Lorca, R.; Martín, M.; Pascual, I.; Astudillo, A.; Díaz Molina, B.; Cigarrán, H.; Cuesta-Llavona, E.; Avanzas, P.; Rodríguez Reguero, J.J.; Coto, E. Characterization of left ventricular non-compaction cardiomyopathy. *J. Clin. Med.* **2020**, *9*, 2524. [CrossRef]

25. Ackerman, M.J.; Priori, S.G.; Willems, S.; Berul, C.; Brugada, R.; Calkins, H.; Camm, A.J.; Ellinor, P.T.; Gollob, M.; Hamilton, R. HRS/EHRA expert consensus statement on the state of genetic testing for the channelopathies and cardiomyopathies: This document was developed as a partnership between the Heart Rhythm Society (HRS) and the European Heart Rhythm Association (EHRA). *Europace* **2011**, *13*, 1077–1109. [CrossRef]
26. Habib, G.; Charron, P.; Eicher, J.; Giorgi, R.; Donal, E.; Laperche, T.; Boulmier, D.; Pascal, C.; Logeart, D.; Jondeau, G. Working Groups 'Heart Failure and Cardiomyopathies' and 'Echocardiography' of the French Society of Cardiology. Isolated left ventricular non-compaction in adults: Clinical and echocardiographic features in 105 patients. Results from a French registry. *Eur. J. Heart Fail.* **2011**, *13*, 177–185. [CrossRef]
27. Lofiego, C.; Biagini, E.; Pasquale, F.; Ferlito, M.; Rocchi, G.; Perugini, E.; Bacchi-Reggiani, L.; Boriani, G.; Leone, O.; Caliskan, K. Wide spectrum of presentation and variable outcomes of isolated left ventricular non-compaction. *Heart* **2007**, *93*, 65–71. [CrossRef]
28. Peters, F.; Khandheria, B.K.; dos Santos, C.; Matioda, H.; Maharaj, N.; Libhaber, E.; Mamdoo, F.; Essop, M.R. Isolated left ventricular noncompaction in sub-Saharan Africa: A clinical and echocardiographic perspective. *Circ. Cardiovasc. Imaging* **2012**, *5*, 187–193. [CrossRef]
29. Jenni, R.; Oechslin, E.; Schneider, J.; Jost, C.A.; Kaufmann, P. Echocardiographic and pathoanatomical characteristics of isolated left ventricular non-compaction: A step towards classification as a distinct cardiomyopathy. *Heart* **2001**, *86*, 666–671. [CrossRef]
30. Chin, T.K.; Perloff, J.K.; Williams, R.G.; Jue, K.; Mohrmann, R. Isolated noncompaction of left ventricular myocardium. A Study Eight Cases. *Circ.* **1990**, *82*, 507–513.
31. Stöllberger, C.; Finsterer, J. Left ventricular hypertrabeculation/noncompaction. *J. Am. Soc. Echocardiogr.* **2004**, *17*, 91–100. [CrossRef] [PubMed]
32. van Dalen, B.M.; Caliskan, K.; Soliman, O.I.; Nemes, A.; Vletter, W.B.; Ten Cate, F.J.; Geleijnse, M.L. Left ventricular solid body rotation in non-compaction cardiomyopathy: A potential new objective and quantitative functional diagnostic criterion? *Eur. J. Heart Fail.* **2008**, *10*, 1088–1093. [CrossRef]
33. Senior, R.; Becher, H.; Monaghan, M.; Agati, L.; Zamorano, J.; Vanoverschelde, J.L.; Nihoyannopoulos, P.; Edvardsen, T.; Lancellotti, P. Clinical practice of contrast echocardiography: Recommendation by the European Association of Cardiovascular Imaging (EACVI) 2017. *Eur. Heart J. Cardiovasc. Imaging* **2017**, *18*, 1205–1205af. [CrossRef] [PubMed]
34. Fusco, F.; Borrelli, N.; Barracano, R.; Ciriello, G.D.; Verrillo, F.; Scognamiglio, G.; Sarubbi, B. Left Ventricular Non-Compaction Spectrum in Adults and Children: From a Morphological Trait to a Structural Muscular Disease. *Cardiogenetics* **2022**, *12*, 170–184. [CrossRef]
35. Dellegrottaglie, S.; Pedrotti, P.; Roghi, A.; Pedretti, S.; Chiariello, M.; Perrone-Filardi, P. Regional and global ventricular systolic function in isolated ventricular non-compaction: Pathophysiological insights from magnetic resonance imaging. *Int. J. Cardiol.* **2012**, *158*, 394–399. [CrossRef]
36. Aras, D.; Tufekcioglu, O.; Ergun, K.; Ozeke, O.; Yildiz, A.; Topaloglu, S.; Deveci, B.; Sahin, O.; Kisacik, H.L.; Korkmaz, S. Clinical features of isolated ventricular noncompaction in adults long-term clinical course, echocardiographic properties, and predictors of left ventricular failure. *J. Card. Fail.* **2006**, *12*, 726–733. [CrossRef] [PubMed]
37. Fazio, G.; Corrado, G.; Novo, G.; Zachara, E.; Rapezzi, C.; Sulafa, A.K.; Sutera, L.; D'angelo, L.; Visconti, C.; Stollberger, C. Ventricular dysfunction and number of non compacted segments in non compaction: Non-independent predictors. *Int. J. Cardiol.* **2010**, *141*, 250–253. [CrossRef]
38. Cheng, H.; Zhao, S.; Jiang, S.; Lu, M.; Yan, C.; Ling, J.; Zhang, Y.; Liu, Q.; Ma, N.; Yin, G.; et al. Comparison of cardiac magnetic resonance imaging features of isolated left ventricular non-compaction in adults versus dilated cardiomyopathy in adults. *Clin. Radiol.* **2011**, *66*, 853–860. [CrossRef]
39. Yin, L. Non-compact cardiomyopathy or ventricular non-compact syndrome? *J. Cardiovasc. Ultrasound* **2014**, *22*, 165–172. [CrossRef]
40. Babes, E.; Babes, V.; Popescu, M.; Ardelean, A. Value of n-terminal pro-b-type natriuretic peptide in detecting silent ischemia and its prognostic role in asymptomatic patients with type 2 diabetes mellitus. *Acta Endocrinol. (1841-0987)* **2011**, *7*, 209–218. [CrossRef]
41. Nemes, A.; Anwar, A.M.; Kaliskan, K.; Soliman, O.I.; Geleijnse, M.L.; van Dalen, B.; Cate, F.J.T. Non-compaction cardiomyopathy is associated with mitral annulus enlargement and functional impairment: A real-time three-dimensional echocardiographic study. *J. Heart Valve Dis.* **2008**, *17*, 31.
42. Petersen, S.E.; Selvanayagam, J.B.; Wiesmann, F.; Robson, M.D.; Francis, J.M.; Anderson, R.H.; Watkins, H.; Neubauer, S. Left ventricular non-compaction: Insights from cardiovascular magnetic resonance imaging. *J. Am. Coll. Cardiol.* **2005**, *46*, 101–105. [CrossRef] [PubMed]
43. Nucifora, G.; Aquaro, G.D.; Pingitore, A.; Masci, P.G.; Lombardi, M. Myocardial fibrosis in isolated left ventricular non-compaction and its relation to disease severity. *Eur. J. Heart Fail.* **2011**, *13*, 170–176. [CrossRef] [PubMed]
44. Oechslin, E.N.; Attenhofer Jost, C.H.; Rojas, J.R.; Kaufmann, P.A.; Jenni, R. Long-term follow-up of 34 adults with isolated left ventricular noncompaction: A distinct cardiomyopathy with poor prognosis. *J. Am. Coll. Cardiol.* **2000**, *36*, 493–500. [CrossRef]
45. Jacquier, A.; Thuny, F.; Jop, B.; Giorgi, R.; Cohen, F.; Gaubert, J.-Y.; Vidal, V.; Bartoli, J.M.; Habib, G.; Moulin, G. Measurement of trabeculated left ventricular mass using cardiac magnetic resonance imaging in the diagnosis of left ventricular non-compaction. *Eur. Heart J.* **2010**, *31*, 1098–1104. [CrossRef] [PubMed]

46. Andreini, D.; Pontone, G.; Bogaert, J.; Roghi, A.; Barison, A.; Schwitter, J.; Mushtaq, S.; Vovas, G.; Sormani, P.; Aquaro, G.D. Long-term prognostic value of cardiac magnetic resonance in left ventricle noncompaction: A prospective multicenter study. *J. Am. Coll. Cardiol.* **2016**, *68*, 2166–2181. [CrossRef]
47. Araujo-Filho, J.A.; Assuncao, A.N., Jr.; Tavares de Melo, M.D.; Bière, L.; Lima, C.R.; Dantas, R.N., Jr.; Nomura, C.H.; Salemi, V.M.; Jerosch-Herold, M.; Parga, J.R. Myocardial T1 mapping and extracellular volume quantification in patients with left ventricular non-compaction cardiomyopathy. *Eur. Heart J. Cardiovasc. Imaging* **2018**, *19*, 888–895. [CrossRef]
48. Dodd, J.D.; Holmvang, G.; Hoffmann, U.; Ferencik, M.; Abbara, S.; Brady, T.J.; Cury, R.C. Quantification of left ventricular noncompaction and trabecular delayed hyperenhancement with cardiac MRI: Correlation with clinical severity. *Am. J. Roentgenol.* **2007**, *189*, 974–980. [CrossRef]
49. Wang, J.-X.; Li, X.; Xu, R.; Hou, R.-L.; Yang, Z.-G.; Zhou, Z.-Q.; Wang, Y.-N.; Guo, Y.-K. Comparison of cardiovascular magnetic resonance features and clinical consequences in patients with left ventricular non-compaction with and without mitral regurgitation—A multi-institutional study of the retrospective cohort study. *Cardiovasc. Diagn. Ther.* **2022**, *12*, 241. [CrossRef]
50. Casas, G.; Rodríguez-Palomares, J.F. Multimodality Cardiac Imaging in Cardiomyopathies: From Diagnosis to Prognosis. *J. Clin. Med.* **2022**, *11*, 578. [CrossRef]
51. Cheng, H.; Lu, M.; Hou, C.; Chen, X.; Li, L.; Wang, J.; Yin, G.; Chen, X.; Xiangli, W.; Cui, C.; et al. Comparison of cardiovascular magnetic resonance characteristics and clinical consequences in children and adolescents with isolated left ventricular non-compaction with and without late gadolinium enhancement. *J. Cardiovasc. Magn. Reson.* **2015**, *17*, 44. [CrossRef] [PubMed]
52. Casas, G.; Limeres, J.; Oristrell, G.; Gutierrez-Garcia, L.; Andreini, D.; Borregan, M.; Larrañaga-Moreira, J.M.; Lopez-Sainz, A.; Codina-Solà, M.; Teixido-Tura, G.; et al. Clinical Risk Prediction in Patients With Left Ventricular Myocardial Noncompaction. *J. Am. Coll. Cardiol.* **2021**, *78*, 643–662. [CrossRef] [PubMed]
53. Halliday, B.P.; Baksi, A.J.; Gulati, A.; Ali, A.; Newsome, S.; Izgi, C.; Arzanauskaite, M.; Lota, A.; Tayal, U.; Vassiliou, V.S.; et al. Outcome in Dilated Cardiomyopathy Related to the Extent, Location, and Pattern of Late Gadolinium Enhancement. *JACC Cardiovasc. Imaging* **2019**, *12*, 1645–1655. [CrossRef] [PubMed]
54. Alba, A.C.; Gaztañaga, J.; Foroutan, F.; Thavendiranathan, P.; Merlo, M.; Alonso-Rodriguez, D.; Vallejo-García, V.; Vidal-Perez, R.; Corros-Vicente, C.; Barreiro-Pérez, M.; et al. Prognostic Value of Late Gadolinium Enhancement for the Prediction of Cardiovascular Outcomes in Dilated Cardiomyopathy. *Circ. Cardiovasc. Imaging* **2020**, *13*, e010105. [CrossRef] [PubMed]
55. Grigoratos, C.; Barison, A.; Ivanov, A.; Andreini, D.; Amzulescu, M.-S.; Mazurkiewicz, L.; De Luca, A.; Grzybowski, J.; Masci, P.G.; Marczak, M.; et al. Meta-Analysis of the Prognostic Role of Late Gadolinium Enhancement and Global Systolic Impairment in Left Ventricular Noncompaction. *JACC Cardiovasc. Imaging* **2019**, *12*, 2141–2151. [CrossRef]
56. Al-Khatib, S.M.; Stevenson, W.G.; Ackerman, M.J.; Bryant, W.J.; Callans, D.J.; Curtis, A.B.; Deal, B.J.; Dickfeld, T.; Field, M.E.; Fonarow, G.C.; et al. 2017 AHA/ACC/HRS Guideline for Management of Patients With Ventricular Arrhythmias and the Prevention of Sudden Cardiac Death: Executive Summary: A Report of the American College of Cardiology/American Heart Association Task Force on Clinical Practice Guidelines and the Heart Rhythm Society. *J. Am. Coll. Cardiol.* **2018**, *72*, 1677–1749. [CrossRef]
57. Huang, W.; Sun, R.; Liu, W.; Xu, R.; Zhou, Z.; Bai, W.; Hou, R.; Xu, H.; Guo, Y.; Yu, L.; et al. Prognostic Value of Late Gadolinium Enhancement in Left Ventricular Noncompaction: A Multicenter Study. *Diagnostics* **2022**, *12*, 2457. [CrossRef]
58. Bennett, C.E.; Freudenberger, R. The current approach to diagnosis and management of left ventricular noncompaction cardiomyopathy: Review of the literature. *Cardiol. Res. Pract.* **2016**, *2016*. [CrossRef]
59. Babes, E.E.; Bustea, C.; Behl, T.; Abdel-Daim, M.M.; Nechifor, A.C.; Stoicescu, M.; Brisc, C.M.; Moisi, M.; Gitea, D.; Iovanovici, D.C. Acute coronary syndromes in diabetic patients, outcome, revascularization, and antithrombotic therapy. *Biomed. Pharmacother.* **2022**, *148*, 112772. [CrossRef]
60. Arbustini, E.; Narula, N.; Dec, G.W.; Reddy, K.S.; Greenberg, B.; Kushwaha, S.; Marwick, T.; Pinney, S.; Bellazzi, R.; Favalli, V.; et al. The MOGE(S) classification for a phenotype-genotype nomenclature of cardiomyopathy: Endorsed by the World Heart Federation. *J. Am. Coll. Cardiol.* **2013**, *62*, 2046–2072. [CrossRef]
61. Heidenreich, P.A.; Bozkurt, B.; Aguilar, D.; Allen, L.A.; Byun, J.J.; Colvin, M.M.; Deswal, A.; Drazner, M.H.; Dunlay, S.M.; Evers, L.R.; et al. 2022 AHA/ACC/HFSA Guideline for the Management of Heart Failure: A Report of the American College of Cardiology/American Heart Association Joint Committee on Clinical Practice Guidelines. *Circulation* **2022**, *145*, e895–e1032. [CrossRef] [PubMed]
62. Cohn, J.N.; Ferrari, R.; Sharpe, N. Cardiac remodeling—Concepts and clinical implications: A consensus paper from an international forum on cardiac remodeling. *J. Am. Coll. Cardiol.* **2000**, *35*, 569–582. [CrossRef]
63. Bonatto, M.G.; Albanez, R.; Salemi, V.M.C.; Moura, L.Z. Use of sacubitril/valsartan in non-compaction cardiomyopathy: A case report. *ESC Heart Fail.* **2020**, *7*, 1186–1189. [CrossRef] [PubMed]
64. Prandi, F.R.; Illuminato, F.; Galluccio, C.; Milite, M.; Macrini, M.; Di Landro, A.; Idone, G.; Chiocchi, M.; Sbordone, F.P.; Sergi, D. A Rare Case of Left Ventricular Non-Compaction with Coronary Artery Anomaly Complicated by ST-Elevation Myocardial Infarction and Subcutaneous Defibrillator Implantation. *Int. J. Environ. Res. Public. Health* **2022**, *19*, 791. [CrossRef] [PubMed]
65. Yang, Y.-W.; Yuan, J.; Xing, J.-F.; Fan, M. Sacubitril-valsartan therapy in a patient with heart failure due to isolated left ventricular noncompaction: A case report and literature review. *Cardiol. Plus* **2022**, *7*, 56–59. [CrossRef]

66. Januzzi, J.L.; Camacho, A.; Piña, I.L.; Rocha, R.; Williamson, K.M.; Maisel, A.S.; Felker, G.M.; Prescott, M.F.; Butler, J.; Solomon, S.D. Reverse Cardiac Remodeling and Outcome After Initiation of Sacubitril/Valsartan. *Circ. Heart Fail.* **2020**, *13*, e006946. [CrossRef]
67. Desai, A.S.; Solomon, S.D.; Shah, A.M.; Claggett, B.L.; Fang, J.C.; Izzo, J.; McCague, K.; Abbas, C.A.; Rocha, R.; Mitchell, G.F. Effect of sacubitril-valsartan vs. enalapril on aortic stiffness in patients with heart failure and reduced ejection fraction: A randomized clinical trial. *JAMA* **2019**, *322*, 1077–1084. [CrossRef]
68. Wang, Y.; Zhou, R.; Lu, C.; Chen, Q.; Xu, T.; Li, D. Effects of the angiotensin-receptor neprilysin inhibitor on cardiac reverse remodeling: Meta-Analysis. *J. Am. Heart Assoc.* **2019**, *8*, e012272. [CrossRef]
69. Mustafa, N.H.; Jalil, J.; Zainalabidin, S.; Saleh, M.S.M.; Asmadi, A.Y.; Kamisah, Y. Molecular mechanisms of sacubitril/valsartan in cardiac remodeling. *Front. Pharmacol.* **2022**, *13*. [CrossRef]
70. McKinnie, S.M.K.; Fischer, C.; Tran, K.M.H.; Wang, W.; Mosquera, F.; Oudit, G.Y.; Vederas, J.C. The Metalloprotease Neprilysin Degrades and Inactivates Apelin Peptides. *ChemBioChem* **2016**, *17*, 1495–1498. [CrossRef]
71. Chatterjee, P.; Gheblawi, M.; Wang, K.; Vu, J.; Kondaiah, P.; Oudit, G.Y. Interaction between the apelinergic system and ACE2 in the cardiovascular system: Therapeutic implications. *Clin. Sci.* **2020**, *134*, 2319–2336. [CrossRef] [PubMed]
72. Liu, Y.; Fan, Y.; Li, J.; Chen, M.; Chen, A.; Yang, D.; Guan, X.; Cao, Y. Combination of LCZ696 and ACEI further improves heart failure and myocardial fibrosis after acute myocardial infarction in mice. *Biomed. Pharmacother.* **2021**, *133*, 110824. [CrossRef] [PubMed]
73. Mazzetti, S.; Scifo, C.; Abete, R.; Margonato, D.; Chioffi, M.; Rossi, J.; Pisani, M.; Passafaro, G.; Grillo, M.; Poggio, D.; et al. Short-term echocardiographic evaluation by global longitudinal strain in patients with heart failure treated with sacubitril/valsartan. *ESC Heart Fail.* **2020**, *7*, 964–972. [CrossRef]
74. Eiringhaus, J.; Wünsche, C.M.; Tirilomis, P.; Herting, J.; Bork, N.; Nikolaev, V.O.; Hasenfuss, G.; Sossalla, S.; Fischer, T.H. Sacubitrilat reduces pro-arrhythmogenic sarcoplasmic reticulum Ca^{2+} leak in human ventricular cardiomyocytes of patients with end-stage heart failure. *ESC Heart Fail.* **2020**, *7*, 2992–3002. [CrossRef] [PubMed]
75. Lyon, R.C.; Zanella, F.; Omens, J.H.; Sheikh, F. Mechanotransduction in Cardiac Hypertrophy and Failure. *Circ. Res.* **2015**, *116*, 1462–1476. [CrossRef]
76. Iborra-Egea, O.; Gálvez-Montón, C.; Roura, S.; Perea-Gil, I.; Prat-Vidal, C.; Soler-Botija, C. Mechanisms of action of sacubitril/valsartan on cardiac remodeling: A systems biology approach. *NPJ Syst. Biol. Appl.* **2017**, *3*, 12. [CrossRef]
77. Liu, J.; Zheng, X.; Zhang, C.; Zhang, C.; Bu, P. Lcz696 Alleviates Myocardial Fibrosis After Myocardial Infarction Through the sFRP-1/Wnt/β-Catenin Signaling Pathway. *Front. Pharmacol.* **2021**, *12*, 724147. [CrossRef]
78. Javadov, S.; Purdham, D.M.; Zeidan, A.; Karmazyn, M. NHE-1 inhibition improves cardiac mitochondrial function through regulation of mitochondrial biogenesis during postinfarction remodeling. *Am. J. Physiol. Heart Circ. Physiol.* **2006**, *291*, H1722–H1730. [CrossRef]
79. Peng, S.; Lu, X.-F.; Qi, Y.-D.; Li, J.; Xu, J.; Yuan, T.-Y.; Wu, X.-Y.; Ding, Y.; Li, W.-H.; Zhou, G.-Q.; et al. LCZ696 Ameliorates Oxidative Stress and Pressure Overload-Induced Pathological Cardiac Remodeling by Regulating the Sirt3/MnSOD Pathway. *Oxidative Med. Cell. Longev.* **2020**, *2020*, 9815039. [CrossRef]
80. Acanfora, D.; Scicchitano, P.; Acanfora, C.; Maestri, R.; Goglia, F.; Incalzi, R.A.; Bortone, A.S.; Ciccone, M.M.; Uguccioni, M.; Casucci, G. Early Initiation of Sacubitril/Valsartan in Patients with Chronic Heart Failure After Acute Decompensation: A Case Series Analysis. *Clin. Drug. Investig.* **2020**, *40*, 493–501. [CrossRef]
81. Pang, Z.; Pan, C.; Yao, Z.; Ren, Y.; Tian, L.; Cui, J.; Liu, X.; Zhang, L.; Chen, Y. A study of the sequential treatment of acute heart failure with sacubitril/valsartan by recombinant human brain natriuretic peptide: A randomized controlled trial. *Medicine* **2021**, *100*, e25621. [CrossRef] [PubMed]
82. Chang, H.-Y.; Chen, K.-C.; Fong, M.-C.; Feng, A.-N.; Fu, H.-N.; Huang, K.-C.; Chong, E.; Yin, W.-H. Recovery of left ventricular dysfunction after sacubitril/valsartan: Predictors and management. *J. Cardiol.* **2020**, *75*, 233–241. [CrossRef] [PubMed]
83. Iovanovici, D.-C.; Bungau, S.G.; Vesa, C.M.; Moisi, M.; Babes, E.E.; Tit, D.M.; Horvath, T.; Behl, T.; Rus, M. Reviewing the Modern Therapeutical Options and the Outcomes of Sacubitril/Valsartan in Heart Failure. *Int. J. Mol. Sci.* **2022**, *23*, 11336. [CrossRef]
84. Peix, A.; Padrón, K.; Cabrera, L.O.; Castañeda, O.; Milán, D.; Castro, J.; Falcón, R.; Martínez, F.; Rodríguez, L.; Sánchez, J. Intraventricular synchronism assessment by gated-SPECT myocardial perfusion imaging in cardiac resynchronization therapy. Does cardiomyopathy type influence results? *EJNMMI Res.* **2020**, *10*, 125. [CrossRef]
85. Qiu, Q.; Chen, Y.-X.; Mai, J.-T.; Yuan, W.-L.; Wei, Y.-L.; Liu, Y.-M.; Yang, L.; Wang, J.-F. Effects of cardiac resynchronization therapy on left ventricular remodeling and dyssynchrony in patients with left ventricular noncompaction and heart failure. *Int. J. Cardiovasc. Imaging* **2015**, *31*, 329–337. [CrossRef] [PubMed]
86. Bertini, M.; Balla, C.; Pavasini, R.; Boriani, G. Efficacy of cardiac resynchronization therapy in patients with isolated ventricular noncompaction with dilated cardiomyopathy: A systematic review of the literature. *J. Cardiovasc. Med.* **2018**, *19*, 324–328. [CrossRef] [PubMed]
87. Minamisawa, M.; Koyama, J.; Kozuka, A.; Miura, T.; Ebisawa, S.; Motoki, H.; Okada, A.; Izawa, A.; Ikeda, U. Regression of left ventricular hypertrabeculation is associated with improvement in systolic function and favorable prognosis in adult patients with non-ischemic cardiomyopathy. *J. Cardiol.* **2016**, *68*, 431–438. [CrossRef]

88. Glikson, M.; Nielsen, J.C.; Kronborg, M.B.; Michowitz, Y.; Auricchio, A.; Barbash, I.M.; Barrabés, J.A.; Boriani, G.; Braunschweig, F.; Brignole, M.; et al. 2021 ESC Guidelines on cardiac pacing and cardiac resynchronization therapy: Developed by the Task Force on cardiac pacing and cardiac resynchronization therapy of the European Society of Cardiology (ESC) With the special contribution of the European Heart Rhythm Association (EHRA). *Eur. Heart J.* **2021**, *42*, 3427–3520. [CrossRef]
89. Akhbour, S.; Fellat, I.; Fennich, N.; Abdelali, S.; Doghmi, N.; Ellouali, F.; Cherti, M. Electrocardiographic findings in correlation to magnetic resonance imaging patterns in African patients with isolated ventricular noncompaction. *Anatol. J. Cardiol.* **2015**, *15*, 550–555. [CrossRef]
90. Lin, T.; Milks, M.W.; Upadhya, B.; Hundley, W.G.; Stacey, R.B. Improvement in systolic function in left ventricular non-compaction cardiomyopathy: A case report. *J. Cardiol. Cases* **2014**, *10*, 231–234. [CrossRef]
91. Eurlings, L.W.; Pinto, Y.M.; Dennert, R.M.; Bekkers, S.C. Reversible isolated left ventricular non-compaction? *Int. J. Cardiol.* **2009**, *136*, e35–e36. [CrossRef]
92. Luckie, M.; Khattar, R.S. Resolution of echocardiographic features of left ventricular non-compaction and systolic dysfunction following treatment for heart failure. *Eur. J. Echocardiogr.* **2010**, *11*, E16. [CrossRef] [PubMed]
93. Vinardell, J.M.; Avila, M.D.; Santana, O. Isolated Left Ventricular Noncompaction Cardiomyopathy: A Transient Disease? *Rev. Cardiovasc. Med.* **2016**, *17*, 80–84. [CrossRef]
94. Gheorghe, G.; Toth, P.P.; Bungau, S.; Behl, T.; Ilie, M.; Pantea Stoian, A.; Bratu, O.G.; Bacalbasa, N.; Rus, M.; Diaconu, C.C. Cardiovascular Risk and Statin Therapy Considerations in Women. *Diagnostics* **2020**, *10*, 483. [CrossRef] [PubMed]
95. Zemrak, F.; Ahlman, M.A.; Captur, G.; Mohiddin, S.A.; Kawel-Boehm, N.; Prince, M.R.; Moon, J.C.; Hundley, W.G.; Lima, J.A.; Bluemke, D.A. The relationship of left ventricular trabeculation to ventricular function and structure over a 9.5-year follow-up: The MESA study. *J. Am. Coll. Cardiol.* **2014**, *64*, 1971–1980. [CrossRef] [PubMed]
96. Priori, S.G.; Blomström-Lundqvist, C.; Mazzanti, A.; Blom, N.; Borggrefe, M.; Camm, J.; Elliott, P.M.; Fitzsimons, D.; Hatala, R.; Hindricks, G.; et al. 2015 ESC Guidelines for the management of patients with ventricular arrhythmias and the prevention of sudden cardiac death: The Task Force for the Management of Patients with Ventricular Arrhythmias and the Prevention of Sudden Cardiac Death of the European Society of Cardiology (ESC). Endorsed by: Association for European Paediatric and Congenital Cardiology (AEPC). *Eur. Heart J.* **2015**, *36*, 2793–2867. [CrossRef] [PubMed]
97. Aung, N.; Doimo, S.; Ricci, F.; Sanghvi, M.M.; Pedrosa, C.; Woodbridge, S.P.; Al-Balah, A.; Zemrak, F.; Khanji, M.Y.; Munroe, P.B. Prognostic significance of left ventricular noncompaction: Systematic review and meta-analysis of observational studies. *Circ. Cardiovasc. Imaging* **2020**, *13*, e009712. [CrossRef]
98. Vaidya, V.R.; Lyle, M.; Miranda, W.R.; Farwati, M.; Isath, A.; Patlolla, S.H.; Hodge, D.O.; Asirvatham, S.J.; Kapa, S.; Deshmukh, A.J. Long-term survival of patients with left ventricular noncompaction. *J. Am. Heart Assoc.* **2021**, *10*, e015563. [CrossRef]
99. Gerard, H.; Iline, N.; Martel, H.; Nguyen, K.; Richard, P.; Donal, E.; Eicher, J.-C.; Huttin, O.; Selton-Suty, C.; Raud-Raynier, P. Prognosis of Adults With Isolated Left Ventricular Non-Compaction: Results of a Prospective Multicentric Study. *Front. Cardiovasc. Med.* **2022**, 1077. [CrossRef]
100. Feng, Y.; Ning, L.; Zhang, J.; Wang, H.; Zhang, H.; Zhang, R.; Deng, Z.; Ni, Y.; Ye, Y.; Ma, A.; et al. Prognosis and subtype analysis of left ventricular noncompaction in adults: A retrospective multicenter study. *Clin. Cardiol.* **2023**, *46*, 390–396. [CrossRef]
101. Sekaran, N.K.; Crowley, A.L.; de Souza, F.R.; Resende, E.S.; Rao, S.V. The role for cardiovascular remodeling in cardiovascular outcomes. *Curr. Atheroscler. Rep.* **2017**, *19*, 23. [CrossRef] [PubMed]
102. Aimo, A.; Gaggin, H.K.; Barison, A.; Emdin, M.; Januzzi, J.L. Imaging, Biomarker, and Clinical Predictors of Cardiac Remodeling in Heart Failure With Reduced Ejection Fraction. *JACC Heart Fail.* **2019**, *7*, 782–794. [CrossRef] [PubMed]
103. Lupón, J.; Gavidia-Bovadilla, G.; Ferrer, E.; de Antonio, M.; Perera-Lluna, A.; López-Ayerbe, J.; Domingo, M.; Núñez, J.; Zamora, E.; Moliner, P.; et al. Dynamic Trajectories of Left Ventricular Ejection Fraction in Heart Failure. *J. Am. Coll. Cardiol.* **2018**, *72*, 591–601. [CrossRef] [PubMed]
104. Valli, F.; Bursi, F.; Santangelo, G.; Toriello, F.; Faggiano, A.; Rusconi, I.; Vella, A.M.; Carugo, S.; Guazzi, M. Long-Term Effects of Sacubitril-Valsartan on Cardiac Remodeling: A Parallel Echocardiographic Study of Left and Right Heart Adaptive Response. *J. Clin. Med.* **2023**, *12*, 2659. [CrossRef]
105. Velazquez, E.J.; Morrow, D.A.; DeVore, A.D.; Duffy, C.I.; Ambrosy, A.P.; McCague, K.; Rocha, R.; Braunwald, E. Angiotensin–Neprilysin Inhibition in Acute Decompensated Heart Failure. *N. Engl. J. Med.* **2018**, *380*, 539–548. [CrossRef] [PubMed]
106. Lupón, J.; Gaggin, H.K.; de Antonio, M.; Domingo, M.; Galán, A.; Zamora, E.; Vila, J.; Peñafiel, J.; Urrutia, A.; Ferrer, E.; et al. Biomarker-assist score for reverse remodeling prediction in heart failure: The ST2-R2 score. *Int. J. Cardiol.* **2015**, *184*, 337–343. [CrossRef]
107. Barison, A.; Aimo, A.; Ortalda, A.; Todiere, G.; Grigoratos, C.; Passino, C.; Camici, P.G.; Aquaro, G.D.; Emdin, M. Late gadolinium enhancement as a predictor of functional recovery, need for defibrillator implantation and prognosis in non-ischemic dilated cardiomyopathy. *Int. J. Cardiol.* **2018**, *250*, 195–200. [CrossRef]

Disclaimer/Publisher's Note: The statements, opinions and data contained in all publications are solely those of the individual author(s) and contributor(s) and not of MDPI and/or the editor(s). MDPI and/or the editor(s) disclaim responsibility for any injury to people or property resulting from any ideas, methods, instructions or products referred to in the content.

MDPI
St. Alban-Anlage 66
4052 Basel
Switzerland
www.mdpi.com

Life Editorial Office
E-mail: life@mdpi.com
www.mdpi.com/journal/life

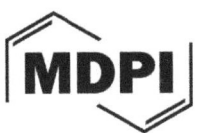

Disclaimer/Publisher's Note: The statements, opinions and data contained in all publications are solely those of the individual author(s) and contributor(s) and not of MDPI and/or the editor(s). MDPI and/or the editor(s) disclaim responsibility for any injury to people or property resulting from any ideas, methods, instructions or products referred to in the content.

www.ingramcontent.com/pod-product-compliance
Lightning Source LLC
LaVergne TN
LVHW070716100526
838202LV00013B/1107